Recent Results in Cancer Research

Fortschritte der Krebsforschung
Progrès dans les recherches sur le cancer

46

Sponsored by the Swiss League against Cancer

Diagnosis and Therapy of Malignant Lymphoma

Edited by

K. Musshoff

With 112 Figures

Springer-Verlag Berlin · Heidelberg · New York 1974

Symposium on "Diagnosis and Therapy of Malignant Lymphoma" to be held at the joint meeting of the Association of Southwest German Radiologists and Specialists in Nuclear Medicine, the Hessian Association for Medical Radiological Therapy and the Association of German Physicans for Radiation Protection and the Union of Nuclear Biology within the German Radiological Society. Freiburg im Breisgau, September 21—23, 1972.

Professor Dr. K. MUSSHOFF, Head of the Department of Radiotherapy, University of Freiburg im Breisgau, Germany

Co-sponsored by
Bundesministerium für Bildung und Wissenschaft der Bundesrepublik Deutschland

ISBN-13:978-3-642-80831-9 e-ISBN-13:978-3-642-80829-6
DOI: 10.1007/978-3-642-80829-6

Softcover reprint of the hardcover 1st edition 1974

Contents

Opening Address. W. Sandritter 1

Introduction. K. Musshoff 2

Anatomy of Lymphoma
Chairman: A. Georgii

The Anatomy of the Lymphatic System. S. Kubik 5

Pathology of Malignant Lymphoma
Chairman: A. Georgii

A Functional Approach to the Classification of Malignant Lymphoma. R. J. Lukes and R. D. Collins 18
The Unspecific Mesenchymal Reaction of the Liver in Patients with Hodgkin's Disease. W. Oehlert 31
Unspecific Mesenchymal Reaction in Bone Marrow in Patients with Hodgkin's Disease. A. Georgii and K. F. Vykoupil 39
The Specific Post-Capillary Venules of Lymphoglandular Tissue in Hodgkin's Disease. N. Söderström 45

Immunopathology of Malignant Lymphoma
Chairman: P. G. Scheurlen

Immunology and Immune Reactions in Malignant Lymphoma. H. D. Flad . . 48
Correlation between EBV Infections and Malignant Lymphomas. H. Schmitz . 55
Epstein-Barr Virus (EBV) in Lymphoid Cells from Patients with Hodgkin's Disease. V. Diehl 59

Investigative Procedures in Malignant Lymphoma and Results
Chairmen: A. Breit and G. W. Löhr

Mediastinoscopy and Thoracoscopy. W. Wolfart and U. Seith 62
Roentgen Anatomy of the Lymphatic System. W. Wirth 64
Lymphographic Differential Diagnosis in Malignant-Lymphomas. K. H. Strickstrock, P. E. Peters, and H. Weissleder 77
Lymphography in Clinical Stage III Hodgkin's Disease. W. A. Fuchs, I. Triller, and M. Haertel 89

Alterations in Pulmonary Diffusion Capacity after Lymphoangiography. K. Kröpelin, L. Baumeister, D. Frey, and W. Wanner 94
The Diagnostic Significance of Laparoscopy in Hodgkin's Disease. W. Dischler and G. Krieger 99
Splenectomy. (Indications, Technique, Complications, Intraoperative Diagnostic Methods). I. Staib, D. Kaiser, and K. Musshoff 107
Changes in Blood Coagulation after Splenectomy. D. Böttcher, J. Blümel, and I. Staib 113
Staging Laparotomy and Splenectomy in Hodgkin's Disease. H. S. Kaplan, R. F. Dorfman, T. S. Nelsen, and S. A. Rosenberg 118
Preliminary Results of Laparotomy with Splenectomy in Patients Previously Treated for Hodgkin's Disease. C. Pauli-Beisel, K. Musshoff, and W. Oehlert 123
Influence of Extensive Biopsy Sampling at Laparotomy on Planning of Radiotherapy in the Non-Hodgkin Lymphoma. R. E. Johnson, P. Chretien, and G. T. O'Conor 128
Bone Marrow Biopsy in Malignant Lymphoma. H. H. Hennekeuser 133
Radioisotope Investigations in Malignant Lymphoma. K. zum Winkel, B. K. Das, and U. Haubold 141
Diagnosis of Malignant Lymphoma with ^{67}Gallium. S. F. Grebe, H. G. Schmidt, F. Dietzel, and M. Römer 148

Primary Extent, Later Extension and Stage as Factors in Therapy of Malignant Lymphoma

Chairmen: K. Hohl and T. M. Fliedner

Presentation and Progression of Hodgkin's Disease. T. Landberg 153
Reticulosarcoma and Lymphosarcoma, Pattern of Relapse and Spread. B. van der Werf-Messing 163
Staging in Malignant Lymphoma (Hodgkin's Disease and Non-Hodgkin Lymphomas). K. Musshoff 167

Therapy of Malignant Lymphoma

Chairmen: B. van der Werf-Messing and R. Gross

.Radiotherapy of Hodgkin's Disease and the Malignant Lymphomas. R. E. Johnson 176
Chemotherapy and Radiotherapy in the Management of the Malignant Lymphomas. A. M. Jelliffe and Y. L. Millett 182
Clinical Trials of the European Organization for Research on Treatment of Cancer (E.O.R.T.C.). B. van der Werf-Messing 190

Therapeutic Results in Malignant Lymphoma

Chairmen: F. Gauwerky and F. Hess

The Curability of Hodgkin's Disease. J. Papillon 195
The Curability of Lympho- and Reticulosarcomas. H. Dancot and W. Feremans 201

Results of Therapy in Hodgkin's Disease: Freiburg i. Br. 1964—1971. K. Musshoff, C. Hartmann, B. Niklaus, and R. Rössner 206
Radiotherapy of Reticulum-Cell Sarcoma: Results and Dose-Time-Relationship. W. Erbe, H. D. Franke, and V. Wiebe 221
Radical Radiotherapy of Hodgkin's Disease. Lund 1944—1956 and 1967—1971. T. Landberg 225
Results of Radiotherapy of Malignant Lymphomas. F. Hess, H. K. Pemsel, and J. W. Plass 229
Present Results in the Treatment of Malignant Lymphomas. Results Obtained in a Series of 317 Cases. K. Hohl 233
Localization and Prognostic Importance of the Post-Radiotherapy Marginal Recurrence of Malignant Lymphomas. H. Bünemann and R. Köster . . . 240

Author Index 241

Subject Index 246

List of Participants

BLÜMEL, I., Dr., University lecturer, Medizinische Klinik der Universität, D 78 Freiburg im Breisgau

BÖTTCHER, D., Dr., Medizinische Klinik der Universität, D 78 Freiburg im Breisgau

BREIT, A., Professor, Strahlenabteilung, Städt. Krankenhaus, D 8390 Passau

BÜNEMANN, H., Dr., Allgemeines Krankenhaus St. Georg, D 2000 Hamburg

DANCOT, H., Dr., Centre Paul-Cogniaux, Institut E. Cavelle-M. Depage, Institut Longchamp, Radiotherapie, B 1180 Bruxelles

DIEHL, V., Dr., University lecturer, Medizinische Klinik, Abteilung für Onkologie der Medizinischen Hochschule D 3 Hannover-Kleefeld

DISCHLER, W., Dr., Medizinische Klinik der Universität, D 78 Freiburg im Breisgau

ERBE, W., Dr., Radiologische Klinik des Universitätskrankenhauses, D 2000 Hamburg-Eppendorf

FLAD, H. D., Dr., University lecturer der Abteilung für klinische Physiologie der Med.-Naturwissenschaftlichen Hochschule der Universität, D 79 Ulm/Donau

FLIEDNER, TH. M., Zentrum für klinische Forschung der Medizinisch-Naturwissenschaftlichen Hochschule der Universität, D 79 Ulm/Donau

FRANKE, H., Professor, Radiologische Klinik und Strahlen-Institut des Universitätskrankenhauses, D 2000 Hamburg-Eppendorf

FUCHS, W. A., Professor, Röntgendiagnostische Abteilung des Zentralen Strahleninstitutes der Universität, CH 3008 Bern

GAUWERKY, F., Professor, Institut für Strahlentherapie und Nuklearmedizin des Allgemeinen Krankenhauses St. Georg, D 2000 Hamburg 1

GEORGII, A., Professor, Pathologisches Institut der Medizinischen Hochschule, D 3 Hannover-Kleefeld

GREBE, S. F., Professor, Nuklearmedizinische Abteilung der Medizinischen Kliniken und Polikliniken der Wilhelm-Conrad-Röntgenklinik der Justus-Liebig-Universität, D 63 Gießen

GROSS, R., Professor, Medizinische Klinik der Universität, D 5000 Köln

HÄRTEL, M., Dr., Malmö Allmänna Sjukhus, Röntgenavdelning, S 214 01 Malmö

HENNEKHEUSER, H. H., Dr., University lecturer, Medizinische Klinik der Universität, D 78 Freiburg im Breisgau

HESS, F., Professor, Strahlenklinik der Universität, D 3550 Marburg/Lahn

HOHL, K., Professor, Röntgenabteilung des Kantonspitals, CH 9006 St. Gallen

JELLIFFE, A. M., MD, F.R.C.P., F.F.R., Meyerstein Institute of Radiotherapy, The Middlesex Hospital, GB London WIN 8 AA

JOHNSON, R. E., MD, Radiation Branch, National Cancer Institute, National Institutes of Health, Bethesda, Maryland 20014 USA

KAISER, D., Dr., Chirurgische Klinik der Universität, D 78 Freiburg im Breisgau

KÖSTER, R., Dr., Institut für Strahlentherapie des Allgemeinen Krankenhauses St. Georg, D 2000 Hamburg

KRÖPELIN, K., Dr., Medizinische Klinik der Universität, D 78 Freiburg im Breisgau

KUBIK, ST., Professor, Anatomisches Institut der Universität, CH 8006 Zürich

LANDBERG, T., Dr., University lecturer, Radiotheraspeutiska Kliniken Konung Gustav V:s Jubileumsklinik Lasarettet i Lund, S 22005 Lund

LÖHR, G. W., Professor, Medizinische Klinik der Universität, D 78 Freiburg im Breisgau

LUKES, R. J., Professor, University of Southern California, School of Medicine, Department of Pathology, Los Angeles, CA 90033 USA

MERTEN, D., Dr., Abteilung für Strahlentherapie, Universität Freiburg, D 78 Freiburg im Breisgau

MUSSHOFF, K., Professor, Abteilung für Strahlentherapie, Universität Freiburg, D 78 Freiburg im Breisgau

OEHLERT, W., Professor, Anatomisches Institut der Universität, D 78 Freiburg im Breisgau

PAPILLON, J., Professor, Faculté Radiologiste des Hopitaux de l'Université, F Lyon

PAULI-BEISEL, CH., Dr., Abteilung für Strahlentherapie der Medizinischen Kliniken der Universität, D 78 Freiburg im Breisgau

SANDRITTER, W., Professor, Pathologisches Institut der Universität. Dean and Speaker of the Joint Commitee of the Medical Facultees at the University of Freiburg, D 78 Freiburg im Breisgau

SCHEURLEN, P. G., Professor, Med. Universitätsklinik und Poliklinik, D 665 Homburg/Saar

SCHMITZ, H., Dr., Hygiene-Institut der Universität, D 78 Freiburg im Breisgau

SEITH, U., Dr., Robert-Koch-Klinik der Chirurgischen Klinik der Universität, D 78 Freiburg im Breisgau

SLANINA, J., Dr., Abteilung für Strahlentherapie, Universität Freiburg, D 78 Freiburg im Breisgau

SÖDERSTRÖM, N., Professor, Department of Internal Medicin A, University Hospital, S Lund

STAIB, I., Professor, Chirurgische Klinik der Universität, D 78 Freiburg im Breisgau

STEINLIN, H. J., Professor, Rector of the University of Freiburg, D 78 Freiburg im Breisgau

STRICKSTROCK, K. H., Dr., Strahleninstitut der Krankenanstalten der Universität, D 79 Ulm/Donau

VAN DER WERF-MESSING, B., Professor, Rotterdamsch Radio-Therapeutisch Instituút NL Rotterdam 5205

ZUM WINKEL, K., Professor, Univ. Strahleninstitut und Klinik Klinikum Westend, D 1 Berlin 19

WIRTH, W., Dr., University lecturer, Röntgenabteilung des Bürgerspitals, CH 6300 Zug

WOLFART, W., Professor, Robert-Koch-Klinik der Chirurgischen Klinik der Universität, D 78 Freiburg im Breisgau

Opening Address

W. Sandritter *

The morphology, immune pathology, and therapy of malignant lymphoma rightly claim the spotlight in a conference of diagnostic and therapeutic radiologists, nuclear radiologists, and radiobiologists. During the last 10 years of research in this field, there has been substantial progress, thanks to the alertness of pathologists on the one hand, and to careful clinical observations of the localization and spread of malignant lymphoma, particularly lymphogranulomatosis, on the other.

It is no accident that a meeting devoted to this theme is being held in Freiburg. The clinical investigation of lymphogranulomatosis has found a focus here in Germany under Dr. K. Musshoff and has gained worldwide recognition. Dr. Lukes, to whom we owe the new histopathological classification of lymphogranulomatosis, has close ties with Freiburg. As a pathologist, he personifies the close cooperation between clinicians and morphologists which is necessary for success in the investigation of this disease.

I wish the convention a successful session.

* Dean and Speaker of the Joint Committee of the Medical Faculties at the University of Freiburg i. Br.

Introduction

K. Musshoff

The group of diseases known as malignant lymphomas are, for a number of reasons, of equal interest to theoretical and clinical medicine. New findings in the fields of virology and immunology could conceivably shed some light on the so far unknown etiology of malignant lymphomas. A viral etiology could explain many of the disparate findings with such a puzzling disease as lymphogranulomatosis, which shows both all the signs of malignancy, such as the characteristic Reed-Sternberg and Hodgkin cells and chromosome abnormalities, and those of an inflammatory disease, i.e. typical changes in the blood count and bone marrow and in the distribution of serum proteins.

So far we have not been able to identify the etiology of this disease. However, clinical observations and pathomorphological investigations involving a joint effort by different branches of medicine have brought us closer to an understanding of the clinical picture.

Descriptive anatomy has given us a clear picture of the regional distribution of the lymphatic system, which has long been neglected in the past. The introductory paper by Dr. S. Kubik (Zurich), who has made valuable contributions to our knowledge of the anatomy of the lymphatic system, deals with this subject.

Histomorphological investigations have shown that in malignant lymphomas there is no one uniform, but a variety of morphological pictures. The morphological type influences the course of the disease and determines the prognosis. We owe the present staging classification of Hodgkin's lymphomas to the work of Dr. R. J. Lukes and his co-workers. Dr. Lukes both discusses this generally accepted classification of Hodgkin's disease and describes some recent work on non-Hodgkin's malignant lymphomas which may further clarify the etiology of this disease.

Here I would like to mention the revealing findings of Dr. Oehlert in Freiburg and of Dr. Georgii in Hannover, who found mesenchymal reactions and damage to the parenchyma in the liver and bone marrow of patients with Hodgkin's disease. Similar changes are found in the spleen and lymph nodes and may be due to the direct action of the etiological agent of Hodgkin's disease and not a sign of actual organ involvement.

Dr. H. F. Flad (Ulm), Dr. Schmitz (Freiburg) and Dr. V. Diehl (Hannover) describe present knowledge and recent findings in the immune pathology of malignant lymphomas.

The new methods of investigation in clinical diagnostic medicine, comprising various radiological and isotope methods and laboratory tests, have enabled us to assess the disease in each individual case with a degree of accuracy previously unattainable. However, most previously used diagnostic procedures gave nonspecific results and could be ambiguous, so more radical endoscopic and surgical measures with tissue biopsies are a really decisive step forward. Such measures as pharyngoscopy, mediastinoscopy, thorascopy, open bone-marrow biopsy, laparoscopy with hepatic and splenic biopsy, and especially laparotomy with splenectomy, are necessary for an exact assessment of the histological type, the degree of malignancy and the extent to which the disease has spread. This is essential for the institution of successful therapy.

A number of colleagues, all with great experience in their particular fields, report on these various methods of investigation. Unfortunately, Dr. DORFMAN of Stanford University Medical Centre was not able to be present. We are very much indebted to Dr. H. S. KAPLAN, who has sent the results and tables from his paper on staging laparotomy in Hodgkin's lymphoma, presented at the International Symposium on Hodgkin's Disease in Stanford, California, March 20—24, 1972.

Further, Dr. R. E. JOHNSON of the Radiation Branch of the National Cancer Institute, Bethesda, Maryland, reports the first results of staging laparotomy in non-Hodgkin's lymphomas. This is an addition to our program.

A large number of very extensive and meticulous clinical investigations in different American and European centers dealing with the site of origin of Hodgkin's lymphomas and the different modes of spread have shown that generally, if not always, Hodgkin's disease originates in one place and spreads from this primary site in a predictable way which is determined by the site of the primary focus and its histological type. These findings have greatly influenced radiotherapeutic methods, which are described by Dr. T. LANDBERG, Lund and Dr. BRIGIT VAN DER WERF-MESSING, Rotterdam. The staging classifications of Rye, New York (1965), and Ann Arbor (1971), in some respects resulting from findings of clinical investigations, will also be discussed.

The malignant lymphomas which were considered incurable only a few years ago can now be cured in a remarkably high percentage of cases thanks to improved methods of diagnostic assessment as a basis for therapy. The indications for radiotherapy or chemotherapy, or a combination of both, are based on the diagnostic findings. The more carefully we assess the pathomorphological type and clinical stage of the disease, the more successful our therapy will be. Dr. R. E. JOHNSON, Dr. A. M. JELLIFFE (London) and Dr. BIRGIT VAN DER WERF-MESSING are going to report on present therapeutic procedures.

Radiotherapy is the main agent in successful therapy, as shown by Dr. J. PAPILLON (Lyon) and Dr. H. DANCOT (Brussels). The results of radiotherapy at some large radiotherapy centres are reported by Drs. W. ERBE, D. FRANKE and W. WEBER (Hamburg), Dr. T. LANDBERG (Lund), Dr. F. HESS (Marburg), and Dr. K. HOHL (St. Gallen), and others. We see, however, that there will eventually be a limit to further increase in the percentage of cures, except for the possible use of X-rays for total body irradiation. Dr. JOHNSON discusses this problem. In Freiburg, we think that chemotherapeutic agents are extremely promising, especially when their effect is enhanced by use in combination.

Perhaps more than in other diseases, diagnostic and therapeutic successes in the treatment and management of malignant lymphoma patients have resulted from a team effort of people in diverse branches of theoretical and clinical medicine. This applies not only to the fundamental investigation of the diseases but also to the management of each case. Since there are so few specially equipped tumor clinics in Germany, good cooperation between the different departments involved in the care of every individual patient is all the more essential.

At this annual meeting of the Vereinigung Südwestdeutscher Röntgenologen und Nuklearmediziner (Association of Southwest German Radiologists and Nuclear Physicians), Hessische Gesellschaft für Medizinische Strahlenkunde (Hessian Society of Medical Radiology), the Vereinigung deutscher Strahlenschutzärzte (Association of German Physicians for Radiation Protection) and the Arbeitsgemeinschaft für Strahlenbiologie in der deutschen Röntgengesellschaft (Working Committee for Radiation Biology in the German Radiology Society) we discuss recent advances in diagnosis and indicate the present possibilities for assessment and therapy of the disease. There can be no doubt that the majority of patients is still inadequately diagnosed and treated at present.

Finally I would like to thank the Federal Ministry for Science and Research (Bundesministerium für Wissenschaft und Forschung) and several commercial firms, particularly those in Freiburg, for their help in making this conference possible. I also thank my colleagues, Dr. SLANINA and Dr. MERTEN, and the secretaries and technicians of the radiotherapy department for their help in the organization.

The Anatomy of the Lymphatic System

S. Kubik

Summary

The lymph flows from a valveless capillary network through collectors with valves into the regional (primary) lymph nodes. The primary, secondary, tertiary etc. lymph nodes form chains and function as filter stations. The spread of a process can be modified by the connections of the collector vessels, – the single nodes respectively, – as well as through by-passes. The lymph of the singular afferent lymph vessels passes through certain node sectors. The number of nodes in the various node groups is determined during embryonic development. In the course of senile involution the lymphatic tissue decreases, but not the number of nodes.

The topography of the lymph nodes, their connections and ways of drainage of the organs are first discussed in areas to be visualized by lymphography (inguinal, iliacal, lumbar nodes). The node groups and the efferent vessels of the abdominal organs, of the thoracic cavity and of the neck area are presented in a brief summary. Connections between lymphatics of the neck area and the thoracic cavity as well as between thorax and abdomen are referred to.

The lymphatic system originates as a valveless capillary network located in the intercellular space. From there the lymph flows through collectors with valves into the lymph nodes. Lymph nodes in which the collecting vessels of an organ or body area terminate are the *regional or primary nodes* of the areas in question. The area drained by a regional lymph node is called its *tributary area* [1]. From the primary nodes to the large lymphatic or, vein trunks the lymph passes through several nodes that form chains. These are secondary or tertiary nodes relative to the regional nodes. The drainage area of a node is enlarged by chain formation according to the central position.

The simple scheme of connections between tributary area and regional node with outflow through a linear chain is changed into a complex and individual system by 1. "segmental passing-over", 2. anastomoses of the efferent vessels and 3. cross-connections between nodes. "Segmental passing-over" means that a collecting vessel bypasses its primary node and runs into a node above, or an efferent vessel of a node "passes over" the nearest station above it [53]. Such vessels can make the lacunar lymph nodes into primary nodes of the leg area, or connect them directly with the common iliac or lumbar nodes (Fig. 1). By means of anastomoses of efferent lymph vessels, the regional lymph nodes of one organ (or part of an organ) can function as additional primary nodes of another organ [25.] Thus, the regional lymph nodes of the cervix can be involved in diseases of the ovary, uterine tube, and corpus uteri (Fig. 2 A). Cross-connections between parallel chains, beside adding defensive stations to the outflow, facilitate the spread of metastases [21].

Normally the lymph of an afferent vessel does not fill the whole of the marginal sinus and intermediate sinuses but passes into the lymph node through a sector area. Because of the spongioid structure of the intermediary sinuses, the outlines of the sector are not sharp; therefore, at least at the beginning of a malignant process, a lymph node is only partly affected [23].

The number and size of the lymph nodes constitute a difficult problem in diagnosis; they are generally inversely proportional. In connection with this question it is necessary to correct the erroneous opinion that the number of nodes declines with increasing age due to physiological senile involution [28]. According to studies of the embryonic development of the nodes, a certain amount of lymphatic tissue is available for the drainage of an area. The later distribution of this quantity of tissue may vary to a great extent: it may form a few large nodes, several small nodes, or a mixture of nodes of different sizes. "Giant nodes" which are only partially subdivided (often with bifurcation nodes) and "micro-nodes" are the two extreme forms [27]. Senile involution primarily affects the medullary substance, the cortex remaining an intact shell. Only the amount of lymphatic tissue is reduced, not the number of nodes [49]. Thus, because of heavy involution, some nodes (mainly small ones) will show no sign of opacification or due to adipose infiltration cannot be distinguished from their surroundings at the time of operation. They exist not withstanding, and they are intercalated in the lymph circulation, which means that they can form metastases. This is very important [40].

From the point of view of diagnosis, a knowledge of the topography of the regional nodes, as well as of their areas and drainage routes is most essential.

Anatomical and lymphographic studies on the inguinal, pelvic and lumbar node groups can be found in: [8, 13, 14, 17, 20, 22, 35, 44, 45, 53, 54].

In Fig. 1 the inguinal nodes and the parietal node groups of the pelvis and the abdomen with their outflow are represented schematically. Some inguinal nodes lie along the inguinal ligament and some around the termination of the great saphenous vein. The external and common iliac nodes together with the lumbar nodes are situated along the blood vessels. They form three chains: lateral, medial, and intermediate. The external and common iliac nodes run along the blood vessels of the same name. They continue along and between aorta and inferior vena cava to the diaphragm, forming the lumbar node group. The internal iliac nodes lie within the angles formed by the branches of the internal iliac artery. Unlike the groups mentioned above, the internal iliac nodes can be only partly visualized by lymphography, if at all.

The direction of flow in the vessels of the lymph nodes and in the collecting vessels is determined by valves. A reverse flow occurs only when the vessels become dilated due to a blockage and the valves do not work properly.

The main outflow routes of the node groups shown in Fig. 1 are marked by broad arrows. Note that:

1. The medial chain is the main channel in the area of the external iliac node group, and the lateral chain in the area of the common iliac group.

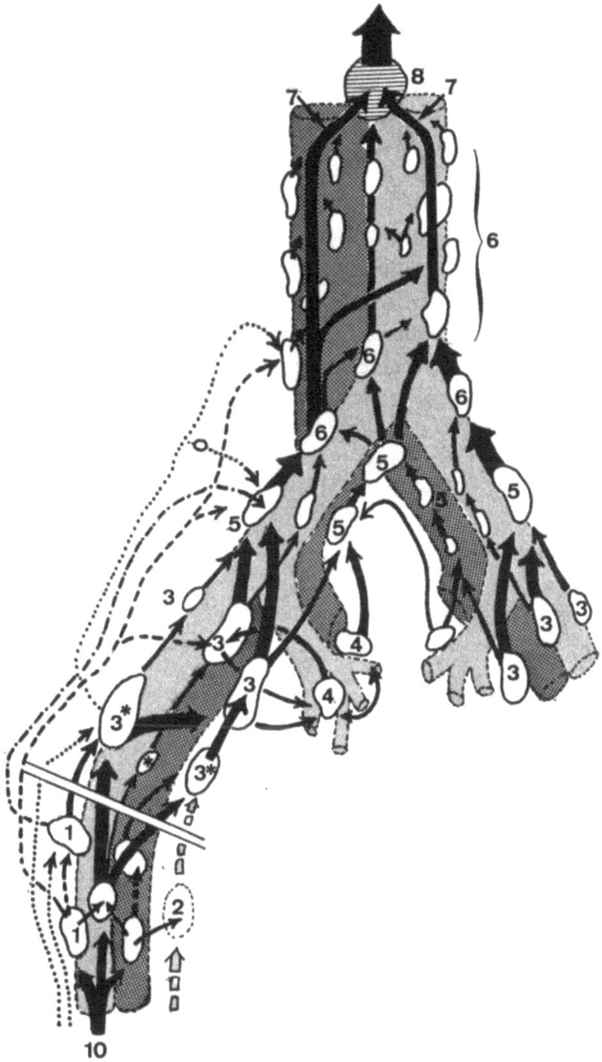

Fig. 1. Scheme of topography and connections of inguinal, iliac, and lumbar node groups. (Broad arrows mark the main outflow, dotted lines the segmental passing-over.) 1. Superficial inguinal nodes. 2. Deep inguinal node. 3. External iliac node group (* lacunar nodes). 4. Internal iliac node group. 5. Common iliac node group. 6. Lumbar nodes. 7. Right and left lumbar lymph trunks. 8. Cisterna chyli and thoracic duct

2. There is a bilateral connection between the external and internal iliac nodes through which some of the internal nodes can very often be visualized by lymphography.

3. The "crossing-over" of the right lumbar cord to the left side makes a connection between the right iliac and left lumbar node chains.

4. There is "segmental passing-over" of single nodes in the node groups of the iliac area (indicated by dotted lines).

Anatomical and clinical investigations into the lymphatic system of the pelvic organs have been made by: [2, 3, 4, 16, 24, 29, 30, 33, 38, 39, 40, 44].

Fig. 2 shows the efferent pathway and the regional lymph nodes of the external genitalia and the pelvic and abdominal organs. The inguinal nodes drain the external genitals and the lowest part of the vagina. The main lymphatic drainage of the bladder, the prostate, and the cervix uteri is into the external iliac nodes. Only accessory pathways enter the common iliac nodes. The vagina drains into all three iliac node groups. Most of the upper part of the vagina is connected with the internal and common iliac nodes and the lower part with the external iliac nodes.

Apart from the urogenital organs mentioned above, the common iliac nodes drain the pelvic portion of the rectum [18]. Most of the collecting vessels of the pelvic organs have direct connections to the regional nodes, although some vessels may be intercepted by visceral nodes (paravesical, parauterine, paravaginal, pararectal nodes). The visceral or intercalated nodes lying in the subperitoneal adipose tissue cannot be visualized by lymphography. The existence of the parauterine and paravaginal nodes described by [14, 16, 44] is questioned by [3].

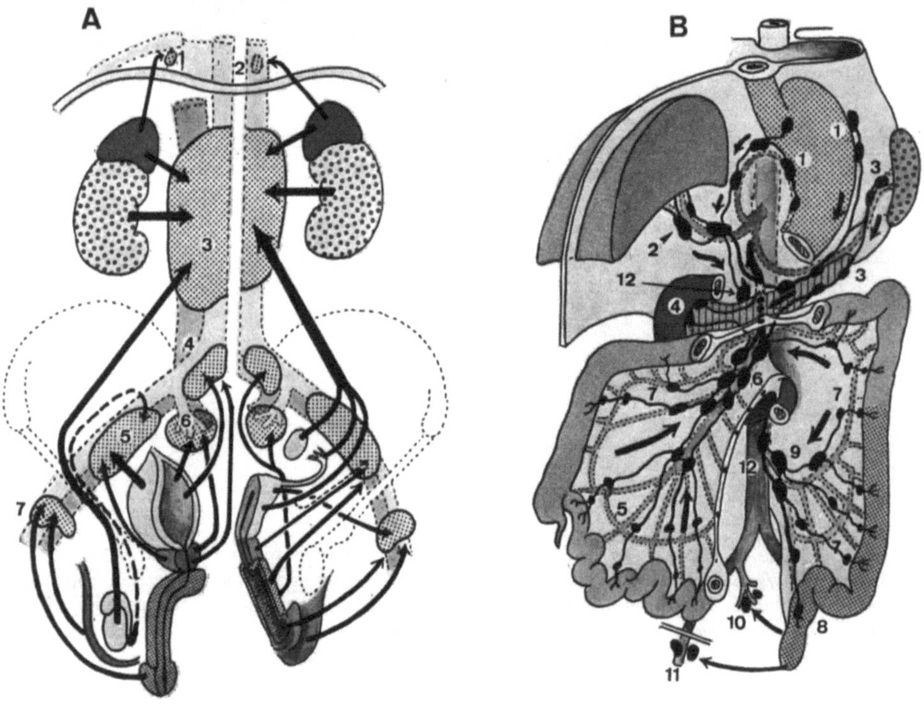

Fig. 2 A. Regional lymph node groups of urogenital organs and adrenal gland. 1. Lowest intercostal lymph node. 2. Retroaortic lymph node. 3. Lumbar lymph node group. 4. Common iliac node group. 5. External iliac node group. 6. Internal iliac node group. 7. Inguinal lymph nodes. B. Lymph nodes and efferents of the gastro-intestinal tract, liver, pancreas, and spleen. (Arrows mark the direction of drainage.) 1. Gastric lymph nodes. 2. Hepatic nodes. 3. Pancreaticolienal node group. 4. Pancreaticoduodenal nodes. 5. Mesenteric nodes. 6. Central mesenteric nodes. 7. Mesocolic nodes. 8. Pararectal node. 9. Inferior mesenteric nodes. 10. Internal iliac nodes. 11. Inguinal nodes. 12. Latero-aortic nodes

The lumbar nodes are the regional nodes of kidneys [36], adrenal glands, testis [5, 7] ovary [6, 9], uterine tube, and corpus uteri [2, 24, 29]. A few ascending lymphatics of the cauda epididymis lead along the artery of the vas deferens to an external iliac node lying in the bifurcation of the common iliac artery. The ascent of the lymphatics of the testicle and of the utero-ovarian *adnexa* is a remainder of the descent of the fetal gonads. The vessels descending from the "tubo-uterine angle" to the inguinal nodes follow Hunter's gubernaculum which later provides the ligamentum teres uteri. The connections between the utero-ovarian cord and the external and common iliac nodes are only secondary and inconstant ways.

Unlike the organs situated in the retroperitoneal area, organs that develop intraperitoneally (gastro-intestinal tube, liver, pancreas, spleen) are drained by lymph nodes lying in mesos, called visceral nodes (Fig. 2 B). The mesenteric nodes form the largest group of nodes in the body, comprising some 100 to 150 nodes. In the area of the small and large intestines the nodes make up three groups: one beside the intestinal wall, one in the mesocolon or mesenterium respectively and one beside the main arterial trunks (central mesenteric nodes). The mesenteric nodes drain the derivatives of the umbilical ansa (jejunum, ileum, cecum, appendix, ascending and transverse colon and the upper part of the descending colon). Their efferent vessels form the intestinal trunk. The lower part of the descending colon and the sigmoid are drained through the inferior mesenteric nodes into the lateral aortic nodes [10]. The collecting vessels of the pelvic part of the rectum end partly in the para-aortic, partly in the internal iliac nodes, whereas the anal part drains into the inguinal nodes [15, 18] (Fig. 2 B).

The regional lymph nodes of the stomach (gastric nodes) [37, 51]; liver (hepatic nodes) [55], duodenum, pancreas [48], and spleen (pancreato-lienal nodes) lie initially in the ventral and dorsal mesogastrium. Due to organ relocation in the course of development, the pancreatic node group becomes secondarily retroperitoneal. It becomes closely associated topographically with the central mesenteric and para-aortic nodes as well as the intestinal trunk with the efferent vessels ending in all three of these. The efferents of the hepatic nodes, though on a different pathway, lead to the intestinal trunk and to the same nodes. The efferents of the gastric nodes differ in that they end in the hepatic and pancreaticolienal nodes (Fig. 2 B).

In addition to the abdominal nodes, efferent lymphatics of the liver and adrenal gland also run into some mediastinal nodes. Efferents of the liver perforate the diaphragm and end in the anterior and posterior mediastinal nodes, whereas those of the adrenal glands end only in the posterior nodes [44] (Fig. 3 A).

The confluence of the efferent channels of the lumbar and visceral nodes, called the intestinal and lumbar trunks, form the thoracic duct (Fig. 3 B).

After passing the thoracic cavity anterior to the vertebral column, the thoracic duct runs into the angle of junction of the left subclavian with the left jugular vein (venous angle) or into one of these venous trunks. The terminal part of the duct may divide into branches and these, if they connect with jugular or subclavian nodes, can cause cervical metastases of abdominal tumors [31]. The most frequent variant of the thoracic duct is a duplication of its upper part. In most such cases one of the divergent channels runs into the left and the other into the right venous angle; a rare variant exhibits a parallel course with common termination at the left venous angle [19]. The formation of islands due to reduplication of the middle thoracic part of the duct is more frequently seen than the production of a plexus due to ramification (Fig. 3 B). The original part of the thoracic duct forms either an ampulla or a plexus in which intercalated nodes are deposited. It is of interest that, where there is lateral displacement of the thoracic duct, the aorta and the azygos vein react in the same manner, thus retaining their parallelity [26].

When internodal connections occur, the intercostal nodes form two chains parallel to the thoracic duct and may function as a collateral pathway (Fig. 3 B). The intercostal nodes drain the pleura. The lowest node can also receive collecting vessels originating in the adrenal gland. The efferent trunk of the 1st and 2nd node group ascends into the cervical region and joins the venous angle. Most of the horizontally flowing efferents of the 3rd to 6th nodes terminate individually in the thoracic duct,

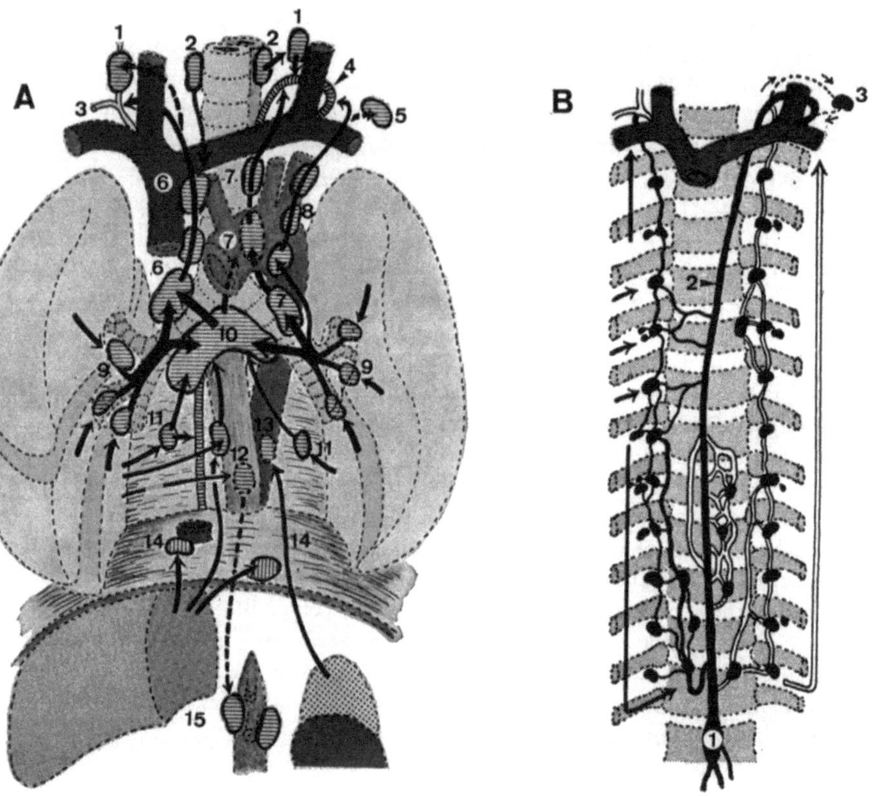

Fig. 3 A. Connections and outflow of the posterior mediastinal and tracheobronchial nodes. 1. Posterior jugular node. 2. Paratracheal node. 3. Right lymphatic duct. 4. Thoracic duct. 5. Supraclavicular node. 6. Right tracheobronchial chain. 7. Left tracheobronchial chain. 8. Left anterior mediastinal nodes. 9. Nodes of the hilus (bronchopulmonary nodes). 10. Node of the bifurcation. 11. Node of the pulmonary ligament. 12. Juxta-esophageal nodes. 13. Retroaortic node. 14. Diaphragmatic nodes. 15. Lumbar nodes (latero-aortic). B. Efferents of the intercostal and paravertebral nodes. (Normal thoracic duct: black; variants of its middle part: white.) Right: Normal situation of drainage. Left: With efferents absent. 1. Cisterna chyli, lumbar and intestinal trunks. 2. Thoracic duct. 3. Inconstant branch of the thoracic duct connected with a supraclavicular node

but the efferents of the 7th to 12th nodes have a common descendent trunk. If the connections to the thoracic duct are absent, the internodal junctions and the efferent trunk of the first node will be utilized as a passage [43] (Fig. 3 B).

In addition to the paravertebral nodes interrupting the intercostal lymph vessels, there are only a few small nodes in the posterior mediastinum (juxta-esophageal, and retro-aortic nodes). They drain the esophagus, the lower lobes of the lungs, the liver, and the adrenal glands. Some of the efferent vessels of these small nodes join with the node of bifurcation and some run directly into the thoracic duct. Descending vessels to the lumbar para-aortic nodes rarely occur (Fig. 3 A).

A large mediastinal group represents the regional nodes of the lungs, the nodes of the hilus, the bifurcation, and the bilateral tracheobronchial chains, which come together at the bifurcation of the trachea [11, 34, 46]. Their efferents join the arch of the thoracic duct and the right lymphatic duct, or run directly into the venous angle. The nodes of the pulmonary ligament draining the lower lobes of the lungs are connected with nodes of the bifurcation and the thoracic duct (Fig. 3 A).

The parasternal and the diaphragmatic nodes, as well as the two chains formed by the anterior mediastinal nodes, lie partly in the anterior and partly in the superior mediastinum. The right anterior mediastinal chain is situated anterior to the superior vena cava, the left chain anterior to the aortic arch. They receive lymphatics not only from the thorax (i. e. heart, pericardium, lungs, thymus and juxtapericardiac nodes), but from the cervical region (thyroid gland and pretracheal nodes) as well. Their efferents ascend to the venous angles (Fig. 4). The pleura and the anterior abdominal wall are drained by the diaphragmatic nodes, the efferent channels of which lead to the anterior mediastinal, juxta-esophageal and parasternal nodes. Parasternal nodes are found primarily in the 1st, 2nd and 6th intercostal spaces. They drain the mammary gland, the pleura, the abdominal wall and anterior chest wall. The efferents of the bilaterally connected chains terminate by opening into the great lymphatic trunks or the venous angles [15].

The above description shows that the efferent trunks of all the mediastinal lymph node groups — with the exception of the 3rd to 12th intercostal nodes — ascend into the cervical region and unite into the bronchomediastinal trunk. This, or the separate trunks, finally open into the right lymphatic duct, or on the left into the thoracic duct. The following variants may occur on both sides: direct opening into the venous angles or into one of the cervical veins, junction with the jugular or subclavian trunk, and connection with a cervical node [42].

The following vessels descend from the thoracic into the abdominal cavity: 1. collecting vessels of the pleura ending in the inferior diaphragmatic nodes; 2. efferent vessels leading from the juxtapericardial nodes to those of the cardia; 3. a rarely occurring connection between a retro-esophageal node and the lumbar nodes (Fig. 4).

The axillary nodes form five groups (Fig. 5). The lateral nodes drain the upper extremity, the subscapular nodes drain the shoulder region, and the pectoral nodes the mammary gland. By intercalation of the central nodes, they send their efferents into the infraclavicular nodes. The main efferent of the latter, the subclavian trunk, opens into the venous angle, but one of their accessory channels leads to the supraclavicular nodes. The most important regional nodes of the mammary gland are the pectoral, infraclavicular, and parasternal nodes, reached by the collecting vessels partly directly, and partly through intercalated nodes (interpectoral, paramammary nodes) [15].

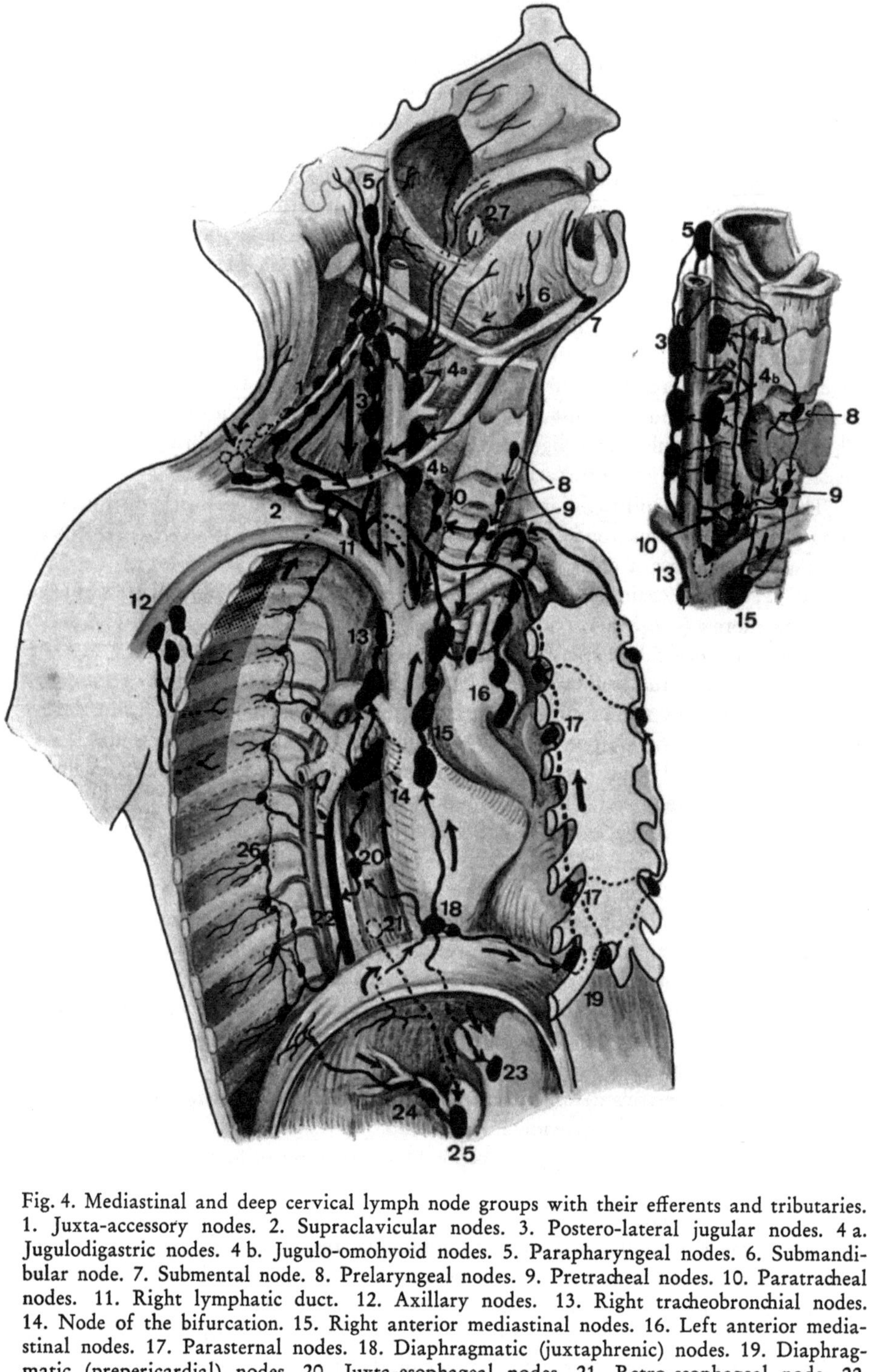

Fig. 4. Mediastinal and deep cervical lymph node groups with their efferents and tributaries. 1. Juxta-accessory nodes. 2. Supraclavicular nodes. 3. Postero-lateral jugular nodes. 4 a. Jugulodigastric nodes. 4 b. Jugulo-omohyoid nodes. 5. Parapharyngeal nodes. 6. Submandibular node. 7. Submental node. 8. Prelaryngeal nodes. 9. Pretracheal nodes. 10. Paratracheal nodes. 11. Right lymphatic duct. 12. Axillary nodes. 13. Right tracheobronchial nodes. 14. Node of the bifurcation. 15. Right anterior mediastinal nodes. 16. Left anterior mediastinal nodes. 17. Parasternal nodes. 18. Diaphragmatic (juxtaphrenic) nodes. 19. Diaphragmatic (prepericardial) nodes. 20. Juxta-esophageal nodes. 21. Retro-esophageal node. 22. Thoracic duct. 23. Gastric (paracardiac) node. 24. Inferior phrenic node. 25. Latero-aortic node. 26. Intercostal nodes. 27. Palatine tonsil

Accessory channels may form connections to the lateral axillary and supraclavicular nodes and via the lymphatic vessels of the abdominal wall to the inguinal nodes. Apart from the areas mentioned, the axillary nodes also receive lymphatics via perforating vessels from the pleura (Fig. 4).

The cervical lymph nodes can be divided into three main groups [12, 47, 50]. The *superior main group,* consisting of the occipital, mastoid, parotid, submandibular, and submental nodes, forms a circle at the junction of the head and neck (Fig. 5). These nodes drain the occipital region, the scalp, the facial region, the orbits, the buccal cavity, the external and middle ear, and the large salivary glands. The *anterior main group* consists of some superficial nodes that drain the skin and the muscle layer (Fig. 5) and a larger number of deep visceral nodes (prelaryngeal, pretracheal and paratracheal nodes) that receive lymph from the larynx, thyroid gland, trachea and esophagus (Fig. 4). The efferents of the prelaryngeal and pretracheal nodes drain into the anterior jugular nodes by intercalation of the paratracheal nodes. Both the pretracheal and the paratracheal nodes are also connected with mediastinal nodes (Fig. 4).

The *lateral main group* contains the greatest number of nodes. It forms three chains consisting of the jugular and supraclavicular nodes and the nodes along the accessory nerve (juxta-accessory nodes) (Figs. 4 and 5). All the lymphatics of the head and neck drain into the lateral main group, either directly from their tributaries, or indirectly after passing through one of the other main groups. The juxta-accessory nodes drain the nuchal area, whereas the supraclavicular nodes receive lymph from the shoulder region, the upper extremity, and the anterior thoracic wall, including the mammary gland (Fig. 5). The internal jugular vein divides the jugular nodes into an anterior and a postero-lateral group. The postero-lateral jugular node group is a chain that forms a triangle together with the juxta-accessory and supraclavicular node groups. It receives efferent lymphatics from the nasal cavity, the middle ear, the thyroid gland and the larynx [32, 52] (Fig. 4). The efferents of the pharynx normally reach the postero-lateral jugular chain through parapharyngeal nodes. Unlike the postero-lateral nodes, the anterior nodes do not form a chain; they are present in two separate groups situated above and below the trunk of the thyrolingual vein. The efferents of the superior, or jugulodigastric group lead to the junction of the juxta-accessory and postero-lateral jugular nodes, and those of the inferior, or jugulo-omohyoid group to the inferior end of the postero-lateral jugular chain. The jugulodigastric nodes drain the efferents of the parotid and submandibular nodes and are connected directly with the efferent vessels of the tongue, palatine tonsil, and nasal cavity. The jugulo-omohyoid nodes represent the secondary stations of the prelaryngotracheal and paratracheal node groups and drain directly the efferents of the larynx and the thyroid gland.

All the lymph from the head and neck area is drained through two main channels (Fig. 4, broad arrows). One of these channels is formed by the jugular node group while the other comprises both the juxta-accessory and supraclavicular chains. At the root of the neck the two channels unite to form the jugular trunk. On the left side, the jugular trunk, like the subclavian and bronchomediastinal trunks, is usually joined by the thoracic duct; however, these trunks can also open independently into the internal jugular or subclavian veins. Similarly, separate endings of the three trunks may also occur on the right side. More frequently, however, they unite to form the right lymphatic duct, which runs into the venous angle (Fig. 5).

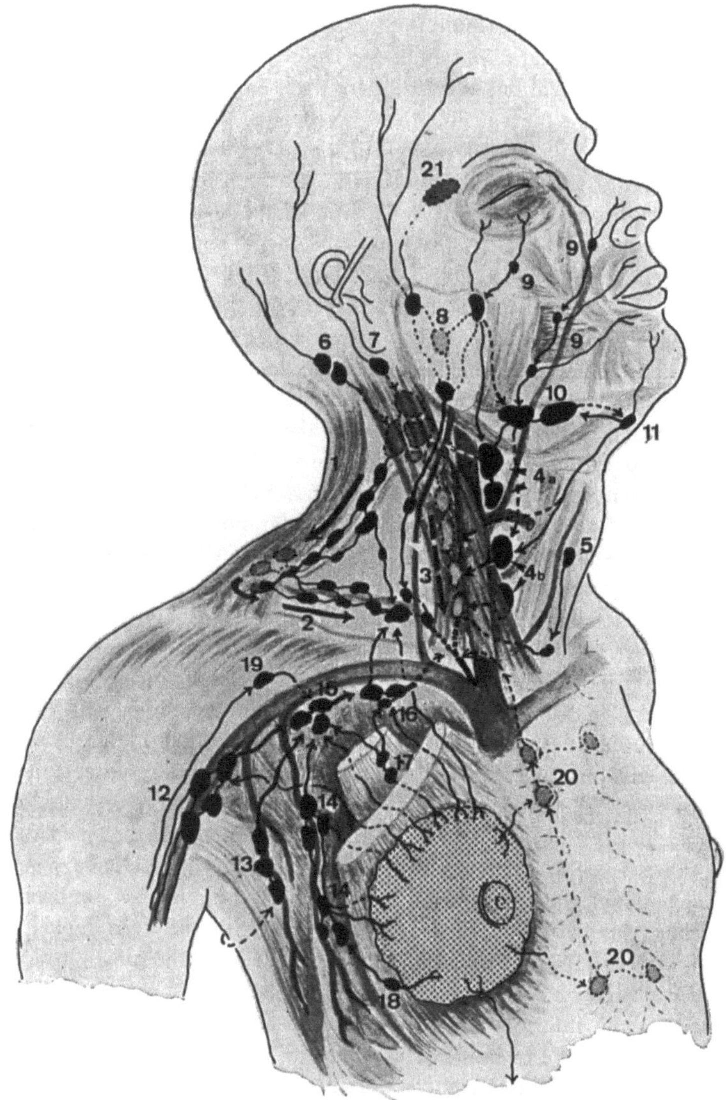

Fig. 5. Cervical, facial, and axillary lymph nodes with their tributaries and efferents. 1. Juxta-accessory nodes. 2. Supraclavicular nodes. 3. Postero-lateral jugular nodes. 4 a. Jugulo-digastric nodes. 4 b. Jugulo-omohyoid nodes. 5. Anterior cervical nodes. 6. Occipital nodes. 7. Mastoid node. 8. Parotid nodes. 9. Facial nodes. 10. Submandibular nodes. 11. Submental node. 12. Lateral axillary nodes. 13. Subscapular nodes. 14. Pectoral nodes (upper and lower groups). 15. Central axillary nodes. 16. Infraclavicular nodes. 17. Interpectoral nodes. 18. Paramammary node. 19. Deltoideo-pectoral node. 20. Parasternal nodes. 21. Lacrimal gland

The fact that no connection exists between the jugulodigastric and jugulo-omohyoid nodes is of great practical importance, as it means that a malignant process originating in the jugulo-digastric nodes (connections as explained above) will spread to all nodes of the lateral main group, whereas the jugulo-omohyoid group reaches only the lowest postero-lateral jugular nodes (Fig. 5).

Only a small number of lymphatics descend from the cervical region into the thoracic cavity. Efferents of the pretracheal nodes and the thyroid gland drain into an anterior mediastinal node lying in the angle at the junction of the right and left brachiocephalic veins [52]; those of the paratracheal nodes, however, join the uppermost member of the tracheobronchial chain (Fig. 4).

This survey of the lymphatic system covers only the most important regional nodes with their connections and outflows. We mentioned some variants in order to make it clear that, because of the aberrations that can occur in a plexus-like system, no single scheme allows an interpretation of each individual case.

References

1. Bartels, P.: Das Lymphgefäß-System. Jena: G. Fischer 1909.
2. Cardis, R., Wettstein, P.: La lymphographie en cancérologie utérine. Méd. et Hyg. (Genève) **25**, 564 (1967).
3. Cherry, C. P., GlueckSmann, A., Dearing, R., Way, S.: Observations on lymph node involvment in carcinoma of the cervix. J. Obstet. Gynaec. Brit. Emp. **60**, 368 (1953).
4. Cervantes, A.: Les lymphatiques de la vessie. Ann. Anat. path. Anat. norm. méd. chir. T. V. (Paris) **3**, 269 (1928).
5. Cooper, J. F., Leadbetter, W. F., Chute, R.: The thoracoabdominal approach for retroperitoneal gland dissection: its application to testis tumors. Surg. Gynec. Obstet. (Chicago) **90**, 486 (1950).
6. Cordier, G., Papamiltiades, Thiounn: Quelques précisions sur l'anatomie des lymphatiques de l'ovaire. C. R. Ass. Anat. (Nancy) **104**, 615 (1959).
7. Cuneo, B.: Note sur les lymphatiques du testicule. Bull. Soc. anat. (Paris) **76**, 105 (1901).
8. Cuneo, M. M. B., Marcille, M.: Topographie des ganglions ilio-pelviens. Bull. Soc. anat. (Paris) **76**, 653 (1901).
9. Czeizel, E., Palkovich, I.: Die ableitenden Lymphgefäße und regionären Lymphknoten des Ovars. Anat. Anz. **111**, 406 (1962).
10. Descomps, P., Turnesco, D.: La circulation lymphatique du gros intestin. Rev. Chir. (Paris) **61**, 329 (1923).
11. Engel, St.: Die Topographie der bronchialen Lymphknoten. Klin. Wschr. (Berlin) **5**, 1136 (1926).
12. Fisch, U.: Lymphographische Untersuchungen über das zervikale Lymphsystem. Fortschr. Hals-Nas.-Ohrenheilk. **14** (1966).
13. Fuchs, W. A., Davidson, J. W., Fischer, H. W.: Lymphography in cancer. Recent Results Cancer Res. (Berlin) **23** (1969).
14. Gerteis, W.: Lymphographie und topographische Anatomie des Beckenlymphsystems. Beilageheft Z. Geburtsh. Gynäk. (Stuttgart) **165** (1966).
15. Haagensen, C. D., Feind, C. R., Herter, F. C., Slanetz, C. A., Weinberg, J. A.: The lymphatics in cancer. Philadelphia: Saunders 1972.
16. Henrichsen, E.: Distribution of metastases in stage I. carcinoma of the cervix. Amer. J. Obstet. Gynec. (St. Louis) **80**, 919 (1960).
17. Hermann, P. G., Benninghoff, D. L., Nelson, J. H.: Roentgen anatomy of the iliopelvic aortic lymphatic system. Radiology (Syracuse) **80**, 182 (1963).
18. Hollinshead, W. H.: Anatomy for surgeons. Vol. 2. New York: Hoeber-Harper Book Co. (1966).
19. Jacobsson, S. J.: Clinical anatomy and pathology of the thoracic duct. Almquist-Wiksell: Stockholm 1972.
20. Jackson, R. J.: Topography of the iliopelvic lymph nodes. Amer. J. Obstet. Gynec. **104**, 1118 (1969).
21. Jossifow, G. M.: Das Lymphgefäß-System des Menschen. Jena: G. Fischer (1930).

22. Koerner, F., Hilpert, K. L.: Lymphographische Untersuchungen zu den Verlaufsformen der retroperitonealen Lymphbahnen. Verh. Anat. Ges. 64. Vers. Homburg 1969. Erg.-Heft Anat. Anz. (Jena) **126,** 297 (1970).
23. Kubik, St., Vizkelety, T., Balint, J.: Die Lokalisation der Lungensegmente in den regionalen Lymphknoten. Anat. Anz. (Jena) **104,** 104 (1957).
24. Kubik, St., Várady, K.: Beiträge zur Frage des Lymphsystems und der Lymphzirkulation im Uterus. Anat. Anz. (Jena) **104,** 18 (1957).
25. Kubik, St.: Die normale Anatomie des Lymphsystems unter besonderer Berücksichtigung der Sammelgebiete der Lymphknoten der unteren Körperhälfte. „Maligne Lymphome", Interdisziplinäre Diskussionen, Dtsch. Röntg. Kongreß. München: Urban & Schwarzenberg 1968.
26. Kubik, St.: Morphologische Grundlagen des Lymphsystems. Diagnostik (Berlin) **4,** 477 (1971).
27. Kubik, St.: Anatomie des Lymphsystems. Radiol. clin. (Basel) **42,** 243 (1973).
28. Laufer, C.: Röntgenanatomische Untersuchungen am Beckenlymphsystem. Diss. Zürich (1971).
29. Lazaro, C.: Connexions ganglionnaires des lymphatiques de l'utérus. Presse méd. **2,** 1487 (1934).
30. Leveuf, J., Godard, H.: Les lymphatiques de l'utérus. Rev. Chir. (Paris) **61,** 219 (1923).
31. Ludwig, J.: Die Lymphgefäßverbindungen zwischen Ductus thoracicus und supraclaviculären Lymphknoten und ihre Bedeutung für die Krebsmetastasierung. Frankfurt Z. Path. **71,** 436 (1961).
32. Mahorner, H. R., Caylor, H .D., Schlotthauer, C. F., Pemberton, J.: Observations on the lymphatic connections of the thyroid gland in man. Anat. Rec. **36,** 341 (1927).
33. Meigs, J. V.: Surgical treatment of cancer of the cervix. New York-London: Grune & Stratton 1954.
34. Nelson, H. P.: The tracheo-bronchial lymphatic glands. J. Anat. (Lond.) **66,** 228 (1934).
35. Nelson, J. H., Masterson, J. G., Herman, P. G., Benninghoff, D. L.: Anatomy of the female pelvic and aortic lymphatic system demonstrated by lymphangiography. Amer. J. Obstet. Gynec. **88,** 460 (1964).
36. Nicolesco, J.: Sur les lymphatiques du rein. Ann. Anat. path. **7,** 503 (1930).
37. Pataky, Z., Kubik, St., Karacsonyi, S., Tömböl, T.: Über den Lymphkreislauf des Magens und seine klinische Bedeutung. Anat. Anz. (Jena) **107,** 1 (1959).
38. Pattillo, R. A., Foley, D.-V., Mattingly, R. F.: Internal pelvic lymphography. Amer. J. Obstet. Gynec. **88,** 110 (1964).
39. Pentl, A. A., Friedman, E. A.: Lymphatic system of the female genitalia. Philadelphia: W. B. Saunders 1971.
40. Reiffenstuhl, G.: Über Involution und Neubildung von Lymphknoten. Arch. Gynäk. **187,** 375 (1956).
41. Reiffenstuhl, G.: Das Lymphsystem des weiblichen Genitale. München-Berlin-Wien: Urban & Schwarzenberg 1957.
42. Rodrigues, A., Pereira, S.: Sur les gros troncs lymphatiques de la base du cou. Ann. Anat. path. **7,** 1019 (1930).
43. Rouvière, H.: De la possibilité d'une circulation lymphatique rétrograde en amont des ganglions du pédicule pulmonaire atteints d'adénite. Ann. Anat. path. **7,** 1109 (1930).
44. Rouvière, H.: Anatomie des lymphatiques de l'homme. Paris: Masson 1932.
45. Ruettimann, A.: Erkrankungen des retroperitonealen Lymphsystems. 6th Ed. In: Lehrb. d. Röntgendiagnostik (Schinz, Baensch, Frommhold, Glauner, Uehlinger, Wellauer, Edit.), Vol. **5,** p. 671. Stuttgart: Thieme 1965.
46. Sukiennikow, W.: Topographische Anatomie der bronchialen und trachealen Lymphdrüsen. Berl. klin. Wschr. **40,** 316, 347, 369 (1903).
47. Taillens, J. P.: Anatomical and clinical studies of the cervical lymph node chains. In: Progress in Lymphology 1966 (Rüttimann, E., Edit.). Stuttgart: Thieme 1970.
48. Tömböl, T., Vajda, J.: Über die Lymphzirkulation des Pankreas. Anat. Anz. (Jena) **110,** 400 (1961).

49. Toendury, G., Kubik, St.: Zur Ontogenese des lymphatischen Systems. In: Handb. d. allg. Path. III/6, 1 (1972). Berlin-Heidelberg-New York: Springer.
50. Trotter, H. A.: The surgical anatomy of the lymphatics of the head and neck. Ann. Otol. (St. Louis) **39**, 384 (1930).
51. Weinberg, J., Greaney, E. M.: Identification of regional lymph nodes by means of a vital staining dye during surgery of gastric cancer. Surg. Gynec. Obstet. **90**, 561 (1950).
52. Welsh, L. W.: The normal human laryngeal lymphatics. Ann. Otol. (St. Louis) **73**, 569 (1964).
53. Wirth, W.: Zur Röntgenanatomie des Lymphsystems der inguinalen pelvinen und aortalen Region. I. Teil: Fortschr. Röntgenstr. (Stuttgart) **105**, 441 (1966). II. Teil: Fortschr. Röntgenstr. (Stuttgart) **105**, 636 (1966).
54. Wirth, W.: Röntgenanatomie des Lymphsystems. Grenzen des Normalen — Variationen — Fehlerquellen. Zürich: Habilitationsschrift 1971.
55. Wolodjko, W. P.: Das Lymphsystem der menschlichen Leber in Beziehung zu ihrer Segmentierung. Z. Anat. Entwickl.-Gesch. (Berlin) **126**, 154 (1967).

A Functional Approach to the Classification of Malignant Lymphoma

R. J. LUKES and R. D. COLLINS

Summary and Conclusions

1. The malignant lymphomas are neoplasms of the immune system. The traditional classifications lack a valid conceptual basis and bear no relationship to our understanding of modern immunology.

2. It now appears possible from our clinical and morphologic studies to propose a functional classification based on the T- and B-cell lymphocytic system in order that we might begin to study the lymphomas from an immunologic standpoint. The lymphomas of lymphocytes frequently appear to involve alterations in lymphocyte transformation, either as a block or a "switch-on" (derepression).

3. A number of functional studies capable of identifying membrane markers that appear relatively specific for T and B cells are presently available and already have indicated that certain malignancies can be classified according to T- and B-cell types.

4. Lymphomas of follicular center cells, either cleaved or noncleaved (transformed cells), are included in the B-cell group and represent the most common cytologic types of lymphoma. They occur in follicular, follicular and diffuse, and diffuse forms, with or without sclerosis, and appear to begin usually, if not always, in follicular centers. The follicular or nodular character of lymphomas relates directly to the nature of the follicular-center-cell proliferation and the basic association of these cells with follicle formation. The favorable prognosis with some lymphomas of follicular pattern reflects the less aggressive nature of cellular proliferation that is still capable of follicle formation.

5. The majority of lymphomas previously classified as reticulum-cell sarcoma or histiocytic lymphoma present features of transformed lymphocytes. Lymphomas of histiocytes as macrophages are rare. Lymphomas of immunoblasts have been included in the reticulum-cell-sarcoma group in the past and have been observed to develop in chronic abnormal immune disorders. It seems likely that a similar neoplasm develops in a variety of immune disorders, including immune deficiencies, alpha-chain disease, immunosuppression of patients for graft rejection, and Sjögren's syndrome.

6. A functional immunologic classification of lymphomas is necessary for a proper understanding of the clinical manifestations of the lymphomas and eventually the development of more appropriate therapeutic approaches. It is believed that the study of malignant lymphomas from an immunologic standpoint, combining sophistic-

ated morphologic and immunologic techniques with in-depth clinical investigation, will establish the classification of lymphomas on a sound conceptual basis in the near future.

The remarkable progress in our understanding of immunology in the past decade has demonstrated that the traditional classifications of malignant lymphomas, the neoplasms of the immune system, bear no relationship to our modern view of immunology. The lack of appreciation of the new lymphocytic systems of B-cell and T-cell types and the remarkable phenomenon of lymphocyte transformation readily accounts for the absence of a sound conceptual basis and the resultant confusion concerning lymphomas. The older classifications of malignant lymphoma were developed principally on the basis of suspected cellular derivation, the degree of apparent differentiation, and the proposed multipotential capability of the reticulum cell to produce a limitless variety of neoplastic lesions.

From our current morphologic studies it now appears possible to identify some of the lymphomas of the thymic-dependent (T-cell) and bursal-equivalent (B-cell) systems and to propose a new functional classification for the lymphomas [1, 13]. These studies suggest that lymphomas of the T- and B-cell systems develop from either a block or "switch-on" (derepression) in lymphocyte transformation rather than from alterations in degree of differentiation [13]. In addition, the lymphomas previously regarded as histiocytic lymphoma or reticulum-cell sarcoma seem, with few exceptions, to be neoplasms of large transformed lymphocytes, most commonly of the B-cell type [13]. A number of functional immunologic techniques that identify membrane markers are being translated rapidly from animal models to the study of human leukemias and lymphomas [6, 19]. These techniques in correlation with morphologic features may in the near future permit the classification of lymphomas to be established on a modern functional immunologic basis.

In this presentation we will review briefly the problems of the traditional classifications, discuss the immunologic basis for our new functional classification of malignant lymphomas, and demonstrate some of the clinical and prognostic implications. This proposal of a functional classification of malignant lymphomas emphasizes the need for a new approach to these neoplasms, with fresh tissue being collected for a variety of functional studies designed to establish a sound conceptual basis for their understanding.

Problems of the Traditional Classifications

Lack of appreciation of the morphologic expressions of lymphocyte transformation and the different behavior of the various lymphocytic systems has unquestionably been responsible for the majority of problems in the classifications of malignant lymphoma over the past decades. In general, lymphomas of lymphocytes previously included cells of small or intermediate size with a limited amount of cytoplasm. The larger cells, including pleomorphic forms that we are presently able to identify as partially or fully transformed lymphocytes, were usually classified in the past within the histiocytic or reticulum-cell sarcoma group. Both lymphosarcoma and reticulum-cell sarcoma appear to have included three or four cell types and these categories were employed in an extremely variable fashion [4, 8, 9]. The result of the variability in the use of the terms lymphosarcoma and reticulum-cell sarcoma in various classifications in general usage in the U.S.A. was that these terms became almost meaningless [8, 9]. Undoubtedly, the absence of specific cytologic techniques and the difficulty of precise cytologic identification in tissue sections contributed significantly to the terminologic problem. The lack of understanding of the lymphocytic systems, and of lymphocyte transformation, combined with limited precision in cytologic identification, produced a peculiar terminologic maze in which terms for the types of lymphoma have been applied in such a variable fashion that it has become impossible either to communicate or compare results from different centers [8, 9].

The classification of RAPPAPORT [20], though recognizing the prognostic significance of nodularity, is based cytologically on differences principally in cell size and in the amount of cytoplasm and is lacking in immunologic relevance.

Lymphocytic Systems and Lymphocyte Transformation

That there are two functional lymphocytic systems has become generally accepted from studies of experimental animals: (a) the thymic-dependent or T-cell system of cellular immunity and (b) the bursal-equivalent (thymic-independent) or B-cell system of humoral immunity. It seems likely that a third lymphocytic system may exist and could account for the marrow stem cell (the non-B or T-cell) for which we suggest the term U cell (undefined cell). A series of studies of congenital immune deficiencies in humans suggest that somewhat parallel B- and T-cell lymphocytic systems exist in man [5]. The cells of these lymphocytic systems have a consistent distribution. Most T cells are situated in the paracortical areas of lymph nodes, the perivascular region of the spleen and small foci in the gastrointestinal tract. B cells are concentrated in the follicular centers of lymph nodes and spleen, are prominent in the lamina propria of the gastrointestinal tract, and are interspersed in the bone marrow. The preferential anatomic distribution results from a highly selective "homing" phenomenon, which is an important factor in the extremely complex daily circulating traffic of lymphocytes.

Under the influence of a variety of stimuli, lymphocytes, apparently of both B- and T-cell types, transform from small or dormant lymphocytes to large metabolically active dividing forms. We think both large and small forms are expressions of lymphocytes and that they represent different metabolic states rather than variations in differentiation. On the basis of this view, many of the morphologic features of lymphocytes which in the past have been related to degrees of differentiation, seem to represent expressions of different states in the transformation phenomenon. The large, completely transformed cell typically is more than four times the size of the normal small lymphocyte. It is primitive in appearance, having a large nucleus with a finely distributed chromatin network, one large or several small nucleoli, and moderate to abundant pyroninophilic cytoplasm. In histologic sections aggregated clusters of normal transformed lymphocytes exhibit wide variations in cell size and resemble a primitive neoplastic process with numerous mitoses. This dramatic experience with histologic sections of normal transformed lymphocytes provided the background stimulus for our search for counterparts in the T- and B-cell lymphocytic systems in disease. The transformed lymphocytes were identified in small numbers in typical benign lymphoid reactions of lymph nodes. At times, however, they present the pathologist with difficult diagnostic problems when they occur in large numbers, as in the regional lymph node of smallpox vaccination or in infectious mononucleosis. In the latter condition we have consistently observed binucleated transformed lymphocytes or immunoblasts that are indistinguishable from the Reed-Sternberg cells of Hodgkin's disease [14, 27].

Lymphomas of T Cells

Evidence is beginning to accumulate of neoplastic proliferation of T cells in Hodgkin's disease, mycosis fungoides, and Sézary's syndrome [3]. There is also some indication that one form of acute lymphocytic leukemia may also involve T cells. We have recently observed a group of patients, primarily adolescents, who presented with mediastinal masses that consisted of a proliferation of distinctive convoluted lymphocytes [1]. Often the marrow is initially uninvolved, only to become diffusely leukemic subsequently. The distinctive proliferating cells are noncohesive, have nuclei with a convoluted appearance, primitive chromatin, small nucleoli, and numerous mitoses. They are steroid- and radiation-sensitive and may represent the immunologically incompetent cell of the thymus. Preliminary functional studies provide some support for the T-cell character of this neoplasm [23]. Cases of this type have been described in the literature as acute lymphocytic leukemia with mediastinal mass [1]. Sternberg reported the association of leukemia with a tumor mass [26]. The group of cases reported, however, included a variety of leukemias, though several were of lymphocytic type. The term *Sternberg sarcoma* [23] seems to us inappropriate for this potential T-cell neoplasm, since it is desirable to emphasize the character and derivation of the neoplastic cell. Therefore, we are proposing the descriptive term, "convoluted lymphocyte, possibly of T-cell type" since at this time the precise nature of the cell is not yet established.

Hodgkin's disease has long been suspected to imply a fundamental lymphocyte abnormality because of the apparent defect in delayed hypersensitivity responsiveness and the tendency for lymphocyte depletion to develop as the disease progresses. Our own approach to the pathologic manifestations of the disease, its natural history, and its histologic types, is based on the suspected critical interrelationship of lymphocytes and Reed-Sternberg cells, or Sternberg cells as they are called in Germany [10, 11, 12]. The mediastinal orientation of the histologic type, nodular sclerosis, provides suggestive evidence of a thymic relationship in Hodgkin's disease. Recently ORDER and HELLMAN [17] presented a hypothesis of the development of Hodgkin's disease on the basis of a defective T-cell surveillance system that permits the development of Reed-Sternberg cells from reticulum cells. From our studies of the morphology of Hodgkin's disease over the past decade [10, 11, 12], *in-vitro* lymphocyte transformation, and the demonstration of Reed-Sternberg-like cells in infectious mononucleosis [14, 27], we have suggested that Reed-Sternberg cells may represent a polyploid expression of transformed lymphocytes or immunoblasts rather than a malignancy of reticulum cells, as long believed. We would modify the ORDER and HELLMAN hypothesis [17] by suggesting that Reed-Sternberg cells develop as polyploid immunoblasts during the transformation of lymphocytes and that this can be initiated by variety of conditions such as viral infections and infectious mononucleosis. In this modified hypothesis, the defective T-cell surveillance proposed by ORDER and HELLMAN [17] would permit the disease to develop by allowing the polyploid immunoblasts or Reed-Sternberg cells to persist and progress in number until they disseminate and produce clinical disease. This hypothesis is consistent with our proposal that the Hodgkin's disease process represents the attempted induction of neoplasia [10] and that the clinical manifestations represent expressions of the struggle between the host (the T cells) and the Reed-Sternberg cells.

Lymphomas of B Cells

The lymphomas of the B-cell lymphocytic system include (a) those associated with abnormal immunoglobulin production and, (b) the lymphomas of precursor cells of the immunoglobulin-producing system, the cells of the follicular center. Chronic lymphocytic leukemia, a closely related process, already appears to be accepted as a B-cell neoplasm [6, 19].

The normal cells of the secondary lymphoid follicle, or follicular center, are regarded as components of the B-cell system on the basis of (a) the ablative experiments of the avian pouch of FABRICIUS that produce agammaglobulinemic animals without follicles or plasma cells, and (b) the immune deficiency of humans, Bruton's agammaglobulinemia, also characterized by an absence of follicles and plasma cells [5]. The normal human follicular center contains four types of cells: (a) a cleaved nucleated cell; (b) a noncleaved nucleated cell with prominent pyroninophilic cytoplasm; (c) the so-called starry-sky phagocyte; and (d) the dendritic reticulum cell [13]. The cleaved and noncleaved cells predominate in the centers and vary in relative frequency with the degree of activity of the follicle. From our camera lucida studies of normal follicular centers we know that both cleaved and noncleaved cells have a wide size range [13]. Nuclear cleavage has similar variations in degree in the cleaved cell. The cytoplasm of both cells is pyroninophilic, but it is scanty in the cleaved cells, and gradually increases in amount in the noncleaved cells with the increase in the size of the nucleus. We have proposed that the normal follicular center is a site of transformation in the B-cell lymphocytic system, possibly associated with exposure to new antigens, the changes progressing from the small lymphocyte through a cleaved-cell phase to the large noncleaved cell, as shown in Fig. 1 [13]. The small B lymphocyte under the influence of antigenic stimulation from the antigen-processing perifollicular cell, as observed by NOSSAL [16], is induced to initiate transformation. The small lymphocyte undergoes nuclear cleaving, gradually enlarges as a cleaved cell, and acquires a small amount of pyroninophilic cytoplasm. In the next phase nuclear cleavage disappears, the nucleus becomes round or oval, and nucleoli appear and enlarge as the amount of pyroninophilic cytoplasm reaches a prominent degree. The noncleaved cell continues to enlarge until it is four or more times as large as the original lymphocyte. The nucleoli are prominent and distinctive, with two typically situated at the nuclear membrane on the short axis of an oval nucleus. The noncleaved cell is the dividing cell of the follicular center, while the cleaved cell appears to be essentially the nondividing form. This proposed *in vivo* transformation of B lymphocytes in the follicular center from small to large cells is in direct contradiction to a commonly held view of differentiation. Our proposal is based on the experience of one author (RJL) with *in vitro* lymphocyte transformation that suggests that the most likely direction is from the small dormant lymphocyte to the large metabolically dividing form. The possibility of a bidirectional transformation or modulation *in vivo* is acknowledged and may account for the differences in views. Our morphologic studies of human malignant lymphomas, however, seem to provide support for the proposed direction, as do the elegant studies of DNA synthesis of follicular center cells in the human tonsil by Mitrou *et al.* [15].

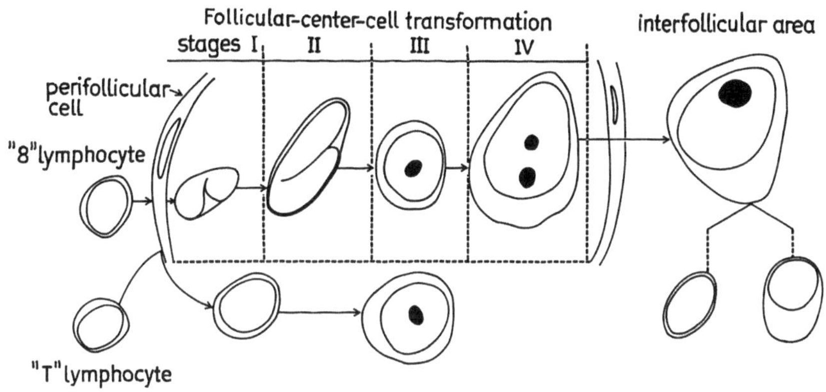

Fig. 1. Schematic representation of transformation of follicular center cells in stages

The majority of nodular and diffuse human lymphomas in our current studies present the cytologic features of the follicular-center-cell (FCC) types. Our camera lucida studies of numerous nodular (follicular) lymphomas revealed that the nodules subjected to light microscopy were composed almost exclusively of cleaved or non-cleaved cells, or varying mixtures of these. Most importantly, these cells were essentially similar to normal follicular-center cells, exhibiting only exaggerations in cell size or degree of nuclear cleavage. The majority of diffuse lymphomas also consist of the same cells, though with a greater range of cell size and frequency of pleomorphism. These proliferations, although always exhibiting some degree of mixture which at times is marked, can be divided into the following four categories, based generally on the size of the two cell types: (a) small cleaved; (b) large cleaved; (c) small non-cleaved; and (d) large noncleaved. All cell types are observed in nodular (follicular) or diffuse patterns, though the majority with the follicular pattern of proliferation are of the small or large cleaved cell type (Fig. 2). The small and large noncleaved cell lymphomas do not commonly exhibit nodularity. The lymphomas of cleaved cells, when diffuse, are usually larger than those with a follicular pattern. The aggressiveness of these lymphomas is a reflection of their normal counterparts. The lymphomas of the noncleaved cells (Fig. 3), regarded as the dividing cells of the follicular center, have numerous mitoses, an apparent high turnover rate with rapidly enlarging masses, and usually a diffuse pattern associated with short median survival times in the range of 3 to 5 months. The small cleaved cell, essentially a nondividing cell, commonly exhibits some attempted follicle formation. It exhibits little or no cellular cohesion, is

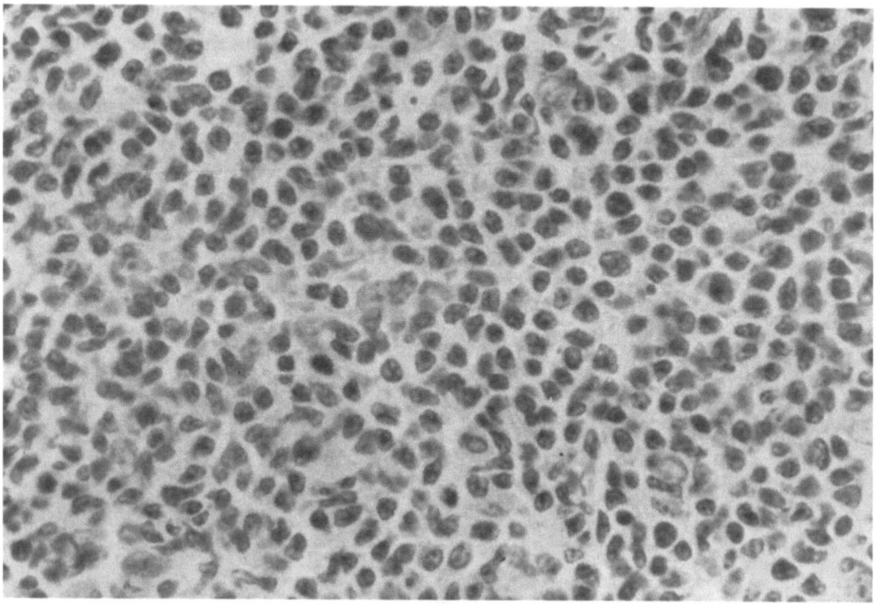

Fig. 2. Small cleaved FCC from lymphomatous follicle. This cytologic type is variable both in size and configuration. Linear subdivisions of nuclei (cleavage) is frequent. RMH No. 1060—71. H & E ×850

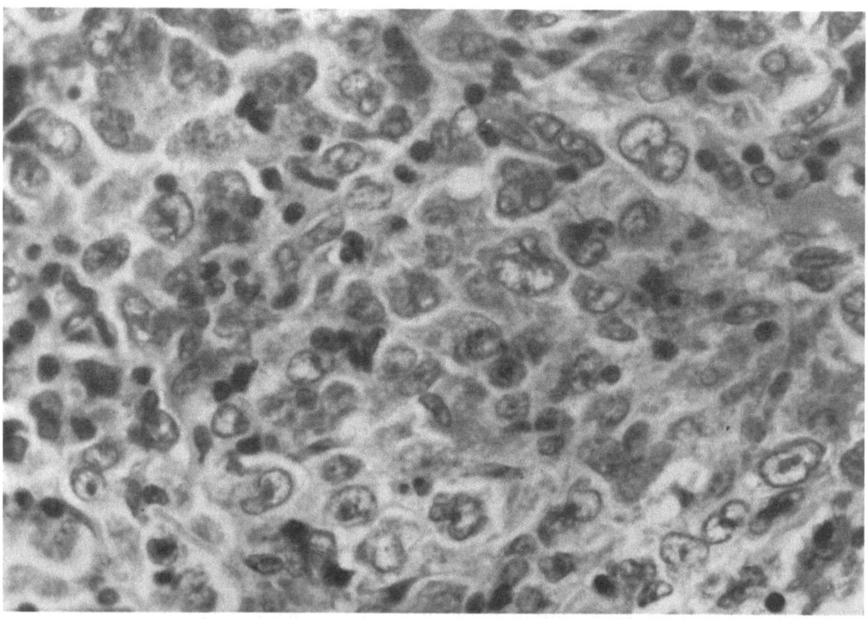

Fig. 3. Large cleaved FCC. This cytologic type exhibit extraordinary variations in nuclear configuration as an expression of a cleavage abnormality. Small cleaved cells are also present. RMH No. 2332—71. H & E ×850

often found in the peripheral blood, and appears to be responsible for widespread "seeding" to the marrow, spleen and liver at a time when the patient may appear well, with limited disease. The process is associated with slow progression and the median survival often exceeds four years, probably depending in part on the stage of development of the process when initially observed. The large cleaved cell (Fig. 4) is associated with the appearance of dividing noncleaved cells, increased aggressiveness and shortened median survival time, even when some degree of follicle formation is evident.

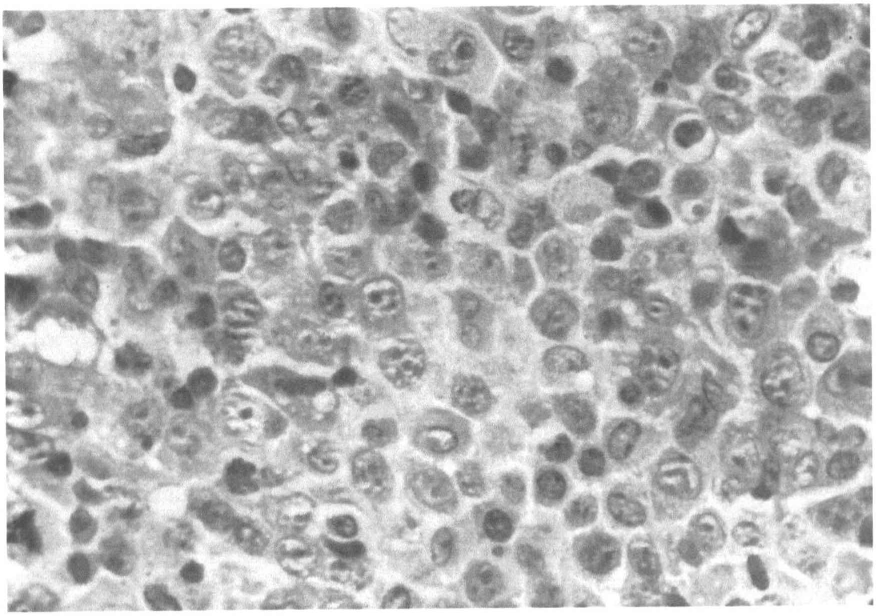

Fig. 4. Large noncleaved FCC. This proliferation varies widely in size, but the nuclei are essentially oval or round, have several nucleoli and the cytoplasm is abundant. RMH No. 489—65. H & E ×850

Our clinical morphologic correlation studies suggest that the majority of lymphomas are of the B-cell type and can be related to the proposed levels of transformation of follicular-center cells (FCC) as shown in Fig. 1. These may develop as either a block or a "switch-on" in transformation, the latter possibly as a manifestation of derepression. In the lymphoma of small lymphocytes, which we regard as the tissue manifestation of chronic lymphocytic leukemia, there appears to be a block at the perifollicular cell with an absence of nodules, apparently due to an inability to form follicles, associated with a lack of plasma cells and the finding of hypo- or agammaglobulinemia. A block at the next stage, i.e. the small cleaved cells, is almost always associated with some degree of nodule or follicle formation; the majority of all follicular or nodular lymphomas are a variation of this type. When the block occurs at the stage of a large cleaved cell, follicle formation at times is found, but the process is often diffuse and rather aggressive. The small noncleaved cell proliferation is typical of the Burkitt lymphoma, as difined in the WHO Conference

Report [2]. The large noncleaved cell represents a "switch-on" of transformation similar to the Burkitt lymphoma, but it occurs in our experience primarily in individuals beyond the fifth decade. This cytologic type of lymphoma is often extremely variable in character, may be associated with abnormal immunoglobulin production, and is closely related to the immunoblastic sarcomas which will be discussed next.

Immunoblastic Sarcoma

Recently we have observed the development of lymphomas of immunoblasts, a monomorphous proliferation of abnormal immunoblasts, in a small group of patients with chronic abnormal immune disorders such as severe rheumatoid arthritis and SLE, for which we are proposing the term "immunoblastic sarcoma". These lymphomas of immunoblasts are interpreted as immunoblastic sarcoma of B-cell type since they commonly exhibit plasmacytoid features (Fig. 5) and may be associated with features of a monoclonal gammopathy. These lymphomas developed abruptly and were associated with rapidly progressive disease that terminated fatally within two to three months. A number of parallel clinical situations have been reported in the literature in recent years as reticulum-cell sarcoma or in related terms; these also seem likely to be immunoblastic sarcomas. These include the reticulum-cell sarcomas reported by Talal to develop in Sjögren's syndrome [25], the group of patients collected by Penn who developed reticulum-cell sarcoma during immunosuppressant therapy for graft rejection [18], and various lymphomas observed in alpha-chain disease [21, 22] and in congenital immune defects [5]. We have also encountered a number of morphologically similar cases in older patients where evidence of an abnormal immune state was not obvious. From these observations it is suggested that immunoblastic sarcoma of B-cell type develops in defective, damaged, or senescent states and follows severe chronic antigenic stimulation. Thus far, all immunoblastic sarcomas appear to be of the B-cell type on the basis of the plasmacytoid features or a monoclonal gammopathy. It seems likely that immunoblastic sarcomas of T cells may also exist, but thus far we have observed none with supportive evidence.

Histiocytic Lymphoma and Reticulum-Cell Sarcoma

Lymphomas of histiocytes regarded as neoplastic macrophages or identifiable reticulum cells have been rare in our recent study of a number of case populations. Lymphomas classified in the past under these terms were based on cell size, amount of cytoplasm, and pleomorphism. Upon review, these lymphomas, with few exceptions, present the features of transformed lymphocytes. The majority of lymphomas of transformed lymphocytes exhibit evidence of follicular-center cells (FCC) as large noncleaved cells, often associated with a component of cleaved cells or with plasmacytoid features. Professor Lennert's group has found abnormal tissue immunoglobulin as evidence of B-cell proliferation in lymphomas classified according to previous criteria as reticulosarcoma [24]. A redefinition of histiocytic lymphoma is needed and in the future positive specific evidence will be required for identification of neoplastic histiocytes.

Functional Studies in Lymphomas

Techniques for identification of lymphocytes of the T- and B-cell systems by means of membrane markers have been developed in the past few years in experimental animal systems. Their rapid application to both normal and neoplastic lymphocytes has yielded important and promising results. Chronic lymphocytic leukemia, with a rare exception, and Waldenström's macroglobulinemia clearly appear to be of the B-cell type, while mycosis fungoides and the closely related Sézary's syndrome appear to be of T-cell type.

Spontaneous rosette formation with sheep erythrocytes appears to identify a membrane receptor in mice T cells while complement is necessary to produce rosette formation with B cells of mice. Similar receptors seem to exist in man though their precise nature is unclear at the present time. Receptors for specific immunoglobulins are also present in membranes of B cells and serve as the most reliable method for their identification since T cells bind relatively minute amounts of immunoglobulins. A specific membrane antigen, the theta antigen, is found on T cells in mice, but as of this date no specific membrane antigen has been identified in human lymphocytes. Attempts have been made to prepare highly specific anti-T-cell serum in man by numerous absorption techniques, but with limited success.

The development of highly specific methods generally applicable for the study of human lymphomas seems likely in the immediate future. The combined use of specific identifying markers, *in-vitro* functional studies, and morphologic features will be the method for the study of human lymphomas in the near future and is the basis of our present investigative approach.

A Functional Classification of Lymphomas

It is now possible to propose a classification of lymphomas on an immunologic basis by combining the new concepts of lymphocytic systems and lymphocyte transformation and our own detailed morphological observations. It is acknowledged that the final classification and determination of the specific lymphomatous types must await detailed functional studies. This proposal, however, is an attempt to provide a working approach on which to study the lymphomas from an immunologic standpoint.

The proposed classification of lymphomas is presented in the Table according to the following major groups: — (a) Undefined (U-Cell); (b) T-Cell; (c) B-Cell; (d) Histiocytic and (e) Unclassifiable. At the present time the U-cell group is hypothetical, but may eventually include proliferations of primitive lymphocytes or stem cells similar to those found in some cases of acute lymphocyte leukemia. The unclassifiable group is reserved for lymphomas that are not classifiable for technical reasons. In the T- and B-cell groups evidence is already available from studies of membrane markers to indicate their exact position, as previously indicated. A recent study [3] of cells from cases of Sézary's syndrome, which is closely related to mycosis fungoides, provided strong evidence of their T-cell nature. The lymphoma of small lymphocytes, the tissue counterpart of chronic lymphocytic leukemia, and the plasmacytoid lymphocytic type associated with IgM monoclonal gammopathy, similarly are of B-cell type [6, 19]. Follicular-center-cell lymphomas of either cleaved or noncleaved type, which may be follicular, follicular and diffuse, or diffuse with or without sclerosis, as lymphomas of plasma-cell precursors would seem conceptually to be of B-cell type, but exhaustive functional studies are necessary to establish their final position. An immunoblastic sarcoma of B-cells appears to exist on the basis of the typical morphologic features of the immunoblasts that are commonly associated with a neoplastic plasmacytoid component and a monoclonal gammopathy. It seems likely that this group will eventually include the majority, if not all, of lymphomas developing in patients with (a) alpha-chain disease [21, 22], (b) Sjögren's syndrome [25], (c) congenital immune defects [5], and (d) on immunosuppressant therapy for graft rejection [18]. A counterpart in the T-cell system seems likely, but we have not yet been able to establish its existence.

Table 1. Classification of malignant lymphomas (LUKES and COLLINS)

I. Undefined cell type

II. T-cell types
   1. Mycosis Fungoides and Sézary's syndrome
   2. Convoluted lymphocytic
   3. ? Immunoblastic sarcoma (of T cells)
   4. ? Hodgkin's disease

III. B-cell types
   1. Small lymphocyte (CLL)
   2. Plasmacytoid lymphocytic
   3. Follicular-center cell (FCC) types
      a) small cleaved
      b) large cleaved
      c) small noncleaved — Burkitt's lymphoma
      d) large noncleaved
   4. Immunoblastic sarcoma (of B cells)

IV. Histiocytic types

V. Unclassifiable

Hodgkin's disease is a strong contender as a T-cell lymphoma, but its unusual character and the unestablished nature of its basic process justify caution in placing it. It is subclassified according to the histologic types we have described [10, 11, 12].

Lymphomas of "true" histiocytes seem rare and will require specific methods for their identification. It may be argued that histiocytic medullary reticulosis should be included in this group on the basis of its accepted malignant histiocytic nature. To some observers the widespread or systemic character of this proliferation without formation of tumor masses provides evidence against its inclusion within the malignant lymphomas. Once we have a sound immunologic basis for understanding proliferations of the lymphoreticular system, it may eventually prove more reasonable to classify all neoplastic proliferations of lymphocytes and histiocytes together and regard their distributional characteristics, now categorized as leukemias and lymphomas, simply as expressions of cellular behavior.

References

1. BARCOS, M. P., LUKES, R. J.: Lymphoproliferative disorder of convoluted lymphocytes. Submitted for publication (1973) Details to follow.
2. BERARD, C., O'CONOR, G. T., THOMAS, L. B., TORLONI, H.: Histopathological definition of Burkitt's tumour. Bull. Wld Hlth Org. **40**, 601—607 (1969).
3. BROUET, J., FLANDRIN, G., SELIGMANN, M.: Thymus-derived nature of the proliferating cells in Sézary's syndrome. New Engl. J. Med. **289**, 341—344 (1973).
4. GALL, E. A.: The reticulum cell, the cytological identity and interrelation of mesenchymal cells of lymphoid tissue. Ann. N. Y. Acad. Sci. **73**, 120 (1958).
5. GOOD, R. A., FINSTAD, J.: The association of lymphoid malignancy and immunologic functions. Proc. of the International Conference on Leukemia-Lymphoma, pp. 185—197, ed. ZARAFONETIS. Philadelphia: Lea and Febiger 1968.
6. GREY, H. M., RABELLINO, E., PIROFSKY, B.: Immunoglobulins on the surface of lymphocytes. IV. Distribution in hypogammaglobulinemia, cellular immune deficiency and chronic lymphocytic leukemia. J. clin. Invest. **50**, 2368—2375 (1971).
7. LENNERT, K.: Follicular lymphoma: A special entity of malignant lymphomas. Plenary Session Papers, First Meeting of the European Division of the International Society of Haematology, Milano, pp. 108—122, ed. E. E. POLLI and A. T. MAIOLO (1971).
8. LUKES, R. J.: A review of the American concept of malignant lymphoma in progress in lymphology, p. 109, ed. A. RUTTIMANN. Stuttgart: Georg Thieme 1967.
9. LUKES, R. J.: The pathological picture of the malignant lymphomas. Proc. of the International Conference on Leukemia-Lymphoma, pp. 333—356, ed. ZARAFONETIS. Philadelphia: Lea and Febiger 1968.
10. LUKES, R. J., BUTLER, J. J., HICKS, E. B.: Natural history of Hodgkin's disease as related to its pathologic picture. Cancer (Philad.) **19**, 317—344 (1966).
11. LUKES, R .J.: Criteria for involvement of lymph node, bone marrow, spleen, and liver in Hodgkin's disease. Cancer Res. **31**, 1755—1767 (1971).
12. LUKES, R. J.: The pathologic manifestations of Hodgkin's disease. Z. Krebsforsch. **78**, 129—136 (1972).
13. LUKES, R. J., COLLINS, R. D.: New observations on follicular lymphoma Gann Monograph on Cancer Research No. 15, Malignant Diseases of the Hematopoietic System, pp. 209—215. Ed. AKAZAKI, K., RAPPAPORT, H., BERARD, C. W., BENNETT, J. M., ISHIKAWA, E. Baltimore: University Park Press 1973.
14. LUKES, R. J., TINDLE, B. H., PARKER, J. W.: Reed-Sternberg-like cells in infectious mononucleosis. Lancet **1969 II**, 1003—1004.
15. MITROU, P. S., QUEISSER, W., LENNERT, K., SANDRITTER, W.: Kombinierte autoradiographischcytophotometrische Untersuchungen von Keimzentrumszellen der menschlichen Tonsille. Virchows Arch. Abt. B. Zellpath. **3**, 156 (1969).
16. NOSSAL, G. J. V., ABBOT, A., MITCHELL, J., LUMMUS, Z.: Antigens in immunity. XV. Ultrastructural features of antigen capture in primary and secondary lymphoid follicles. J. exp. Med. **127**, 277—289 (1968).
17. ORDER, S. E., HELLMAN, S.: Pathogenesis of Hodgkin's disease. Lancet **1972 I**, 571—573.
18. PENN, I., HALGRIMSON, C. G., STARZL, T. E.: De novo malignant tumors in organ transplant recipients. Transp. Proc. **3**, 773—778 (1971).
19. PREUDHOMME, J. L., KLEIN, M., VERRAUST, P., SELIGMANN, M.: Immunoglobules monoclonales de membranes dans les leucemies lymphoides chroniques. Rev. Eur. Etud. Clin. Biol. **16**, 1025—1031 (1971).
20. RAPPAPORT, H.: Tumors of the hematopoietic system. Atlas of Tumor Pathology, Section III, Fascicle 8, Armed Forces Institute of Pathology 1966.
21. RAPPAPORT, H., RAMOT, B., HULU, N., PARK, J. K.: The pathology of so-called mediterranean abdominal lymphoma with malabsorption. Cancer (Philad.) **29**, 1502—1511 (1972).
22. SELIGMANN, M., MIHAESCO, E., FRANGIONE, B.: Alpha chain disease. Ann. N. Y. Acad. Sci. **190**, 487—500 (1971).

23. SMITH, J. L., CLEIN, G. P., BARKER, C. R., COLLINS, R. D.: Characterization of malignant mediastinal lymphoid neoplasm (Sternberg Sarcoma) as thymic in origin. Lancet **1973 I**, 74—76.
24. STEIN, H., LENNERT, K., PARWARESCH, M. R.: Malignant lymphomas of B cell type. Lancet **1972 II**, 855—857.
25. TALAL, N., SOKOLOFF, L., BARTH, W. F.: Extrasalivary lymphoid abnormalities in Sjögren's syndrome (reticulum cell sarcoma, "pseudolymphoma", macroglobulinemia). Amer. J. Med. **43**, 50—65 (1967).
26. STERNBERG, G.: Leukosarcomatose und Myeloblastenleukämie. Beitr. Anat. etc. Ohr **61**, 75 (1916).
27. TINDLE, B. H., PARKER, J. W., LUKES, R. J.: "Reed-Sternberg Cells" in infectious mononucleosis? Amer. J. clin. Path. **58**, 607—617 (1972).

The Unspecific Mesenchymal Reaction of the Liver in Patients with Hodgkin's Disease

W. OEHLERT

Summary

In 84% of patients with Hodgkin's disease we could detect a mesenchymal reaction in the liver with or without liver involvement by laparoscopical and histological examination. The activation of mesenchymal cells extended from a diffuse proliferation (stage I) to the formation of histiocytic nodules (stage II) partially with atypical reticulum cells and with eosinophilic granulocytes (stage III). A similar reaction could be found in spleens after staging laparotomy with splenectomy with or without enlargement of the spleen. There was a positive correlation between the involvement of liver or spleen and the severity of the mesenchymal reaction but no correlation with the histological type or the clinical stage of Hodgkin's disease.

We conclude that the mesenchymal reaction in liver and spleen is an unspecific proliferating reaction of the reticular-histiocytic system in patients with Hodgkin's disease, similar to the reactions in patients with the immuncell-proliferating syndrome or with plamocytoma.

Laparoscopic examination of patients with Hodgkin's disease in whom liver involvement is suspected, detects liver infiltrates in only very few cases. A few prominent greyish-white nodules are usually seen.

The histological picture is characterized by Hodgkin and Sternberg-Reed cells and eosinophilic granulocytes in a fibrous stroma (Fig. 1).

In cases in which there is no clear liver involvement, a fibrous reaction of the liver capsule with ectatic lymph vessels can be observed laparoscopically. These alterations correspond to those observed in inflammatory liver alterations. In such cases, unspecific activation of the RES with a diffuse increase of Kupffer cells with very few nodular histiocytes is found histologically. We designated these alterations "unspecific mesenchymal reaction Stage I" (Figs. 2 and 3). In other cases we have found the development of larger nodular reactions with histiocytes, plasma cells and eosinophilic granulocytes; we call this "unspecific mesenchymal reaction Stage II" (Figs. 4 and 5).

Finally, there is a group of patients with mainly periportal, but also intralobular localized granulomatous infiltrates with histiocytes, plasma cells, eosinophilic granulocytes and isolated atypical reticulum cells with large nuclei. These large cells, however, cannot be classified as Hodgkin or Sternberg giant cells. We designated these

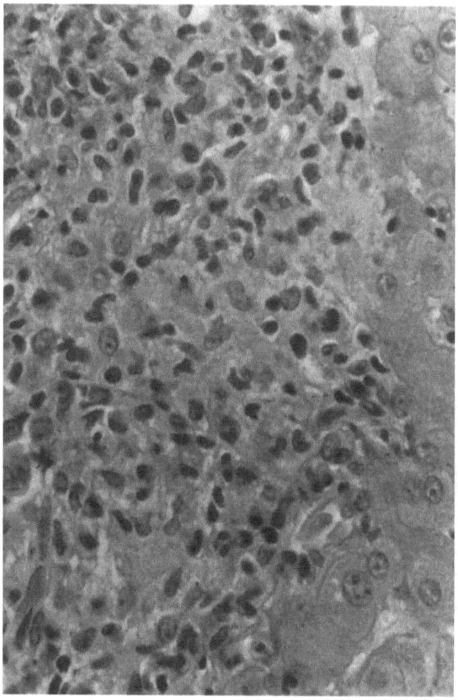

Fig. 1. Liver involvement of Hodgkin's disease. The large granuloma is built up from lymphocytes, Hodgkin and Sternberg-Reed cells

Fig. 2. Mesenchymal reaction Stage I of the liver in a patient with Hodgkin's disease. Diffuse activation and increase of mesenchymal cells with multiple mononuclear cells in the sinusoids, forming small granulomas

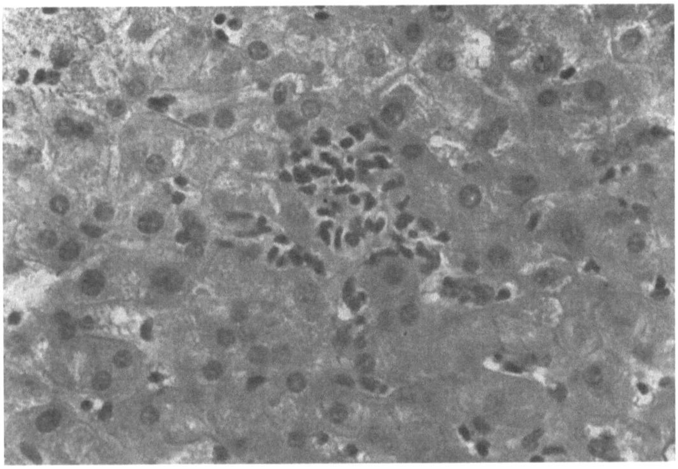

Fig. 3. Mesenchymal reaction Stage I at a higher magnification. Lymphocytes and histiocytes have formed a vaguely delineated granuloma

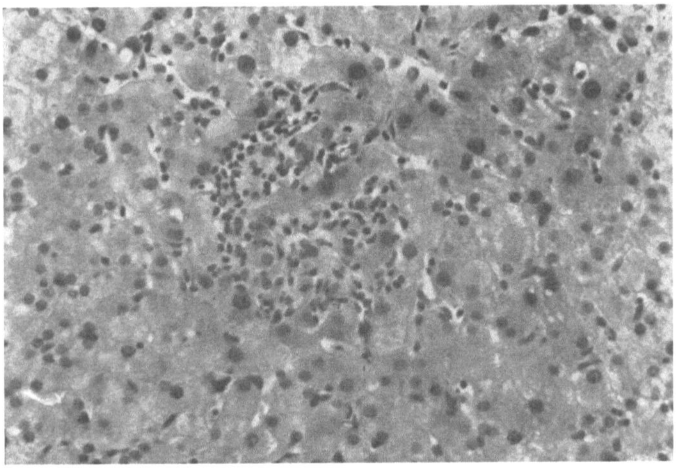

Fig. 4. Mesenchymal reaction Stage II with a larger granuloma consisting lymphocytes and histiocytes. Enlarged Kupffer cells in a diffuse distribution

changes as "unspecific mesenchymal reaction Stage III" (Figs. 6 and 7). In nearly all cases with mesenchymal reactions, we found accompanying degenerative changes in liver parenchymal cells, which could also be classified in three stages on the basis of the number and distribution of liver-cell necroses, degree of intrahepatic cholestasis and mitotic activity of the liver parenchyma. In many cases, glycogen nuclei were found mainly in the periphery of liver lobules (see Fig. 6); however, this showed no positive correlation with glucocorticoid treatment. In one case without liver involvement we found one Sternberg-Reed Cell with deformed nucleus in a sinusoid (Fig. 8).

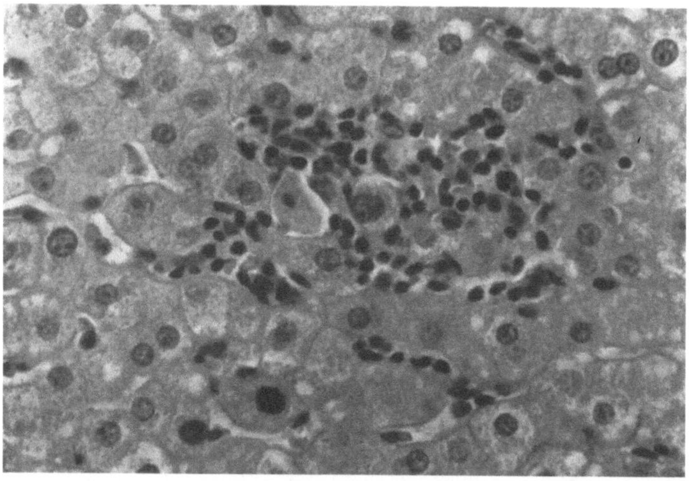

Fig. 5. Mesenchymal reaction Stage II with significant parenchymal lesions. Cellular infiltration of the liver parenchyma with lymphocytes and histiocytes (upper right corner). Parenchymal damage with "Councilman bodies". Diffuse increase of enlarged Kupffer cells

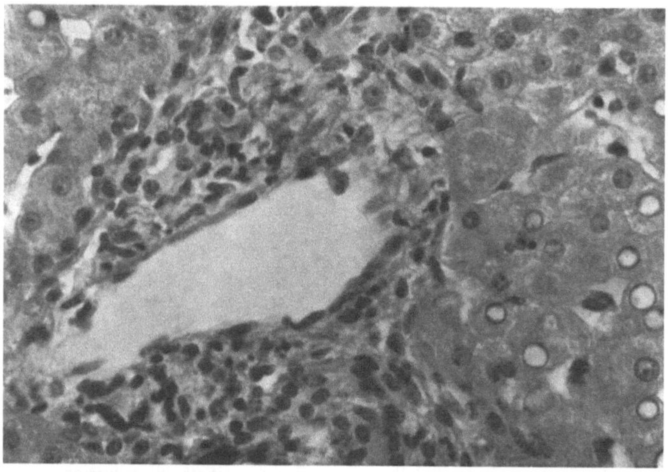

Fig. 6. Mesenchymal reaction Stage III. A large nodular infiltration with lymphocytes, histiocytes, eosinophils and reticulum cells with enlarged nuclei. In the surrounding liver parenchyma are many so-called glycogen nuclei

The material so far examined includes histological specimens of liver tissue from 161 patients with Hodgkin's disease and 67 splenectomized patients. Table 1 shows that liver involvement was detected laparoscopically in 24 out of 161 patients with Hodgkin's disease. These 24 patients all showed unspecific mesenchymal reaction Stage III. Of patients without liver involvement, 84.6% showed unspecific mesenchymal reaction Stages I—III.

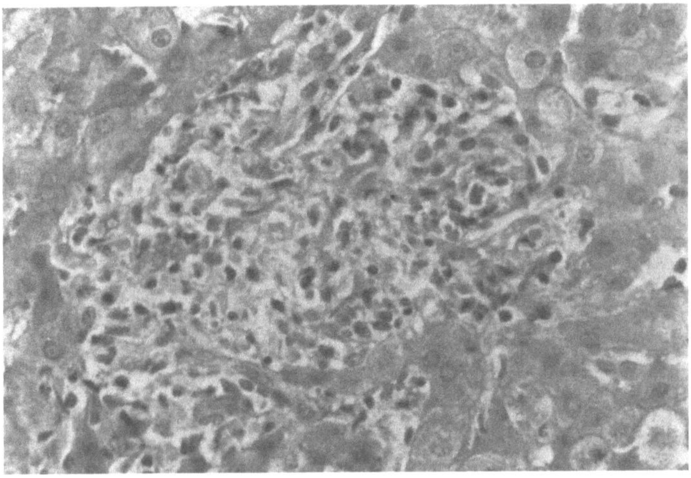

Fig. 7. Mesenchymal reaction Stage III. A sharply delineated granuloma with lymphocytes, eosinophils and reticulum cells with large nuclei. Hodgkin or Sternberg-Reed cells could not be found in the serially investigated liver specimen

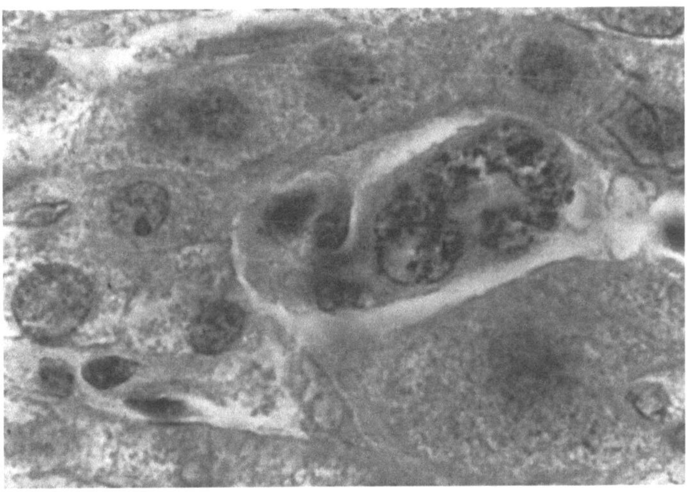

Fig. 8. A Sternberg-Reed cell inside a sinusoid of a Hodgkin's disease case without liver involvement

As Table 2 shows, there is no positive correlation between the histological form of Hodgkin's disease and the incidence and stage of mesenchymal reaction of the liver. The incidence of the various histological forms in these 161 patients is exactly the same as in the larger group of 508 patients in an earlier series [4]. No correlation was found between the clinical stage of the disease and incidence of liver mesenchymal reactions (Table 3).

Table 1. Unspecific mesenchymal reaction of the liver in 161 patients with Hodgkin's disease

Stages of the mesenchymal reaction	without liver involvement of Hodgkin's disease	with liver involvement of Hodgkin's disease
0	21 (15.4%)	—
I	30 (21.9%)	—
II	47 (34.4%)	—
III	39 (28.3%)	24 (100%)

Table 2. Histologic classification of Hodgkin's disease in patients with unspecific mesenchymal reaction of the liver

Stages of the mesenchymal reaction and liver involvement	n	Histological form in lymph nodes			
		lymphocytes & histiocytes	nodular sclerosis	mixed	lymphocyte depletion
0	21	2	10	4	5
I—III	116	29	44	25	18
liver involvement	24	4	8	10	2

Table 3. Unspecific mesenchymal reaction in the various clinical stages of patients with Hodgkin's disease

Stages of the mesenchymal reaction in the liver	Clinical stages of Hodgkin's disease				
	I	II	III	IV	n
0	8	4	9	—	21
I	2	10	13	5	30
II	2	6	28	11	47
III	—	4	17	18	39
liver involvement	—	—	—	24	24

A splenectomy was performed on 61 of the Hodgkin's disease patients. Liver and lymph node biopsies were taken at the same time. The spleen was enlarged in nearly all cases, but only in 20 cases could Hodgkin's granuloma of the spleen be detected by serial macroscopic and microscopic investigations. In many cases the reason for the enlargement of the spleen was an activation of endothelial and reticulum cells with a marked eosinophilia. An increase of the plasma cells could also be observed and small granulomas had developed out of reticulum cells, but without Hodgkin and Sternberg-Reed cells. The liver specimens were not sufficient in all cases for grading of the mesenchymal reaction, but where an examination was possible, spleen involvement was combined with a liver reaction of Stage II or III (Table 4).

Similar mesenchymal reactions in the liver were observed by other investigators who performed systematic laparotomy in patients with Hodgkin's disease [1, 2, 6].

Table 4. Unspecific mesenchymal reaction in the liver in patients with Hodgkin's disease after splenectomy

		Mesenchymal reaction			Not classified
		I	II	III	
Spleen without liver involvement	47	10	15	9	13
Spleen with liver involvement	20	—	10	8	2

They also discovered that involvement of the liver in the early stage of the Hodgkin's disease is rare. They consider that a nodular reaction like Stage III of our classification is of value in the diagnosis of Hodgkin's disease [7].

On the other hand we know that in other diseases, such as the chronic immune proliferative syndrome [12], cases of medullar plasmocytoma, Brill-Symmers lymphoblastoma or Waldenström disease, nodular mesenchymal reactions in the liver are quite common [11]. A similar mesenchymal reaction is also found in patients with hypernephroma [5].

Popper and Schaffner [10] consider that small granulomas consisting of reticulum cells and Kupffer cells develop into Hodgkin's granulomas. If this is so, granulomas of Stage III of our classification could be precursors of the Hodgkin involvement of the liver.

Present evidence does not yet confirm this opinion. We have reported [8, 9] about control biopsies of patients with Hodgkin's disease, where a regression from nodular mesenchymal reaction Stage III to Stage II or I had taken place.

We conclude that the mesenchymal reactions of both the liver and the spleen which we observed during our studies and classified in 3 stages are unspecific reactions of the reticular histiocytic system in patients with Hodgkin's disease: these changes have no direct connection with the histological classification and the stage of the disease. Perhaps these mesenchymal reactions observed not only in the spleen and liver but also in the bone marrow [3], are the morphological expression of a disturbance in the immune proliferative system.

Our results lead us to conclude that a laparoscopy for liver and spleen biopsy is an essential diagnostic procedure in all Hodgkin's disease cases, whether or not splenectomy is performed.

References

1. Barge, J., Potet, F.: Etude anatomo-pathologique du foie dans la maladie de Hodgkin. Presse méd. **79**, 565 (1971).
2. Diebold, J., Camilleri, J. G.: La biopsie hépatique au cours des laparotomies systématiques pour maladie de Hodgkin. Valeur diagnostique et signification des lésions observées. Path. europ. **6**, 299 (1971).
3. Georgii, A., Vykoupil, K. F.: Unspecific mesenchymal reaction in bone marrow in patients with Hodgkin's disease. This symposium (p. 39).

4. HAMANN, W., OEHLERT, W., MUSSHOFF, K., NUSS, A., SCHNELLBACHER, B.: Histologische Einteilung des Lymphoma malignum Hodgkin und seine Bedeutung für die Prognose. Dtsch. med. Wschr. **95**, 112 (1970).
5. LINHART, P., HEILMANN, K., WEITZEL, A.: Reversible Leberfunktionsstörung bei Patienten mit Hypernephrom. Dtsch. med. Wschr. **96**, 29 (1971).
6. LUKES, R. J.: Criteria for involvement of lymphnode, bone marrow, spleen, liver in Morbus Hodgkin. Cancer Res. (1972), in press.
7. MACLEOD, M., STALKER, A.: Diagnosis of Hodgkin's disease by liver biopsy. Brit. med. J. **1972 II**, 1449.
8. OEHLERT, W., DISCHLER, W.: Unspezifische Mesenchymreaktion und Parenchymschäden der Leber bei Patienten mit Morbus Hodgkin. Dtsch. med. Wschr. **97**, 323 (1972).
9. OEHLERT, W., MUSSHOFF, K., WUNSCH, B., WILLMANN, H., BECK, K.: Unspezifische Mesenchymreaktionen und Parenchymschäden der Leber bei Patienten mit Morbus Hodgkin. Klin. Wschr. **48**, 126 (1970).
10. POPPER, H., SCHAFFNER, F.: The liver. Structure and function. New York: McGraw-Hill 1957.
11. THALER, H.: Leberbiopsie. Berlin-Heidelberg-New York: Springer 1969.
12. WESTERHAUSEN, M., OEHLERT, W.: Chronisches pluripotentielles immunoproliferatives Syndrom. Dtsch. med. Wschr. **97**, 1407 (1972).

Unspecific Mesenchymal Reaction in Bone Marrow in Patients with Hogdkin's Disease

A. Georgii and K. F. Vykoupil

Summary

For 72 patients with Hodgkin's disease with no evidence of bone marrow infiltration, the intensity of tumour-myelopathy is compared to the histological classification of lymphnodes (Rye classification), clinical findings and therapy. Tumour-myelopathy is defined as a lesion of the haematopoetic parenchyma and vascular mesenchyma which is thought to be a direct consequence of Hodgkin's disease. These alterations were also seen in 24 other malignant lymphomas (lymphosarcomas, giant follicular lymphomas or germinoblastomas, and reticulosarcomas). In contrast, the bone marrow of patients with carcinomas and sarcomas did not demonstrate analogous lesions. Similarities and differences in the histological findings of tumour-myelopathy due to malignant lymphomas are discussed in relation to autoimmune diseases such as Lupus erythematosus and rheumatoid arthritis.

Since Glatstein [5] introduced exploratory laparotomy, increased efforts to establish an exact staging of Hodgkin's disease have led to a growing interest in the morphology of both the spleen and the bone marrow. In the past 4 years more than fifty papers mainly on the frequency of marrow involvement have been published. The main purpose of these studies was to determine whether the bone marrow is directly involved in Hodgkin's disease. There is a general agreement that only closed needle biopsy of the bone marrow yields satisfactory results, whereas aspiration techniques followed by cytological study of the smear have been abandoned by most authors [6, 8]. Despite the number of papers, none deals in detail with the mesenchyma and parenchyma of bone marrow. In Hodgkin's disease we found characteristic lesions in the bone marrow which were completely independent of neoplastic growth. Immunological alterations must be seriously considered as a possible cause for these lesions.

Studies of this kind require a sophisticated and therefore expensive technique of section preparation. Morphological studies of bone marrow slides are only of value when the nondecalcified biopsy specimen has been embedded in epoxy resin and sectioned by milling. After a nine-year comparison of paraffin and plastic embedding of specimens, we finally discarded the conventional paraffin technique in favor of resin, which yields a far more accurate cytomorphological impression, particularly of mesenchymal structures, e.g. walls of capillaries or other vessels.

During our routine diagnosis of bone marrow biopsy specimens from patients with neoplastic diseases, especially Hodgkin's disease, we found characteristic lesions of the bone marrow that we would like to term *tumor myelopathy*. These clearly affect the reticuloendothelial component of the bone marrow with its vessels and adventitial cells. The lesions consist of a swelling of the wall and the endothelial layer of the vessels, a proliferation of plasma and mast cells in the adventitia, and spotty edema of the marrow cavity. Protein deposits including Russel bodies are found in very close proximity to the vessels. A further very typical feature is an excessive nucleophagocytic activity in the histiocytes, resembling lupus erythematosus. However, the parenchyma of the bone marrow space with its three maturing cell series is also affected. There is a disturbance of maturation: erythropoiesis is inhibited while granulo- and megakaryocytopoiesis are accelerated.

We define "tumor myelopathy" as mesenchymal and parenchymal lesions of the bone marrow caused by a remote effect of a lymphoproliferative tumor located outside the marrow space. This definition implies that tumor myelopathy will be seen frequently in malignant lymphomas and not so often in carcinomas and sarcomas.

Our series included 72 patients with Hodgkin's disease who had been myelotomized in accordance with the method of BURKHARDT (Table 1). Twelve had Hodgkin infiltrates of the bone marrow, mostly of the lymphocyte-depleted sclerosing type. This 17% marrow involvement lies at the upper limit of the percentage range indicated in the literature [10]. Patients with any marrow involvement were not considered further, since bone marrow changes might be due to the direct effect of the infiltrates. Of the remaining 60 cases, only 3 were free of tumour myelopathy. This means that only 0.4% of the total number of patients had normal bone marrow.

Table 1. Survey of histological findings in bone marrow of the patients examined

Histology	Cases	%
Myelotomies of Hodgkin patients	72	100
Hodgkin infiltration	12/72	17
Myelopathy without Hodgkin infiltration	57/60	95
Bone marrow with no abnormalities	3/72	4,0

The described lesions may be graded into four degrees according to their histological appearance and intensity. The semi-schematic Table 2 represents the possible lesions in the reticuloendothelial system and the parenchyma and at the site at which they probably begin. Most of these lesions are of the chronic type. The involvement of the vessels induces vascular and perivascular sclerosis and fibrosis with disappearance of vessels, which results in partial atrophy of the bone marrow.

We observed proliferation of plasma and mast cells, stimulated granulopoiesis, nucleophagocytosis, edema of the bone marrow space with its protein deposits and Russell bodies, swelling of the walls of capillaries and veins with plasma-cell invasion of the adventitia, and finally sclerosing atrophic mesenchyma. Despite advanced

Table 2. Histology of myelopathy

Histology		Intensity of meyolopathy			
Structure	Appearance	I	II	III	IV
Capillaries	Edema				
Larger vessels	Edema				
Plasmocytosis	Pericapillary Diffuse				
Mastocytosis	Perivascular Perisinous				
Histiocytosis	With protein storage With siderin storage				
Nucleophagocytosis					
Reticulin fibers	Sclerosing edema				
Erythropoiesis	Inhibition				
Granulopoiesis	Stimulation				
Megakaryocytopoiesis	Stimulation				
Marrow atrophy					

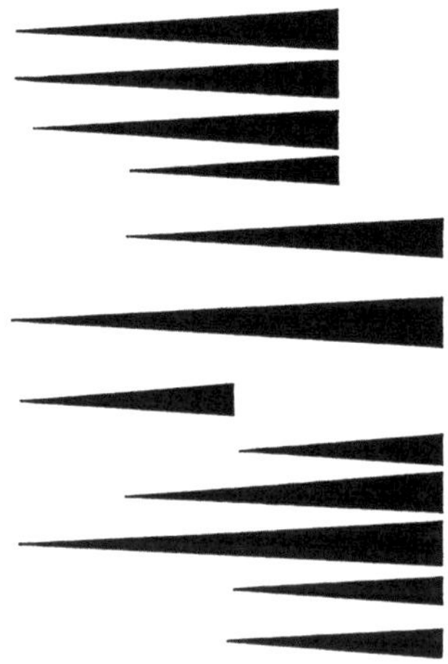

myelofibrosis, the mesenchyma still displays swelling of the vessel walls with surrounding plasma- and mast-cell proliferation.

Here we leave the topic of myelopathy to mention briefly an apparently unrelated observation relating to an early stage in the development of a Hodgkin granuloma. Kadin [7] describes isolated small granulomas. Their occurrence and specificity have been discussed [3]. Among our patients we found isolated granulomas in 5 of 60 Hodgkin-negative bone-marrow biopsies. These display normal epitheloid cells without formation of reticular fibers and without necrosis or any anaplastic reticulum cells. These epitheloid cells and sarcoidlike minimal lesions correspond exactly to the early lesions we saw in the Malpighian bodies of the spleen in Hodgkin patients, as mentioned in a recent paper by Farrer-Brown [4]. Therefore we define them as Hodgkin-specific lesions and agree with the interpretation of Kadin [7]. In connection with these findings, we find there are certain parallels in the observations of Oehlert [9], who have demonstrated granuloma-like lesions in the portal fields of liver biopsies; these are not absolutely specific for Hodgkin's disease.

We consider these observations and the very distinct indications for their specificity important since they again call attenion to the problems of proving autochthononous origin for Hodgkin's disease.

As we have hitherto presented only a purely morphological description of these bone marrow lesions, questions arise concerning their relationship to the clinical picture, that is, between histological classification, clinical staging and finally the specificity of these lesions. Comparison of primary histological findings in the four staging groups demonstrates that tumor myelopathy can be found in all four histological subgroups (Table 3). The clinical classification shows that the intensity of myelopathy is completely independent of the staging of the disease (Table 4).

Separating more recent, untreated cases from advanced, treated cases, we found that, while the two cases not displaying any tumor myelopathy had not been treated at all (Table 5), most of the more recent untreated cases do display myelopathy.

Finally the question of the specificity of our tumor myelopathy arises. First we have to study its frequency in lymphoproliferative disease of other types. A comparison with three other types of malignant lymphomas clearly shows that myelopathy is often present in all other cases (Table 6). Although the number of bone marrow biopsies of patients with malignant lymphomas we have examined is still small, all results indicate that myelopathy occurs more frequently in patients with Hodgkin's disease, in which these lesions are also more accentuated on our graded scale of severity.

The question of specificity includes the possibility that bone lesions can arise even in the absence of a tumor. This is possible in view of our earlier findings in patients with lupus erythematosus. But there are certain differences compared to the myelo-

Table 3. Histological subtypes and myelopathy

Initial histology of lymph nodes (Rye)		Grades of myelopathy				
		0	I	II	III	IV
LP = Lymphocytic Predominance	9	0	4	4	1	0
NS = Nodular Sclerosis	10	0	3	5	1	1
MC = Mixed Cellularity	12	2	5	4	0	1
LD = Lymphocyte Depletion	6	0	1	1	4	0

Table 4. Clinical stage and grades of myelopathy

Assessment at myelotomy			Grades of myelopathy				
Stage	Cases	%	0	I	II	III	IV
I	1	2	—	—	1	—	—
II	19	37	1	8	9	0	1
III	22	42	1	10	7	4	0
IV′	10	19	—	2	2	4	2
Total	52	100	2	20	19	8	3

Table 5. Myelopathy and therapy

Stage	Cases at onset (not treated)		Cases advanced (treated)	
	Negative	Positive	Negative	Positive
I+II	1	10	0	9
III	1	7	0	14
IV	0	3	0	7

Table 6. Myelopathy in malignant lymphomas

Types	Ratio	Intensity of myelopathy			
		I	II	III	IV
Reticulum cell sarcoma	17/14	12	2		
Lymphosarcoma	7/4	4			
Germinoblastoma	2/2	2			
Hodgkin's disease	60/57	23	23	8	3

pathy of Hodgkin patients: L.E. patients show hyaline necrosis of the blood-vessel walls in their bone marrow and more inflammatory cell proliferation requiring use of the term vasculitis (see also BURKHARDT [1]). Finally, arteries are also affected in lupus erythematosus.

To summarize, we believe that myelopathy in malignant lymphomas, especially in Hodgkin patients, is a typical lesion of the bone marrow and directly indicative of fundamental immunological changes in these patients [2]. The morphology of this myelopathy is so characteristic that in combination with other clinical symptoms it is a clear sign of the underlying disease. Progression of myelopathy with vascular obliteration, mesenchymal sclerosis, and resulting cessation of hematopoiesis seems to offer a clear-cut morphological explanation for the anemia, thrombocytopenia, granulocytopenia with susceptibility to hemorrhage and infection frequently present in advanced stages of Hodgkin's disease.

Reasoning that such lesions might also be present in the mesenchyme outside the bone-marrow space, we discovered some support for this assumption in the spleen, and the lesions seen by OEHLERT in the mesenchyme of the liver might be interpreted in a similar way. There may thus be a connection with the general clinical symptoms, especially the recurrent fever typical of Hodgkin patients.

Our results suggest it is tumor myelopathy rather than direct Hodgkin infiltration of the bone marrow which is the crucial lesion. We consider that our study throws some light on the etiology of this lymphoproliferative disease.

References

1. BURKHARDT, R.: The mesenchymal reaction of the bone marrow in hypersensitive mesenchymal diseases. Klin. Wschr. **43**, 1299 (1965); **44**, 1 (1966).
2. CHASE, M. W.: Delayed-type hypersensitivity and the immunology of Hodgkin's disease, with a parallel examination of sarcoidosis. Cancer Res. **26**, 1097 (1966).
3. DUHAMEL, G.: Les localisations a la moelle osseuse de la maladie de Hodgkin. Presse méd. **79**, 2305 (1971).
4. FARRER-BROWN, G., BENNETT, M. H., HARRISON, C. V., MILLETT, Y., JELLIFFE, A. M.: The diagnosis of Hodgkin's disease in surgically excised spleens. J. clin. Path. **25**, 294 (1972).
5. GLATSTEIN, E., GUERNSEY, J. M., ROSENBERG, S. A., KAPLAN, H. S.: The value of laparatomy and splenectomy in the staging of Hodgkin's disease. Cancer (Philad.) **24**, 709 (1969).

6. GRAAN, V., POOL, J. L., MAYER, K.: Comparative study of bone marrow aspiration and biopsy in patients with neoplastic disease. Cancer (Philad.) **19**, 1898 (1966).
7. KADIN, M. E., DONALDSON, S. S., DORFMAN, R. F.: Isolated granulomas in Hodgkin's disease. New Engl. J. Med. **283**, 859 (1970).
8. LIAO, K. T.: The superiority of histologic sections of aspirated bone marrow in malignant lymphomas. Cancer (Philad.) **27**, 618 (1971).
9. OEHLERT, W., DISCHLER, W.: Unspezifische Mesenchymreaktion und Parenchymschäden der Leber bei Patienten mit Morbus Hodgkin. Dtsch. med. Wschr. **97**, 323 (1972).
10. ROSENBERG, S. A.: Hodgkin's disease of the bone marrow. Cancer Res. **31**, 1733 (1971).

The Specific Post-Capillary Venules of Lymphoglandular Tissue in Hodgkin's Disease

N. SÖDERSTRÖM

Summary

High endothelium post-capillary venules, a specific detail in the structural organization of normal lymph nodes, were looked for in lymph nodes invaded by different types of malignant lymphoma. Such venules proved completely absent in lymphosarcoma and reticulosarcoma tissue; they were usually absent in chronic lymphatic leukemia (present in specimens from one of six cases studied) but constantly and sometimes even abundantly present in the specific lymphoma tissue of Hodgkin's disease (9 cases representing lymphocyte predominance, mixed cellularity and nodular sclerosis). The absence of a perivenular cuff of lymphocytes, especially striking in a case of nodular sclerosis, made the author doubt the concept of Gowans that the intraendothelial lymphocytes represent *parenchyma-bound* immigrant lymphocytes from blood.

The *post-capillary high endothelium (HE) venules* are a curious and highly specific feature in the structure of mammalian lymph nodes. They are characterized by very high and bulky endothelium cells, often bulky enough to obturate the venular lumen completely. Still more impressive is the presence of *numerous viable lymphocytes within the cytoplasm of these endothelium cells.* There is also overrepresentation of lymphocytes within the lumen of these venules, which sometimes stick to the endothelium cells as in the formation of an immunological "rosette".

The reduced diameter of the lumen and its infiltration with lymphocytes tend to obscure the vascular pattern of HE venules in the thick sections used in routine histopathology; this may explain why they appear to have been completely overlooked by histopathologists. In thin sections (1 μ or less) and especially after silver or osmium impregnation, HE venules are a very conspicuous and typical feature of diffuse cortex of *lymph nodes* and *tonsils.* They are still present, though less numerous, in gut-associated lymphoid tissue, but they are not seen in the spleen or in the *normal* thymus (though sometimes seen in the "thymitis" of myasthenia and other conditions). Abnormal *ectopic* lymphatic tissue does not contain typical HE venules, even when this tissue is well-differentiated (e.g. Hashimoto goiters).

HE venules are not seen in secondary nodules, and they lose their high endothelium in the medullary cords. They have thus been said to supply an intermediate region of lymph nodes, the so-called *paracortical zone.* PARROT et al. labeled this *thymus-dependent zone* the "homing" region of thymus-derived lymphocytes.

HE venules have long attracted the curiosity of histologists and there has been much discussion as to their function. This problem seemed to have been solved by the experiments of Gowans *et al.* in the early sixties, which suggested that the intraendothelial lymphocytes were *blood* lymphocytes passing *through* the endothelial cells *into the lymphoglandular parenchyma.* Since then it seems to have become generally accepted that long-lived, *recirculating* lymphocytes (today they would be called T lymphocytes) use the HE venules as immigration ports for their passage through the lymph node parenchyma. HE venules might thus be regarded as a local morphological expression of *cellular immunity.*

This concept leaves to the future the problem of the role of the lymphocytes *within* the endothelium cells. The starting point for the present study was a vague hypothesis presented by Gunz *et al.* in 1970 that the endothelium cells might regulate the numbers of circulating lymphocytes by counting the inflowing cells. The high lymphocyte counts in lymphatic leukemia might be the result of a failure of the endothelium cells to recognize (and count) leukemic lymphocytes.

Since little was known of the prevalence of HE venules in chronic lymphatic leukemia (CLL), I examined thin sections of lymph nodes from 6 cases of CLL, and found that in 5 cases the HE venules were either absent altogether or very scanty. In the sixth case, they were apparently normal. I shall not discuss these potentially significant findings at present; in any case, the HE venules could hardly be expected to function according to the hypothesis of Gunz in those lymph nodes where they were no longer present.

In addition, however, I obtained a number of lymph node specimens from 4 non-leukemic cases diagnosed as *lymphosarcoma* and *reticulum cell sarcoma.* Here the situation was quite clear: HE venules were always completely absent from the tumor tissue, but in two specimens they could still be seen in remnants of normal lymph node tissue found outside the tumor. This was, of course, the expected finding: the lymphoma tissue expanded like a true tumor, destroying the normal lymph node tissue together with its typical constituents, the HE venules.

Finally, some *Hodgkin* nodules turned up in the series. I had expected HE venules to be absent or at least reduced in number in this type of lymphoma too; cellular immunity is known to be depressed in Hodgkin's disease and it would be an attractive explanation to attribute this to an elimination of the entrance ports for T lymphocytes. However, to my surprise, apparently typical HE venules were abundantly present all through the specimens examined, a total of 9 cases representing lymphocyte preponderance, mixed cellularity and nodular sclerosis. In the cases of mixed cellularity and lymphocyte preponderance, the lesions gave the impression of an expanded paracortical zone containing more or less numerous Sternberg-Reed cells.

The HE venule morphology was not completely normal. The normal HE venule is surrounded by a cuff of small lymphocytes which is especially conspicuous when it separates the venule from adjacent intraparenchymal sinuses. In my Hodgkin specimens, this lymphocyte cuff sometimes appeared to be absent. This was especially apparent in the nodular sclerosis case, where HE venules appeared to be absent, until I noticed that small lymphocyte foci still present in the broad acellular scars were actually typical HE venules with numerous (in part intraendothelial) lymphocytes within the venule but virtually no lymphocytes outside the basement membrane. This was also apparent in some other specimens where HE venules were seen to protrude into the lumen of lymph sinuses without a trace of the lymphocyte sheath which normally separates the sinus endothelium from the wall of the venule.

The first conclusion to be drawn from these observations is that the Hodgkin lesion does not behave like a neoplastic lymphoma. When localized to lymph nodes, the Hodgkin tissue retains such specific details of the functional structure of lymph nodes as the HE venules, as would be expected in a reactive transformation of ordinary lymph node tissue, but not in a tumor.

Another consideration must be mentioned. In the Hodgkin tissue the lymphocytes appear to have reached their goal when they have entered the venular endothelium, and the relations between lymphocytes and endothelium cells mimic the curious phenomenon of emperipolesis in lymphocyte culture. The picture is similar in the normal lymph node; the only difference is the presence in the node of a perivenular cuff of lymphocytes containing the labeled lymphocytes which GOWANS regarded as immigrants from the venular lumen. They might, however, as well have travelled through the capillaries of the parenchyma. Their presence in the perivenular space may be explained by the same attraction to the high endothelial cells which makes blood lymphocytes stick to them on the lumen side.

References

1. GOWANS, J. L., KNIGHT, E. J.: The route of recirculation of lymphocytes in the rat. Proc. Roy. Soc. (Biol.) **159**, 257—282 (1964).
2. PARROT, D. M. V., DE SOUSA, M. A. B., EAST, J.: Thymus-dependent areas in the lymphoid organs of neonatally thymectomized rats. J. Exper. Med. **123**, 191—201 (1966).
3. VINCENT, P. C., GUNZ, F. W.: Control of lymphocyte numbers in blood. Lancet **1970 II**, 342—344.

Immunology and Immune Reactions in Malignant Lymphoma

H.-D. FLAD

Summary

The immunological findings in Hodgkin's disease and chronic lymphocytic leukemia are reviewed and described on the basis of the concept of thymus-derived (T) and bone-marrow-derived (B) lymphocytes. Environmental and genetic factors appear to be involved in the pathogenesis of Burkitt lymphoma and Hodgkin's disease respectively. The pathogenesis of malignant lymphoma in general is discussed on the basis of a recently developed hypothesis.

There is considerable experimental and clinical evidence for the existence of two populations of lymphocytes, a thymus-derived or thymus-dependent (T) population mediating cellular immunity, and a bone marrow-derived (B) population mediating humoral immunity [1]. This concept has proved helpful in the characterization of primary and secondary immune deficiences. Impairment of cell-mediated immunity results in a decreased ability of the organism to express delayed skin reactivity, homograft rejection and defense against viral infections. Defects in humoral immunity are characterized by impairment of antibody production and low levels of one or several classes of immunoglobulins. The purpose of this study is 1) to describe immunological features of malignant lymphomas on the basis of the concept of T and B cells and 2) to collate immunological phenomena with hypotheses for pathogenetic mechanisms of malignant lymphoma.

1. Hodgkin's Disease (HD)

A variety of immunological phenomena have been described in Hodgkin's Disease (HD) (Table 1). There is no doubt that cell-mediated immunity is impaired in this disease [2], although the extent of the deficiency of T cells has recently been debated [3, 4]. Generally, patients with the lymphocyte-depleted form of HD have a poorer prognosis and appear to be considerably depressed in their cellular immune reactivity. However, not only quantitative but also qualitative changes of the lymphocytes are found in patients with HD. A higher percentage of blood lymphocytes in these patients synthesize DNA and are PAS-positive [5]. *In vitro* these cells respond poorly to phytohemagglutinin, antigen or allogeneic cells [6]. Their capacity to stimulate normal lymphocytes, which is based on histocompatibility differences, is reduced [7].

Table 1. Immunological findings in Hodgkin's Disease

Cell-mediated immunity		
Delayed cutaneous hypersensitivity		
primary (DNCB, DNFB)	(↓)	
secondary (PPD, Candida etc.)	(↓)	
Tranplantation reactions	↓	
Normal lymphocyte transfer reaction (NLT)	↓	
Transfer of tuberculin sensitivity to patients	negative	
Response to "transfer factor"	negative	
Humoral immunity		
primary response	normal or	↓
secondary response	normal	
Antibodies against EB virus		↑
Antibodies against herpes virus hominis	normal	
Antibodies against other viruses	normal or	↓
Immunoglobulins	normal	(↓)
Autoantibodies	+ or −	
Cold-reacting C-fixing lymphotoxins	+ or −	
Lymphocytes *in vitro*		
% DNA synthesizing cells in peripheral blood	↑	
Lymphocyte response to PHA	↓	
Lymphocyte response to antigens and allogeneic cells	↓	
Performance as stimulator cells in MLC	↓	
Production of mediators of cellular immunity (MIF, MF)	↓	
Response to mediators	↓	
Cytotoxic activity on target cells	↓	
Nonspecific defense mechanisms		
Serum complement (C3)	normal, or	↑
Phagocytosis of RES	normal, or	↑
Abnormal serum proteins (α3 globulin, monoclonal γ globulins)	+ or −	

Cell-mediated immunity cannot be transferred from normal hypersensitive individuals to patients with HD, a finding that indicates the necessity for participation of host cells in the expression of transferred delayed hypersensitivity [8]. The transfer of delayed hypersensitivity involves the elaboration of transfer factor by sensitized lymphocytes [9]. This low molecular weight substance confers *in vivo* and *in vitro* specific immunological reactivity on nonsensitized lymphocytes, which start to proliferate and participate in a delayed skin reaction. We investigated why transfer of delayed hypersensitivity is unsuccessful in HD patients [10]. It could be shown that lymphocytes from patients with HD do not proliferate *in vitro* after stimulation with "antigen-induced mitogenic factor" of normal lymphocytes (Fig. 1). Thus, the mechanism of clonal proliferation, by which sensitization of the host occurs, is blocked in patients with HD and in patients with chronic lymphocytic leukemia (CLL).

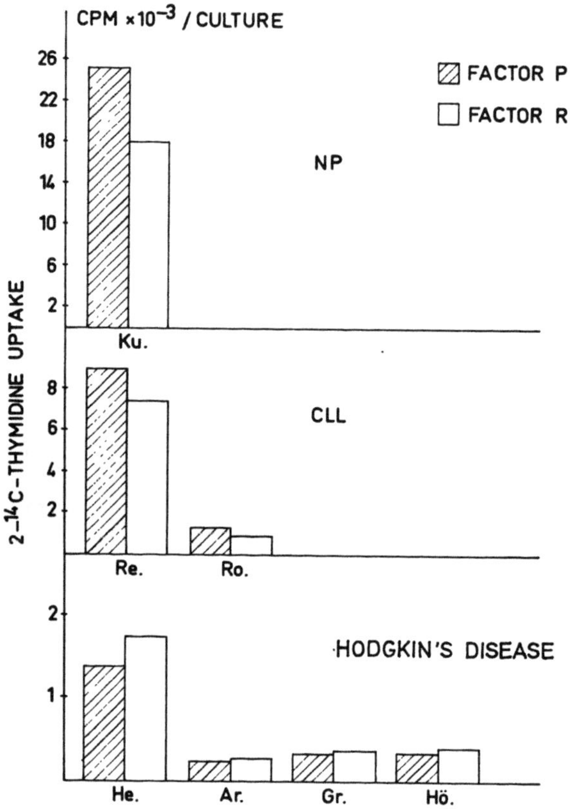

Fig. 1. Failure of lymphocytes of patients with chronic lymphocytic leukemia (CLL) and Hodgkin's disease to respond to antigen-induced mitogenic factor derived from normal lymphocytes of a Mantoux-positive donor. Lymphocytes of a normal individual (NP) and of patients are cultured with 0.3 ml factor P (culture supernatant of normal lymphocytes "pre-incubated" with 10 μg/ml Tuberculin for 36 hr) or 0.3 ml factor R (culture supernatant of normal lymphocytes "reconstituted" after 36 hr with 10 μg/ml Tuberculin). Response is given as counts/min/culture on day 5

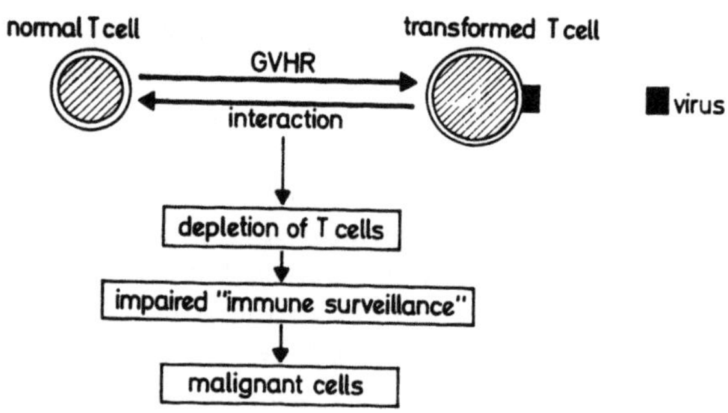

Fig. 2. Hypothesis for the pathogenesis of Hodgkin's disease (after ORDER and HELLMAN [11]). For further explanation see text

Why are cellular immune functions so considerably and systematically impaired even when HD is still a localized disease involving only lymph nodes in one region? It has been proposed that a virus may transform T cells and a chronic graft-versus-host reaction may be going on between normal and transformed T cells ([11]; Fig. 2). This may lead to a depletion of T cells and a loss of their functional capacity. The most important function of T cells is immune surveillance [12]. As a consequence of the loss of immune surveillance, malignant transformation of reticulum cells occurs, giving the histological appearance of malignant HD with an abundance of reticulum cells and Sternberg-Reed cells.

2. Lymphosarcoma and Chronic Lymphocytic Leukemia

In these conditions, cell-mediated immunity is intact in the early course of the disease. Progressive disease is characterized by a marked diminution of serum immunoglobulins, indicating a defect of B lymphocytes. There is now experimental and clinical evidence for the presence of two populations of lymphocytes in CLL, one normal and one leukemic [13, 14]. A relative diminution of normal T lymphocytes results in an impairment of cell-mediated immunity only when the absolute number of leukemic cells increases.

Three findings suggest the presence of normal and leukemic cells in CLL:

1. Lymphocytes of the thoracic duct respond better to phytohemagglutinin stimulation *in vitro* than do lymphocytes of the peripheral blood [14]. In normal individuals, no difference is noted between blood and lymph lymphocytes.

2. Studies with ^{3}H-cytidine-labeled lymphocytes suggest that the capacity of CLL lymphocytes to recirculate from blood to lymph is less than that of normal lymphocytes [15].

3. In CLL, blood lymphocytes show a higher percentage of cells bearing surface immunoglobulin determinants than do thoracic duct lymphocytes [16]. From these findings it may be concluded that the majority of leukemic cells remains intravascular and that only a minority of cells (the normal subpopulation) recirculates from blood to lymph. Whether CLL lymphocytes lack a specific "surface receptor" necessary for their passage from blood to lymph through the post-capillary venules remains to be determined [17].

3. Environmental and Genetic Factors

Burkitt lymphoma (BL) should be mentioned very briefly here. There is direct evidence that both Epstein-Barr (EB) virus *and* malaria are involved as environmental factors in the pathogenesis of BL. Host defense against BL tumor antigens has been demonstrated by skin testing with saline extracts of tumors [18]. In recent years histocompatibility testing has been used to study associations between tissue antigens and diseases. Thus, a significantly higher frequency of the antigenic specifities W 5 and HL-A 11 was found in HD ([19]; Table 2). This suggests that Hodgkin patients may develop their disease because of a genetic predisposition. There are two possible mechanisms by which antigen might predispose a patient:

Table 2. HL-A antigenic frequencies in normals and in patients with Hodgkin's Disease [Forbes and Morris J. clin. Invest. **51**, 1156 (1972)]

	Frequency (%)	
	HL-A 11	W 5
Hodgkin's disease (n=127)	28.4	32.3
Normals (n=273)	13.6	12.1

1. Antigenic determinants of oncogenic viruses could cross-react with the HL-A antigen W 5 in such a way that the virus is not recognized as foreign and so is able to produce the disease. The antigen W 5 might represent a favorable receptor site for viral attachment. Since not all people with W 5 develop HD, other factors must be involved.

2. The presence of the antigen W 5 could be associated with a predisposition to HD (or carcinogenesis in general) if the genes controlling the production of tissue antigens were linked to the genes controlling immune responsiveness, as has been shown to be the case in mice and guinea pigs [20, 21] and which was proposed by Burnet in his theory on immunosurveillance [12]. According to this view, transplantation antigens represent reference markers to identify tumor antigens and also reflect a profile of immune responsiveness. In fact, there is some indication that patients with a certain antigenic pattern reject kidney transplants earlier than others.

4. Hypothesis of the Development of Malignant Lymphomas

The described immunological deficiencies and the evidence for genetic predisposition in malignant lymphoma are summarized in a hypothesis which has been put forward recently [22]: Any long-lasting immune response, whether it is directed against surface antigens of microorganisms, against alloantigens in transplantation, or against autologous cells in autoimmunity, may lead to an activation of latent oncogenic viruses, which then induce malignant transformation and proliferation (Fig. 3). This hypothesis helps the understanding of several important clinical problems: i) the development of malignancies in recipients of renal allografts [23]; ii) the high incidence of malignant lymphomas in patients with autoimmune disease; iii) the association between malaria and Burkitt's lymphoma. The EB virus may function as a "passenger", only infecting the tumor cells secondarily.

The common mechanism in these three situations is faulty immunoregulation in which feedback control of the antibody production (primarily of the IgG class) in the lymphoid tissue is disturbed [24]. The described immune deficiencies in malignant lymphoma are characteristic of the disease and also play a causative role in their pathogenesis. Research in the next few years will be directed to substantiating this concept and preventing the development of malignant lymphoma by blocking the inductive immune response resulting in defective feedback control which leads to activation of oncogenic viruses.

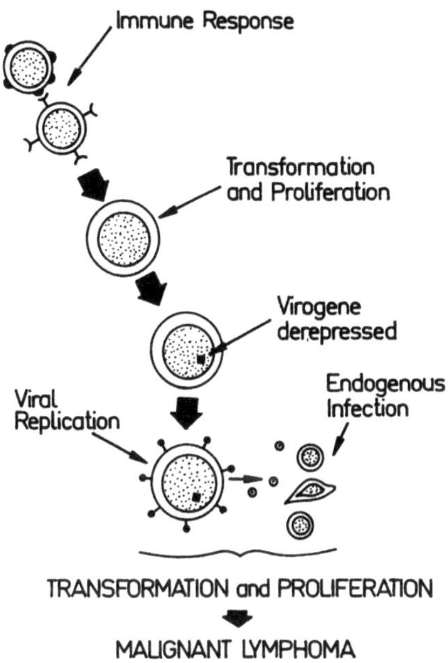

Fig. 3. Schematic hypothesis for the development of malignant lymphomas (after SCHWARTZ [22]). For further explanation see text

References

1. ROITT, I. M., GREAVES, M. F., TORRIGIANI, G., BROSTOFF, J., PLAYFAIR, J. H. L.: The cellular basis of immunological responses. A synthesis of some current views. Lancet **1969 II,** 367.
2. AISENBERG, A. C.: Manifestations of immunological unresponsiveness in Hodgkin's Disease. Cancer Res. **26,** 1152 (1966).
3. BROWN, R. S., HAYNES, H. A., FOLEY, H. F., GODWIN, H. A., BERARD, C. W., CARBONE, P. P.: Hodgkin's Disease. Immunologic, clinical and histological features in 50 untreated patients. Ann. intern. Med. **67,** 291 (1967).
4. YOUNG, R. C., CORDER, M. P., HAYNES, H. A., DE VITA, V. T.: Delayed hypersensitivity in Hodgkin's Disease. A study in 103 untreated patients. Ann. intern. Med. **52,** 63 (1972).
5. CROWTHER, D., FAIRLEY, G. H., SEWELL, R. L.: Significance of changes in the circulating lymphoid cells in Hodgkin's Disease. Brit. med. J. **1969 II,** 473.
6. HERSH, E. M., OPPENHEIM, J. J.: Impaired in vitro lymphocyte transformation in Hodgkin's Disease. New Engl. J. Med. **273,** 1006 (1965).
7. TWOMEY, J., DOUGLASS, C., NORRIS, S.: Failure of leucocytes in Hodgkin's Disease to stimulate a mixed leucocyte reaction (MLR). In: Proc. 7th leucocyte Culture Conference (FRITZ DAGUILLARD, editor). New York: Academic Press 1973.
8. MÜFTÜOGLU, A. Ü., BALKUV, S.: Passive transfer of tuberculin sensitivity to patients with Hodgkin's Disease. New Engl. J. Med. **277,** 126 (1967).
9. LAWRENCE, H. S.: Transfer factor. Advanc. Immunol. **11,** 195 (1969).
10. FLAD, H.-D., HUGET, R. P.: Effect of mitogenic factor on lymphocytes from patients with primary and secondary immune deficiencies. Paper presented at the 3rd Meeting of the Gesellschaft für Immunologie. Marburg, 1971.
11. ORDER, S. E., HELLMANN, S.: Pathogenesis of Hodgkin's Disease. Lancet **1972 I,** 571.
12. BURNET, F. M.: Immunological surveillance. Elmsford, N. Y.: Pergamon Press 1970.

13. HERSH, E. M., GUINN, G. A., ROSSEN, R., WALLACE, S., ROSE, R., FREIREICH, E. J.: Two populations of lymphocytes in chronic lymphocytic leukaemia. In: Proc. IV Leukocyte Culture Conference. (Ed.: O. R. MCINTYRE.) New York: Appleton Century Crofts 1970.
14. FLAD, H.-D., HUGET, R. P., BREMER, K., BRUCH, CHR.: Two populations of lymphocytes in chronic lymphocytic leukaemia (CLL). Europ. J. clin. Invest. **2**, 284 (1972).
15. BREMER, K., SCHICK, P., WACK, O., THEML, H., BRASS, B., HEIMPEL, H.: Rezirkulation von Lymphozyten bei Patienten mit malignen lymphatischen Erkrankungen. Blut **24**, 215 (1972).
16. FLAD, H.-D., HUBER, C., BREMER, K., MENNE, H. D., HUBER, H.: Impaired recirculation of B lymphocytes in chronic lymphocytic leukemia. Europ. J. Immunol. **3**, 688 (1973).
17. VINCENT, P. C., GUNZ, F. W.: Control of lymphocyte level in the blood. Lancet **1970 II**, 342.
18. FASS, L., HERBERMANN, R. B., ZIEGLER, J.: Delayed cutaneous hypersensitivity reactions to autologous extracts of Burkitt lymphoma. New Engl. J. Med. **282**, 776 (1970).
19. FORBES, J. F., MORRIS, P. J.: Analysis of HL-A antigens in patients with Hodgkin's Disease and their families. J. clin. Invest. **51**, 1156 (1972).
20. MCDEVITT, H. O., BENACERRAF, B.: Genetic control of specific immune responses. Advanc. Immunol. **11**, 31 (1969).
21. ELLMAN, L., GREEN, I., MARTIN, W. J.: Histocompatibility genes, immune responsiveness and leukaemia. Lancet **1970 I**, 1104.
22. SCHWARTZ, R. S.: Immunoregulation. Oncogenic viruses and malignant lymphomas. Lancet **1972 I**, 1266.
23. PENN, J., HAMMOND, W., BRETTSCHNEIDER, L., STARZL, T. E.: Malignant lymphomas in transplantation recipients. Transplant. Proc. **1**, 106 (1969).
24. UHR, J. W., MÖLLER, G.: Advanc. Immunol. **8**, 81 (1968).

Correlation between EBV Infections and Malignant Lymphomas

H. Schmitz

Summary

Epstein-Barr virus (EBV) IgM antibodies can be demonstrated for only few weeks after onset of infectious mononucleosis (IM). Thus EBV IgM antibodies indicate a recent EBV infection. We looked for EBV IgM antibodies in persons with recently diagnosed Hodgkin's disease. Only 2 of 6 patients showed EBV IgM antibodies. The EBV seems to be involved in Hodgkin's disease in single cases only.

Recent observations in animals, particularly monkeys, imply a viral etiology for human lymphomas [1].

Epidemiological investigations of both the Burkitt lymphoma and Hodgkin's disease support the infection theory. For oncological effects of viruses to be manifested, penetration of the viruses into the cells, i. e. an infection, is required.

In tumor formation there is no replication of virus leading to the death of the affected cell. A so-called transformation takes place instead, and the new genetic material alters the cellular characteristics. New antigens appear on the cell surface of transformed human cells, and the cells become able to divide indefinitely *in vitro.* The new surface antigens of transformed cells lead to an immunological reaction by the organism. The possible role of both RNA and DNA viruses in human lymphomas is currently being discussed. Among DNA viruses, the herpes viruses in particular have revealed strong indications of etiological involvement in human lymphomas. Thus the *saimiri* herpesvirus was the first tumor virus discovered which causes lymphosarcoma consistently within a few weeks in marmoset monkeys.

One herpes virus identified with great regularity in human Burkitt tumors is the Epstein-Barr virus (EBV), which has also become causally implicated in mononucleosis. Cells cultured from Burkitt tumors reveal transformations due to EBV. They have new antigenic qualities and multiply indefinitely *in vitro.* Since patients with such tumors reveal high antibody titers to the whole virus, EBV must reproduce in human tumor patients, although it cannot be detected in transformed tumor cells *in vivo.* There are three indications for the etiological involvement of EBV in the Burkitt tumor: 1. identification of EBV-transformed lymphoblastoid tumor cells, which mostly contain viral nucleic acid; 2. the fact that all tumor patients have EBV antibodies; 3. it is primarily children who may have had no previous EBV infection who develop Burkitt tumors.

It is true that cells transformed by EBV are also found in infectious mononucleosis (IM) patients, i. e. people who have no diagnosed malignant disease; high antibody titers to EBV can also be obtained in healthy people. There is thus no conclusive evidence that EBV is in some way responsible for the Burkitt tumor. Hodgkin's disease has also been considered in connection with EBV. Our investigations carried out in 1971 reveal that particularly high antibody titers were very frequently found in sera from patients who had Hodgkin's disease compared with statistics for the corresponding age group of leukemia patients. In the case of leukemia patients, antibodies to the related cytomegalo virus (CMV) were obtained with conspicuous frequency. In some Hodgkin's disease patients who synthesize no antibodies to EBV [2] it is probably difficult to invoke an EBV etiology.

The EBV IgG antibodies identified by Henle's method can be demonstrated over a period of many years in the serum and occur in 60—80% of all healthy adults. Therefore the Henle test cannot be used to determine whether these antibodies were formed prior to onset of the disease, during the disease, or afterwards. Consequently, we have tried to determine the exact point of EBV infection in lymphoma patients by means of our EBV IgM antibody test [3]. As in the Henle test, these EBV IgM antibodies are determined by immunofluorescence. Fig. 1 shows fluorescence of EBV-infected tumor cells in the presence of fluorescent-labeled IgM antibodies. The individual virus-infected lymphocytes are luminous and clearly visible. These IgM antibodies can be determined in the sera of patients who have been infected with EBV for only a few weeks. As the acute infection regresses and the virus is eliminated from the blood, the EBV IgM antibodies also disappear. Fig. 2 shows changes in the EBV

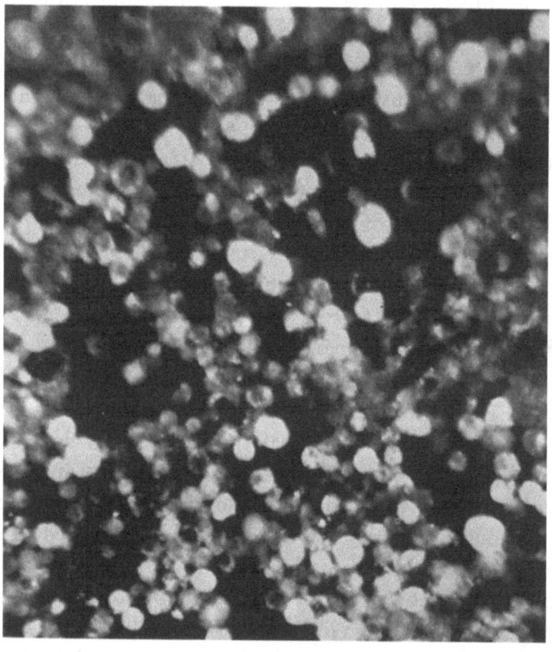

Fig. 1. Specific fluorescence of EBV-infected HR1K cells in the EBV IgM test

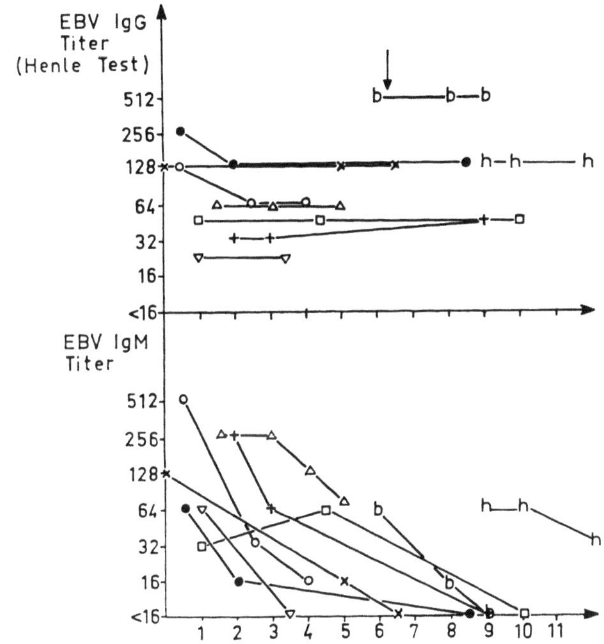

Fig. 2. Kinetics of the EBV IgG and IgM antibodies in 7 infectious mononucleosis patients, in a boy with Burkitt's lymphoma (b-b-b-), and in a Hodgkin patient (h-h-h-)

IgM antibody titer and, for comparison, EBV IgG antibodies in various patients. In IM-patients there is a rapid decrease in EBV IgM antibodies, so identification of IgM antibodies reveals a florid infection of only a few weeks' duration. IgM antibodies, which can be demonstrated only in florid infections, were also found in an 11-year-old boy (marked b-b-b-) with a Burkitt lymphoma of the left cheek which had a relatively short history. The arrow marks the date of tumor excision. If these EBV IgM antibodies could be identified in all Burkitt tumors of recent origin, the postulation of EBV etiology in Burkitt tumors would receive support, for the coincidental occurrence of acute EBV infection and tumor formation in many cases would be statistically quite improbable. Unfortunately, new Burkitt tumor cases were not available.

We therefore turned to Hodgkin's disease. As. Fig. 2 shows, EBV IgM antibodies were also determined in a young female patient with a brief Hodgkin history. Similar observations were made in another case. However, there were 4 patients with a similarly brief history in whom no EBV IgM antibodies were found, though in these patients, the EBV IgM antibodies may have already decreased below detectable limits. Various etiological factors rather than one single factor may be responsible for the development of Hodgkin's disease.

To investigate whether EBV infection is causal or fortuitous in Hodgkin's disease by identification of EBV IgM antibodies, it is necessary to have serum samples taken from Hodgkin patients in the earliest possible stage of the disease.

References

1. KLEIN, G.: Herpesvirus and oncogenesis. Proc. nat. Acad. Sci. (Wash.) **69**, 1056 (1972).
2. OBRECHT, P., SCHMITZ, H., WESTERHAUSEN, M.: Untersuchungen über Antikörper gegen das Epstein-Barr-(EB) und Cytomegalievirus (CM) bei Hämoblastosen und malignen Tumoren. Verh. dtsch. Ges. inn. Med. **77**, 754 (1971).
3. SCHMITZ, H., SCHERER, M.: IgM-antibodies to Epstein-Barr virus in infectious mononucleosis. Arch. ges. Virusforsch. **37**, 332 (1972).

Epstein-Barr Virus (EBV) in Lymphoid Cells from Patients with Hodgkin's Disease

V. Diehl

Summary

Long-term growth of peripheral lymphocytes from patients with Hodgkin's disease was related to clinical, immunological and pathological parameters of the tumor patients. Establishment of continuously growing lymphoblastoid cultures depended on a positive serological EBV reactivity of the cell donor and an intact cellular immune reaction. It is suggested that the established lymphoblastoid cells resemble immunologically reactive cells and not Hodgkin-specific tumor cells.

Growth of lymphocytes from Hodgkin patients was observed in 47%, whereas control lymphocytes commenced growth only in 18,2% of the culture attempts; umbilical cord blood cells failed to grow.

A large number of lymphoblastoid cell lines have been established *in vitro* in recent years. They were derived from peripheral blood or biopsy cells, both from healthy individuals and from patients with lymphoproliferative diseases.

The success rate of cultivation of lymphocytes *in vitro* seemed to depend on the culture technique used and varied between 0 and 100%. Despite this variation it was possible to compare the growth rates in standardized conditions of lymphocytes from various donor groups.

[1] showed that lymphoid cells grow *in vitro* only if the donor had been exposed to EBV, i. e. when the donor serum contained EBV-specific antibodies. EBV-associated antigens were later demonstrated in nearly all continuously growing cell lines during maintenance in culture, if tested early enough. Furthermore, [2] demonstrated EBV-specific nucleic acid sequences in all lymphoblastoid lines thus far examined by DNA-RNA hybridization studies. These results, combined with serological findings, suggested a close relationship between EBV and lymphoproliferative diseases.

A brief account is given here of the *in vitro* growth of peripheral lymphocytes of Hodgkin patients in relation to clinical and pathological parameters and EBV reactivity in lymphoid lines derived from Hodgkin patients.

Earlier investigations indicated that EBV is not transmitted via the placenta. In cooperation with [3] we were able to show that DNA derived from umbilical-cord leukocytes does not hybridize with EBV-specific mRNA (Table). DNA derived from primary leukocytes of healthy individuals or Hodgkin patients occasionally shows slightly elevated hybridization rates in nucleic acid homology studies. This may indicate the presence of latent EBV genomes in these cells (unpublished results). Established lymphoblastoid lines derived from these donors generally show increased hybridization rates, indicating the presence of EBV DNA in these cells. Attempts to culture peripheral lymphocytes from various donor groups were in agreement with these findings.

Table 1. Hybridization of cellular DNA with EBV-specific mRNA. Note the elevated hybridization rate in lymphoblastoid lines derived from peripheral blood of Hodgkin patients, in comparison to DNA from umbilical cord leukocytes

Cells	Donor	Counts per minute hybridized
Ri	Umbilical-cord leukocytes	86.81
Mü	Umbilical-cord leukocytes	124.128
Sa	Umbilical-cord leukocytes	96.79
Kl	Umbilical-cord leukocytes	101.151
Kr	Umbilical-cord leukocytes	102.112
S 118	Hodgkin, peripheral blood	357.364
S 131	Hodgkin, peripheral blood	257.355
S 77	Hodgkin, peripheral blood	390.324
S 84	Hodgkin, peripheral blood	940.957
S 95	Hodgkin, peripheral blood	771.787
Adenovirus-12-Transformed Hamster cells	Hamster kidney cells	138.112

Forty-nine attempts to establish umbilical-cord lymphocytes *in vitro* failed. Twelve out of 66 culture attempts with lymphocytes from healthy donors were successful. This corresponds to a success rate of about 18.2%. By means of the same technique, 16 out of 34 (47%) cultures were established from peripheral blood cells of untreated patients with Hodgkin's disease. In the treated group, the success rate was 2 out of 26, i. e. 7.7%; this low rate could reflect the influence of immunosuppressive therapy or be due to the advanced stage of the disease.

The outgrowth of peripheral lymphocytes in the untreated group of Hodgkin patients depended on some clinical and pathological parameters, though patients with a favorable histology (Lymphocytic Predominance, Nodular Sclerosis) did not differ from the unfavorable group (Mixed Cellularity and Lymphocytic Depletion); the rate of cell-line establishment for both groups was 47%.

Lymphocytes from patients with localized disease (stages I and II) grew better (55%:36%) than cells from patients with disseminated disease (stages III and IV). Similar differences were noted for active (58%) and inactive (33%) disease. A striking difference was observed by comparing patients with an intact Mantoux reaction against tuberculin antigen and those who did not react. In the tuberculin-positive group, 15 out of 21 culture attempts yielded permanent cell lines (71%) compared to 1 out of 31 attempts (7.7%) in the negative one. The absolute number of lymphocytes (above or below $1500/mm^3$) had no influence on the establishment rate, provided the total number of leukocytes did not decrease below $2000/mm^3$.

The presence of large mononuclear cells in the peripheral blood did not increase the rate of establishment *in vitro:* only 3 out of 12 cultures (25%) were established in the presence of these reactive cells, compared to 13 out of 22 attempts (59%) in their absence.

[4] have described large mononuclear cells in patients with Hodgkin's disease or infectious diseases and in patients after immunization. The increase in these cells seems to parallel the progression of the disease.

The influence of the cellular immunity reaction on growth of lymphocytes *in vitro* is further demonstrated by the observation that successive culture attempts in one patient were successful only when the Mantoux reaction was positive and signs of active disease were absent. With progression of disease, the tuberculin reaction became negative and three further culture attempts failed.

These findings agree with those of [5], who could only induce *in-vitro* transformation of lymphoid cells with EBV in PPD-reactive donors in the presence of the specific antigen.

The serological EBV reactivity titers of the Hodgkin patients showed values of 1:10 to 1:320 with a geometric mean of 1:79. EBV-associated antigens could be demonstrated in all but one of the cultures established.

To sum up:

1. Peripheral lymphocytes of patients with Hodgkin's disease were established *in vitro* in long-term cultures with a higher success-rate than cells from normal individuals (47% against 18.2%).
2. The outgrowth apparently depended on integrity of the cellular immunity reaction of the donor.
3. Reactive, large lymphoid cells and active disease, mostly present in mutual association, seemed to inhibit the capacity of the cells to grow *in vitro.*
4. All patients had antibodies against EBV-specific antigens (EA, VCA, MA).
5. EBV-specific antigens could be detected in all but one long-term culture.
6. It is suggested that the established lymphoblastoid cells are immunologically reactive cells and not Hodgkin-specific tumor cells.

References

1. Nilsson, K., Klein, G., Henle, W., Henle, G.: The establishment of lymphoblastoid lines from adult and fetal human lymphoid tissue and its dependance on EBV. Int. J. Cancer **8**, 443—440 (1971).
2. zur Hausen, H.: Epstein barr virus in human tumor cells. Int. Rev. of Exper. Path., Vol. 11. Academic Press 1972.
3. zur Hausen, H., Diehl, V., Wolf, H., Schulte-Holthausen, H., Schneider, U.: Occurance of Epstein barr virus genomes in human lymphoblastoid cell lines. Nature (Lond.) New Biol. **237**, 189—190 (1972).
4. Crowther, D., Hamilton Fairley, G., Sevell, R. L.: Desoxyribonucleic acid synthesis in the lymphocytes of patients with malignant disease. Europ. J. Cancer **3**, 417—421 (1967).
5. Baumal, R., Bloom, B., Scharff, M. D.: Induction of long term lymphocyte lines from delayed hypersensitivity donors, using specific antigen plus Epstein barr virus. Nature (Lond.) **230**, 20—21 (1971).

Mediastinoscopy and Thoracoscopy

W. Wolfart and U. Seith

Summary

With the aid of the mediastinoscopy, diseased lymph nodes can be removed for accurate histological determination. This investigation is practicable not only for the primary diagnosis but for the control of the development after X-irradiation too. Complication rates reported in the medical literature vary between 1,4% and 1,7% and fatalities between 0,04% and 0,08%.

The requirement for a successful application of the thoracoscopy, i. e. for a complete examination of the total pleural cavity, is a free pleural space. We have found only localized areas paravertebrally and in the mediastinal pleura, which are not difficult to remove. Our observations raise the question of whether generalized disease of the pleura is indicated bei pleural effusion. Thoracoscopy is almost free of complications and can also be performed with intubation narcosis, if the use of pneumothorax might be fatal for a patient with reduced breathing.

The two investigative procedures discussed can aid diagnosis as well as follow-up observation of lymphadenomatosis.

1. Mediastinoscopy

The frontal tracheal wall is exposed by means of a 3-cm incision in the fossa jugularis. The mediastinum can then be opened between the trachea and the vena brachicephalica, enabling the forward and lateral wall of the trachea, the bifurcation angle and the main bronchi to be reached without difficulty.

The percentage of complications resulting from this investigative procedure is very small. We had the following results with 850 cases: 4 serious hermorrhages, all of which could be controlled through tamponment; 1 pneumothorax; 1 paresis of the recurrent nerve; 2 perforations of the esophagus; 1 mediastinal abscess resulting from an accidental puncture of the trachea; and no deaths. Complication rates reported in the medical literature vary between 1.4% and 1.7% and fatalities between 0.04% and 0.08%.

The diseased lymph nodes can be removed totally, thereby allowing the pathologist enough material to make a very accurate histological determination of the type of lymphatic disease.

At first, mediastinoscopy was used only for primary diagnosis, but we have shown that this investigative procedure can be repeated even after X-irradiation of the mediastinum.

Surgery is slightly more difficult in this case, but the lymph nodes can be prepared to provide enough material for a thorough histological diagnosis.

2. Thoracoscopy

After a pneumothorax has been induced, a light carrier with a small ocular attached by means of a trocar is directed into the pleural cavity. When effusion is present, it is drawn off through a drainage tube before the light carrier is inserted. The effusion will be used for differential diagnostic, cytological and bacteriological investigations. Tissue particles can be removed with a small tongs for histological investigation.

Successful application of this procedure requires a free pleural space. Therefore it should be carried out as soon as possible after the first signs of pleural effusion and before adhesion of the pleural membranes takes place. Even a partial adhesion is extremely undesirable, for it hinders a complete examination of the total pleural cavity. This seems to be important, because in the few cases of lymphogranulomatosis we have investigated thoracoscopically, we have never found generalized changes in the pleural membranes. We have found only localized areas located mainly paravertebrally and in the mediastinal pleura. There are usually small lumps, approximately 2 mm in diameter, in adjacent groups, each group covering an area of up to 1—2 cm². We have never found such areas in more than two or three places in the whole pleural cavity. It is not difficult to remove them for histological investigation. These lumps are very flat, and they can be covered by deposits of fibrin after prolonged pleural effusion.

Our observations on the use of thoracoscopy raise the question of whether generalized disease of the pleura is indicated by pleural effusion. In many instances, disease seems to be localized to the mediastinal pleura, the visceral pleura adjacent to the hilus and the mediastinum, and the pleura near the paravertebral lymph nodes, caused by infiltration from diseased mediastinal lymph nodes. Here we must ask whether the effusion caused by the diseased pleura should be treated by irradiation of the mediastinal or paravertebral lymph nodes. To answer this question, we recommend that thoracoscopy should be used at the first sign of a pleural effusion in a large number of cases to determine whether the disease of the pleura is generalized or only localized.

Thoracoscopy is a surgical method which is almost free of complications if aseptic procedure is followed. Even with patients whose breathing has been so reduced that the use of a pneumothorax might be fatal, this investigative procedure can be used with intubation narcosis. After thoracoscopy, immediate re-expansion of the lung is achieved through drainage of the thorax, so that there is no interference with ventilation. So long as a patient can safely be anesthetized, there are practically no contraindications.

Roentgen Anatomy of the Lymphatic System

W. Wirth

Summary

The anatomy of the inguino-pelvic-lumbar lymphatic system as well as of the thoracic duct can be well demonstrated by lymphography of the foot. The radiographic findings correlate with the classical anatomic descriptions. Variations and difficulties in the differentiation between "normal" and "abnormal" are especially mentioned.

The *exact* definition and naming of various groups of lymph nodes in a lymphogram is possible radiologically only by simultaneous visualization of the blood vessels. A simpler method is to use specific *skeletal reference lines*, which are adequate for most purposes (Fig. 1). (The X-ray beam is directed vertically through a point 5 cm below the navel.)

The *obturator line* corresponds to a horizontal line drawn through the middle of the obturator foramen. It divides the upper from the lower inguinal nodes.

The *acetabular line* represents a vertical line drawn through the medial part of the hip joint. This marks the division between the outer and inner group of the upper inguinal nodes.

The *inguinal line* joins the anterior superior iliac spine with the pubic tubercle and corresponds to the course of the inguinal ligament. This line forms the border between the inguinal and foremost iliac nodes.

The *iliosacral line* corresponds to a horizontal line drawn through the middle of the sacro-iliac joint and marks the dividing angle of the common iliac artery and therefore the border between the anterior and posterior iliac nodes.

The *iliolumbar line* is a horizontal at the level of the iliac crest or through the middle of the 4th lumbar vertebral body. This is an average indicator of the aortic bifurcation and marks the border between the posterior iliac and the lumbar nodes.

Generally the lumbar lymph node group ends at the level of the lumbar vertebrae 1 or 2, where the lymph empties via the lumbar trunks or the cisterna chyli into the thoracic duct [15, 46, 49].

The reference lines illustrated can also be applied to oblique projections [46, 49].

The lymph nodes stationed in the lymphatic circulation act as filters and defence posts, and are remote sites for the formation of lymphocytes. They generally lie embedded in fatty tissue near the blood vessels. Usually they are arranged in groups (especially in the inguinal region) or in chains (especially in the pelvic region) [24, 25, 42, 49].

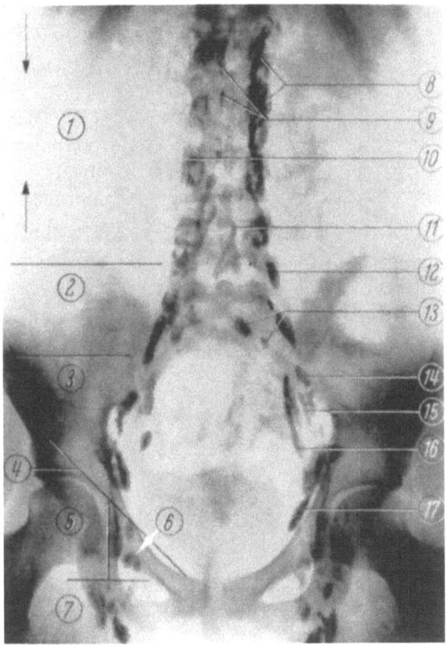

Fig. 1. Skeletal orientation lines according to WIRTH in the antero-posterior projection with perpendicular X-rays. 1 lnn. lumbales, 2 lnn. iliaci communes, 3 lnn. iliaci externi, 5 lnn. inguinales superolaterales, 6 lnn. inguinales superomediales et profundi, 7 lnn. inguinales inferiores, 8 lnn. aortales, 9 lnn. interaorticocavales, 10 ln. cavalis, 12 ln. iliacus communis lat., 13 lnn. iliaci communes med., 14 ln. iliacus externus lat., 15 ln. iliacus externus intermed., 16 ln. iliacus externus med., 17 ln. lacunaris med.

The *shape and size* of the lymph nodes varies considerably; they can be round, oval, or kidney-shaped. Their size depends upon the age and constitution of the individual, among other factors, and fluctuates according to the functional load. In adults the size can vary from 0.5×0.5 cm for circular shapes, and 1—3 cm for elongated shapes. In areas (particularly in the pelvic region) where the original lymph nodes have not divided, they may reach a length of 5—7 cm (Fig. 2 a, b). The *number* of nodes also varies considerably. An abdominal lymphogram can contain from 60 to 130 nodes [13, 19, 35, 46].

A certain *relationship exists between size and number* of the nodes: the fewer the nodes, the bigger they are, and vice versa, which means the total volume of lymph nodes is relatively constant. This also applies, with some exceptions, to individual regions. The number of nodes in the lymphogram decreases with increasing age. However, this appearance is illusory because the smaller nodes become radiologically invisible due to involution and fat accumulation [13, 46].

A slight *increase in volume* occurs following lymphography due to accumulation of the contrast medium and the consequent exudative and cellular reaction; nodal volume returns to normal after two to three weeks. An apparent *decrease in volume* seen in the lymphogram is caused by the disappearance, over weeks or months, of the contrast medium from the marginal sinus of the lymph nodes which causes the

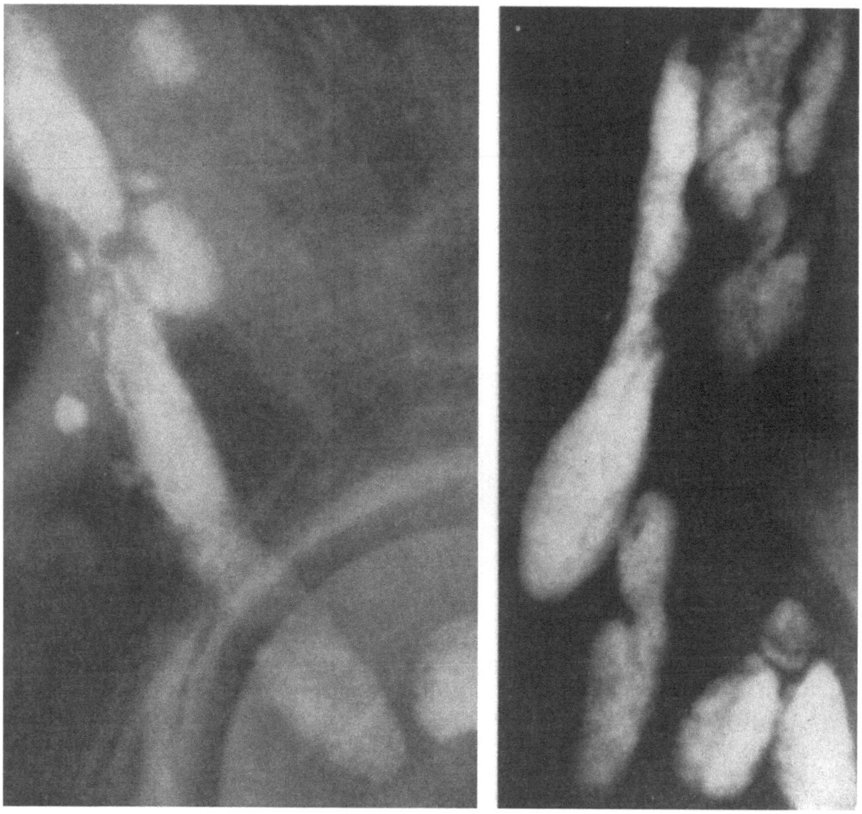

a b

Fig. 2 a and b. Unseparated and therefore very long lymph nodes

delineation of the nodes to become irregular. These changes in size must be considered when assessing the results of treatment [49].

The lymph nodes are surrounded by a connective tissue capsule. The bands of connective tissue — trabeculae — penetrating the inner node from the capsule and hilum produce the gross organic structure. In the intertrabecular spaces reticular connective tissue forms a fine meshwork, mostly filled with lymphatic tissue. The rest remains open and forms a system of sinuses through which the lymph passes. This intermediate sinus system is connected with the marginal sinus and with the terminal sinus. The primary and secondary nodules, which are spherically arranged groups of lymphocytes, lie in the periphery of the lymph nodes [49].

The lymph is brought to the nodes by the vasa afferentia (Fig. 3), which are distributed over almost the whole node surface, often branching before entering the marginal sinus. The lymph trickles from the marginal sinus through the labyrinth of the intermediate sinus toward the hilum and thence into the terminal sinus, where the vasa efferentia have their origin. The efferent vessels, confined to the hilum are therefore fewer in number than the afferent vessels; however, they are thicker and have

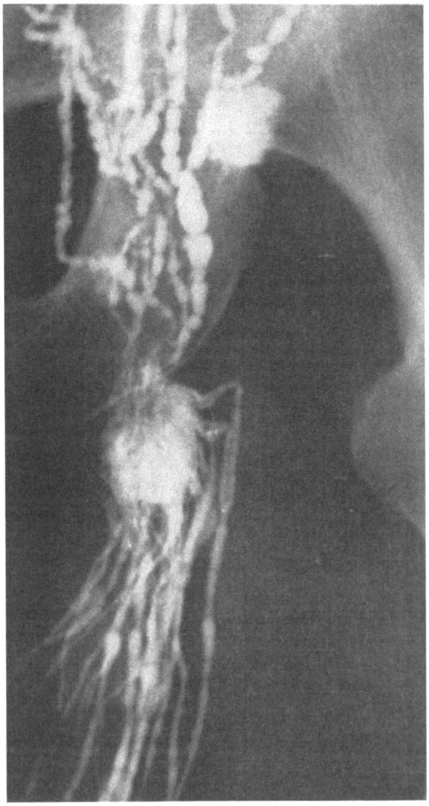

Fig. 3. Vasa afferentia and efferentia

more valves. They carry the lymph centrally toward the next group of lymph nodes [1, 11, 13, 46, 49].

In the *lymphangiogram* (i. e. during the filling phase) the nodes are so densely filled with contrast medium that it is almost impossible to see local differences in the retention of contrast material by the reticulum such as might be caused by hyalinosis, lipomatosis or fibrosis (Fig. 4 a). After the excess contrast medium has drained away, local differences become visible (Fig 4 b). When the hilum lies on the anterior or posterior surface, it causes a thinning or even a defect in the lymphadenogram, especially when perihilar lipomatosis is present (Fig. 5 a, b) [1, 5, 17, 27, 32, 37, 39, 41, 45, 46].

Degenerative changes are mostly found in the inguinal region and in anterior pelvic nodes. Generally they lie centrally and sometimes also marginally. Defects can only be called central when they lie centrally in two projections [46]. Degenerative areas look like small metastases; larger ones are more often marginal and cause swelling and circulatory disturbances. This is recognizable in 24- or 48-hour X-rays of unemptied lymph vessels. Differentiation can be extremely difficult in the early stages of development [41, 42, 45, 49].

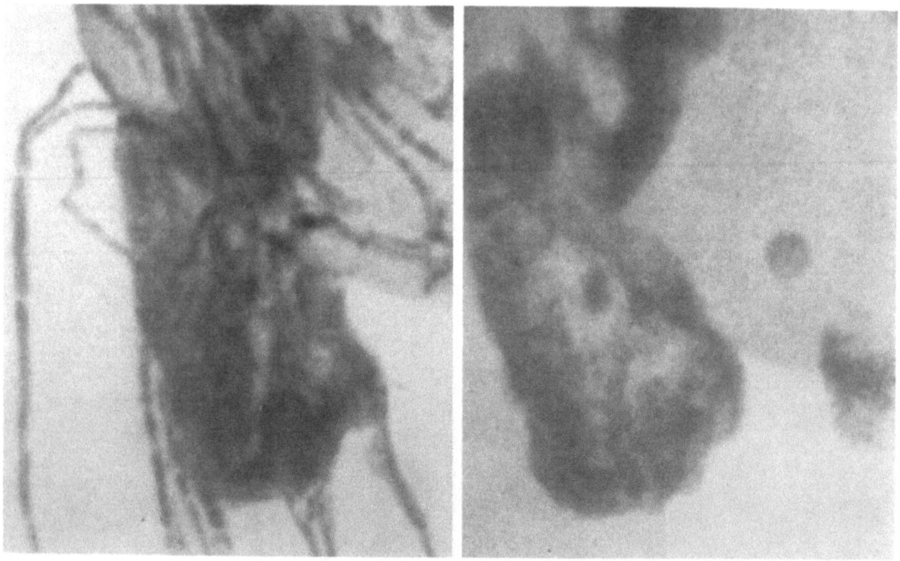

a b

Fig. 4. a Lymphangiogram (early phase). The lymph node contains too much contrast material; differences in the pattern are therefore not visible, b Lymphadenogram (late phase). Filling defect due to fibrosis

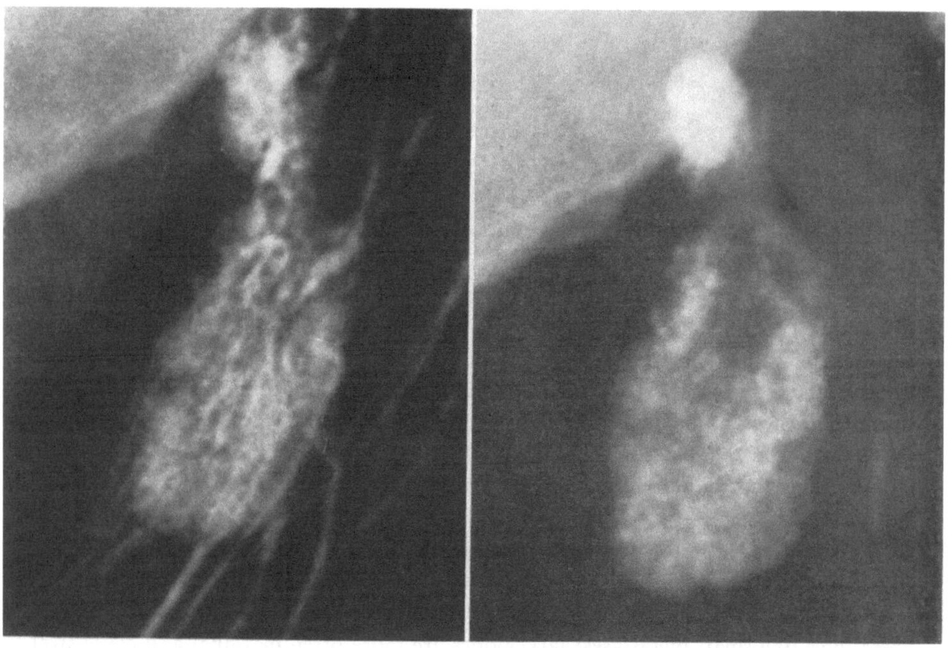

a b

Fig. 5. a Lymphangiogram. Hilum projected on the ventral or dorsal border of the lymph node, b Lymphadenogram. Filling defect caused by the hilum

In the *lymphadenogram* (i.e. after emptying of the vessels) the normal lymph node shows an even reticular or slightly spotted homogeneous appearance (Figs. 2, 7a). This reflects, on the one hand, the lymph node structure, especially the lymph follicle and the sinus reticulum, the finely stained contrast medium being better defined in the periphery of the node due to the clustering of follicles. On the other hand, the summation effect of the different sized drops of contrast medium could also account for the speckled appearance of the lymphogram (Figs. 2, 7 a) [13, 41, 42, 49].

Fig. 6 shows the arrangement in a histological section of drops of contrast medium of various sizes released through the depositing process and appearing as empty areas [2, 33, 41, 42].

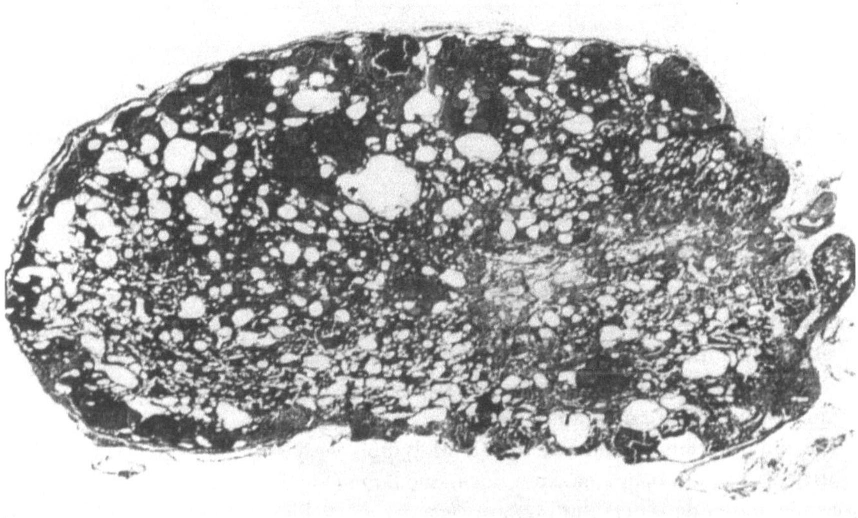

Fig. 6. Histological section through a lymph node after lymphography

In normal nodes the *border* appears lined or finely notched due to the equal distribution of the contrast medium in the marginal sinus (Figs. 2, 7 a).

The contrast medium disappears from all the lymph nodes of each patient at about the same rate. The *speed of disappearance,* however, differs considerably from patient to patient and may last weeks or many months. When there are uncertain lymphographic results or new clinical symptoms, or in order to monitor therapeutic success, it is initially sufficient to take an *abdominal picture* only.

When the marginal sinus is empty of contrast medium and the node structure is no longer visible, lymphography must be repeated. Small amounts of contrast medium remaining in the nodes do not preclude a *2nd, 3rd or 4th lymphography* [49].

Reactionary swelling, e. g. postoperative, *acute* (Fig. 7 b) or *chronic inflammatory disease* (Fig. 7 c); produces only slight alterations in the lymphogram: a slight to moderate increase in size and a looser arrangement of contrast medium (cf. the normal node; Fig. 7 a). However, the nodes are intact in form, coarser copies of normal nodes [40]. The initial stage of a *malignant lymphoma* may present a similar picture in the

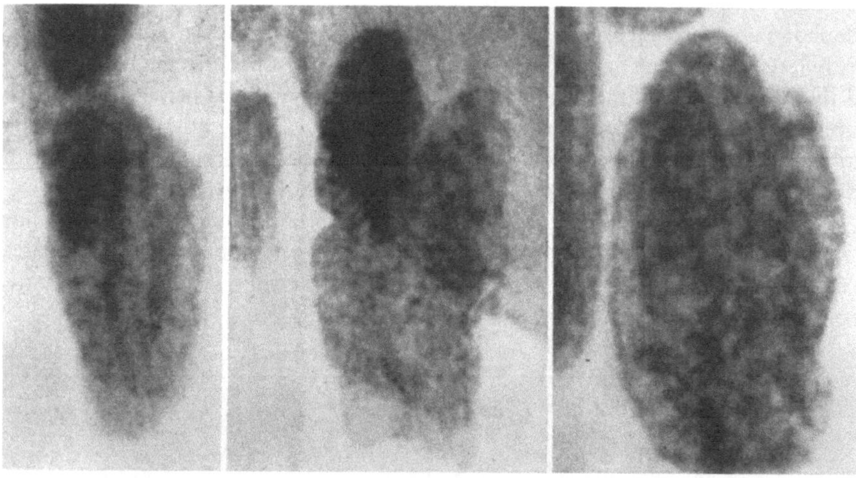

a b c

Fig. 7. a Normal lymph node pattern, b Acute inflammation, c Chronic inflammation

lymphogram. The transitions of the normal nodes through the various stages of inflammation to the initial form of the diffusely growing malignant lymphoma are discrete; differentiation in the lymphogram is correspondingly difficult.

Some peculiarities of the normal anatomy and topography which could lead to false interpretation are mentioned below.

The lymph from the medial bundle of lymph vessels of the thigh drains, in the majority of cases, into two medium sized, one large (Fig. 5) or one large and one small lower inguinal node. These findings are very constant (Fig. 8 a) [46].

The upper inguinal nodes vary considerably. This is because some of the upper outer and upper inner nodes are not stained when the injection is made in the foot (Figs. 1, 3, 8) [7, 13, 25, 46, 49].

Lymph vessels of the medial bundle occasionally join an upper inguinal lymph node directly, by-passing the lower ones (Fig. 8 b). The outer lacunar node rarely forms the first station. By-passing of lymph-node groups also occurs in other regions [46, 49].

The lymph from the superficial and deep inguinal nodes flows in the classical case into three lacunar nodes, i. e. the first stations of the pelvic lymph nodes (Fig. 9). The very constant outer lacunar lymph node is mostly large and round, while the inner one is elongated. The middle one is often absent (Fig. 9) [46].

Generally, the total iliac region as far as the promontorium comprises three main channels. They are interlinked by cross-connections of band or mesh form (Fig. 9). One of these three channels may be missing, frequently the middle one [6, 7, 8, 9, 13, 15, 27, 32, 35, 37, 38, 46].

The pelvic lymph nodes along the external and common iliac artery are usually long and always visible. In contrast to this, the small round nodes in the area of the internal iliac artery and its ramifications are seen only occasionally (Fig. 9) [13, 28, 46].

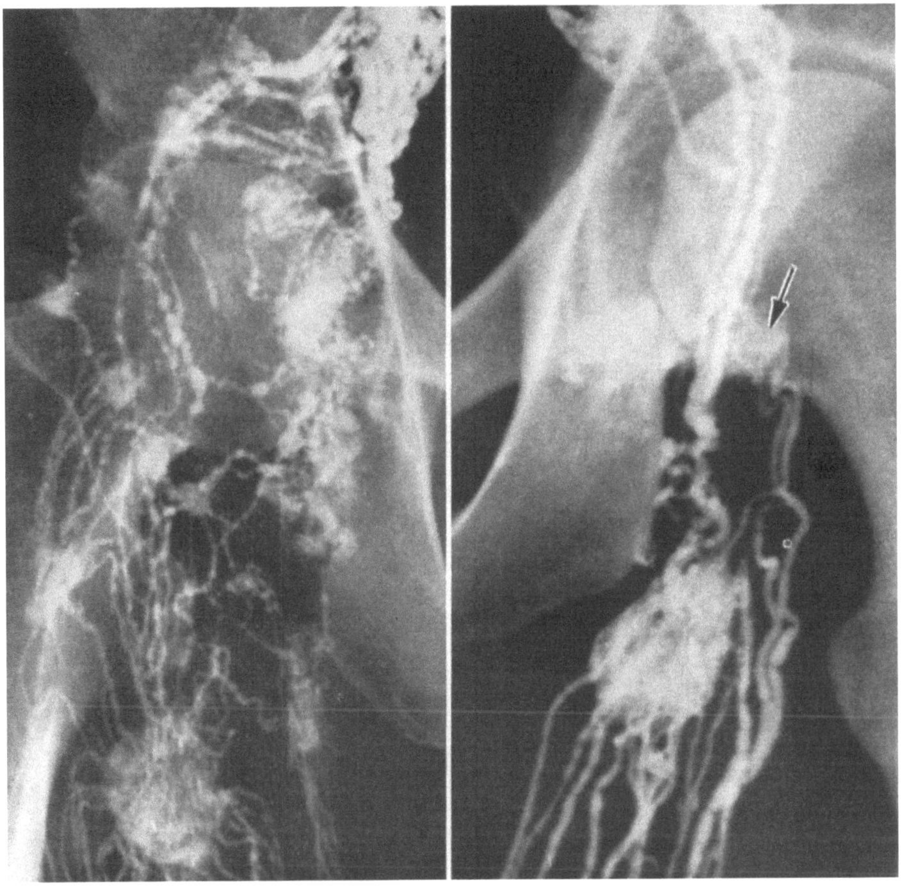

a b

Fig. 8. a Filling phase, inguinal region, b Lymphatics of the thigh leading directly to an upper inguinal node (→)

The three iliac chains described meet in the region of the aortic bifurcation. At this level the lymph from the two sides mixes, because of cross-connections in the lumbar region (Fig. 10) [13, 46].

Generally one finds three channels in the lumbar region, the left one around the aorta, the middle one between the aorta and vena cava and the right one around the vena cava. The middle one is often missing (Fig. 10). The lymph nodes are mostly oval [19, 35, 46, 49].

The principal organs influencing the course of the lymph vessels and the corresponding position of the lymph nodes are the aorta and pelvic arteries. If they are tortuous, the lymph vessels and nodes change their position accordingly, giving the appearance of a displacement of the lymph system by a tumor mass [46, 49].

An occasional variation is a direct connection between the iliac and lumbar nodes, a so-called pelvic shovel vessel. It is often interrupted by 1 or 2 small lymph nodes.

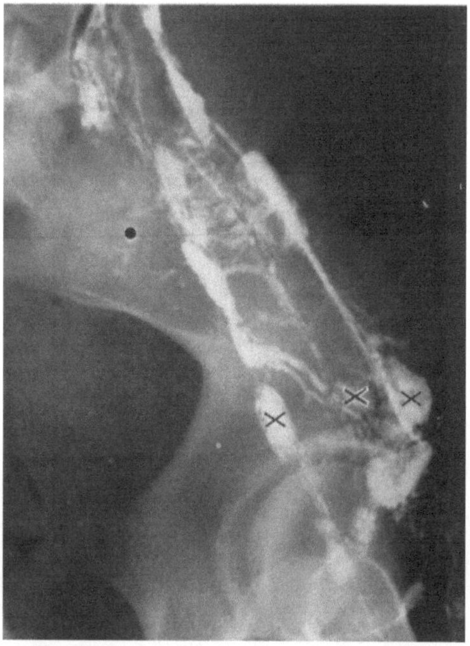

Fig. 9. Lnn. lacunares (×), first station of the three pelvic chains. Lnn. iliaci interni (●)

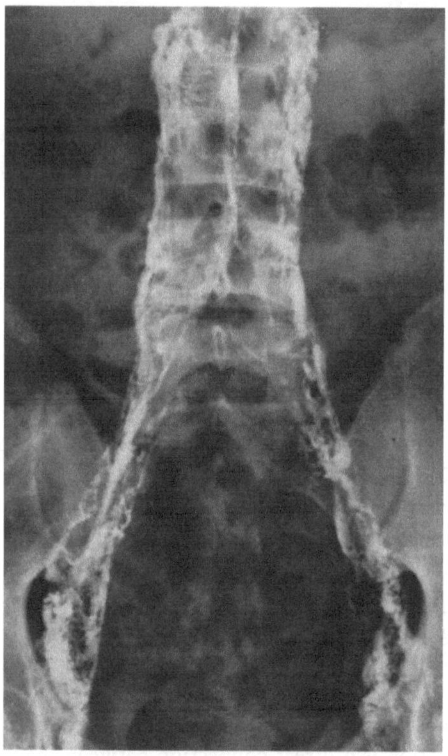

Fig. 10. Communication of the two pelvic sides in the region of the aortic bifurcation. Typical position of the three lumbar chains

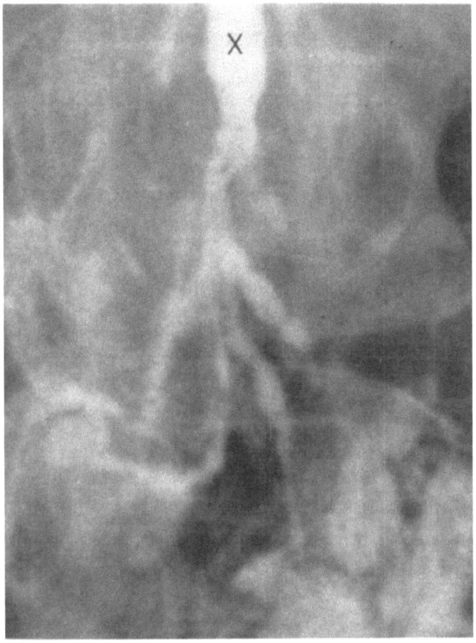

Fig. 11. Trunci lumbales and cisterna chyli (×) (magnified)

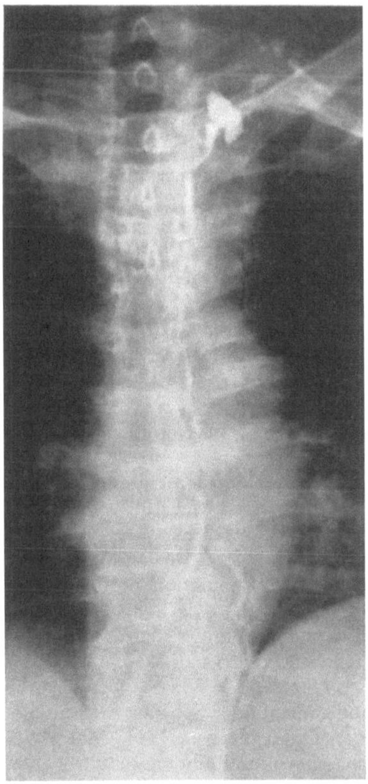

Fig. 12. Ductus thoracicus with enlargement before entering the vein on the left side. Supraclavicular lymph nodes

This variation should not be interpreted as a collateral in drainage disturbances [46, 49].

Over the lumbar trunks and, when present, the cisterna chyli (Fig. 11), the lymph flows into the thoracic duct, which can be divided into 3 parts: a short abdominal section, a long thoracic one, and a shorter cervical section (Fig. 12 [16, 18, 19, 31, 35, 46, 47, 49].

About 0.8—1.6 ml of lymph per minute flows into the venous system through this, the largest lymph trunk of the body. In contrast to the smaller lymph vessels, the duct possesses only a few valves. The duct empties mostly into the left venous angle where, in 50% of cases, a few supraclavicular lymph nodes are filled with contrast medium. Occasionally a right-sided or double-sided opening is found [36, 47, 49].

Variations of the thoracic duct are frequent, e. g. partial doubling or splitting. Besides such variations, mediastinal lymph nodes were visible in about 5% of a group of 500 patients with healthy thoraxes. In such cases it is possible, albeit seldom, to visualize a mediastinal malignant lymphoma by lymphography of the foot [30, 35, 47, 49].

References

1. Arvay, N., Picard, J. D.: La lymphographie. Étude radiologique et clinique des voies lymphatiques normales et pathologiques. Paris: Masson 1963.
2. Bourquin, J.: Histologische Grundlagen des Lymphadenogrammes. Radiologe **8**, 150 (1968).
3. Casley-Smith, J. R.: The structure of normal large lymphatics; how this determines their permeabilities and their ability to transport lymph. Quart. J. exp. Physiol. **51**, 96 (1966).
4. Casley-Smith, J. R., Florey, H. W.: The structure of normal small lymphatics. Quart. J. exp. Physiol. **46**, 101 (1961).
5. Collette, J. M.: Envahissements ganglionnaires inguino-pelviennes par lymphographie. Acta radiol. (Stockh.) **49**, 154 (1958).
6. Cunéo, B., Marcille, M.: Topographie des ganglions ilio-pelviens. Bull. Soc. anat. (Paris) 653 (1901).
7. Desprez-Curely, J. P., Bismuth, V., Laugier, A.: L'exploration radiologique des ganglions ilio-lombaires par lymphographie. Nouv. Rev. franç. Hémat. **2**, 91 (1962).
8. Ditchek, T. R., Blahut, J., Kittleson, A. C.: Lymphadenographie in normal subjects. Radiology **80**, 175 (1963).
9. Fischer, H. W., Lawrence, M. S., Thornbury, J. R.: Lymphography of the normal adult male. Radiology **78**, 399 (1962).
10. Frischbier, H. J.: Studies on the effect on the tissues of oily contrast media. In: Progress in Lymphology, Vol. I, p. 331. Stuttgart: Thieme 1967.
11. Fuchs, W. A., Davidson, J. W., Fischer, H. W.: Lymphography in Cancer. Berlin-Heidelberg-New York: Springer 1969.
12. Gergeley, R.: The roentgenological examination of the lymphatics in man. Radiology **71**, 59 (1958).
13. Gertels, W.: Lymphographie und topographische Anatomie des Beckenlymphsystems. Z. Geburtsh. Gynäk. Suppl. 165. Stuttgart: Enke 1966.
14. Heinzel, F., Rösler, H., Rüttimann, A., Wirth, W.: Kinetische Untersuchungen nach intralymphatischer Applikation radioaktiver Substanzen. Radiologe **8**, 154 (1968).
15. Hermann, P. G., Benninghoff, D. L., Nelson, J. H., Mellins, H. Z.: Roentgenanatomy of the ilio-pelvic-aortic lymphatic system. Radiology **80**, 182 (1963).
16. Idanov, D. A.: Anatomie du canal thoracique et des principaux collecteurs lymphatiques du tronc chez l'homme. Acta anat. (Basel) **37**, Suppl. 35 (1959).

17. JACKSON, L., WALLACE, S., SCHAFFER, B., GOULD, I., KRAMER, S., WEISS, A.: The diagnostic value of lymphography. Ann. intern. Med. **54**, 870 (1961).
18. JACOBSSON, S.: Clinical anatomy and pathology of the thoracic duct. Stockholm: Almqvist & Wiksell 1972.
19. JOSSIFOW, G. M.: Das Lymphgefäßsystem des Menschen. Jena: G. Fischer 1930.
20. KAINDL, F. K., MANNHEIMER, E., PFLEGER-SCHWARZ, L., THURNHER, B.: Lymphangiographie und Lymphadenographie der Extremitäten. Stuttgart: Thieme 1960.
21. KINMONTH, J. B.: Lymphangiography by radiological methods. J. Fac. Radiol. (Lond.) **5**, 13 (1955); **6**, 217 (1955).
22. KOEHLER, P. R., MEYER, W. A., SKELLEY, D. F., SCHAFFER, B.: Body distribution of ethiodol following lymphangiography. Radiology **82**, 866 (1964).
23. KOEHLER, P. R., WOHL, G. T., SCHAFFER, B.: Lymphangiography — a survey of its current status. Amer. J. Roentgenol. **91**, 1216 (1964).
24. KUBIK, ST.: Farbphoto-Atlas der topographischen Anatomie, Vol. III. Stuttgart: Thieme 1968.
25. KUBIK, ST.: Die normale Anatomie des Lymphsystems unter besonderer Berücksichtigung der Sammelgebiete der Lymphknoten der unteren Körperhälfte. Strahlentherapie, Suppl. **69**, 8 (1969).
26. KUBIK, ST., TÖNDURY, G., RÜTTIMANN, A., WIRTH, W.: Nomenklature of the lymph nodes of the retroperitoneum, the pelvis and the lower extremity. In: Progress in Lymphology, Vol. I, p. 52. Stuttgart: Thieme 1967.
27. LAMARQUE, P., PAGES, A., PUJOL, H., GINESTIE, J. F., COMBES, C.: Anatomie radiologique et valeur semiologique des images ganglionnaires en lymphographie. J. Radiol. Électrol. **48**, 253 (1967).
28. LAUFER, C.: Röntgenanatomische Untersuchungen am Beckenlymphsystem. Thesis. In press.
29. LUDWIG, J.: Die Lymphgefäßverbindungen zwischen Ductus thoracicus und supraclaviculären Lymphknoten und ihre Bedeutung für die Krebsmetastasierung. Frankfurt. Z. Path. **71**, 436 (1961).
30. LÜNING, M., ROMANUIK, P. A.: Die Darstellung der mediastinalen Lymphknoten nach Lymphographie des retroperitonealen Systems. Radiol. diagn. (Berl.) **9**, 605 (1968).
31. MALEK, P., BELAN, A., KOLC, J.: Der Ductus thoracicus in der Röntgenkinematographie. Experimentalstudie. Fortschr. Röntgenstr. **93**, 806 (1960).
32. MOULONGUET-DOLÉRIS, O., ARVAY, N., PICARD, J. C., MANLOT, G.: La lymphographie: Technique, indications et résultats (Conclusions partant sur 230 explorations). J. Radiol. Électrol. **42**, 281 (1961).
33. PAGES, A.: Aspects histo-pathologiques des ganglions après lymphographie récente. Arch. Anat. path. **13**, 3 (1965).
34. ROO, I. DE, THOMAS, P., KROPHOLLER, W.: The Importance of Tomography for the Interpretation of the lymphographic picture of lymph node metastasis. Amer. J. Roentgenol. **94**, 924 (1965).
35. ROUVIÈRE, H.: Anatomie des lymphatiques de l'homme. Paris: Masson 1932.
36. RUSZNYAK, J., FÖLDI, M., SZABO, G.: Physiologie und Pathologie des Lymphkreislaufes. Jena: G. Fischer 1957.
37. RÜTTIMANN, A.: Die Lymphographie. In: Lehrbuch der Röntgendiagnostik, Vol. I (SCHINZ, BAENSCH, FROMMHOLD, GLAUNER, UEHLINGER, WELLAUER, Eds.) 6th Ed. Stuttgart: Thieme 1965.
38. RÜTTIMANN, A. (Ed.): Progress in Lymphology, Vol. I. Stuttgart: Thieme 1967.
39. RÜTTIMANN, A., BUONO, M. S. DEL: Die Lymphographie mit öligem Kontrastmittel. Fortschr. Röntgenstr. **97**, 662 (1962).
40. RÜTTIMANN, A., WIRTH, W.: Möglichkeiten und Grenzen der Lymphographie mit öligem Kontrastmittel. Radiologe **8**, 140 (1968).
41. TJERNBERG, B.: Lymphography. An animal study on the diagnosis of V x 2 carcinoma and inflammation. Acta Radiol. Suppl. 214 (1962).
42. VIAMONTE, M., ALTMAN, D., PARKS, R., BLUM, E., BEVILAQUA, M., RECHER, L.: Radiographic — Pathologic Correlation in the Interpretation of Lymphangioadenograms. Radiology **80**, 903 (1963).

43. VON KEISER, D., ZUM WINKEL, K., FRISCHBIER, H. J.: MÜLLER, H.: Vergleich zwischen röntgenologischer und szintigraphischer Darstellung. Fortschr. Röntgenstr. 100, 557 (1964).
44. WALLACE, S., JACKSON, L., DODD, O. D., GREENING, R. R.: Lymphatic dynamics in certain abnormal states. Amer. J. Roentgenol. 91, 1187 (1964).
45. WEISSLEDER, H., OBRECHT, P.: Diagnostische Probleme bei der Lymphangioadenographie. Fortschr. Röntgenstr. 100, 81 (1964).
46. WIRTH, W.: Zur Röntgenanatomie des Lymphsystems der inguinalen, pelvinen und aortalen Region. Fortschr. Röntgenstr. 105, 441, 636 (1966).
47. WIRTH, W., FROMMHOLD, H.: Der Ductus thoracicus und seine Variationen. Lymphographische Studie. Fortschr. Röntgenstr. 112, 23 (1970).
48. WIRTH, W., HAFNER, E.: Changes in body temperature and white blood count after lymphography with oily contrast medium. In: Progress in Lymphology, Vol. II, p. 218. Stuttgart: Thieme 1970.
49. WIRTH, W., KUBIK, ST.: Anatomie und Röntgenanatomie des Lymphsystems. In: Atlas der Lymphographie (RÜTTIMANN, A., VIAMONTE, V., Eds.). Stuttgart: Thieme. In press.

Lymphographic Differential Diagnosis in Malignant Lymphomas

K. H. Strickstrock, P. E. Peters, and H. Weissleder

Summary

The most important reason for lymphography as routine method in the diagnosis of malignant lymphomas is staging in histologically proven cases. In 205 patients with Hodgkin's disease the stage had to be changed in 45,3%. "Undetermined" cases at the time of lymphography will be finally staged by radiographic monitoring of the opacified lymph-nodes at short time intervals. These results now must be confirmed by laparotomy with open lymph-node biopsy. In cases without histological verification where clinical findings are suspicious of malignant lymphoma, differential diagnosis by means of lymphography is possible to a limited extent by analysis of the sum of several lymphographic symptoms, above all in Hodgkin's disease. Computer analysis of 121 lymphograms in Hodgkin's disease with differential histological subgroups demonstrates that in the subgroups, too, there is a certain correlation between predominant combinations of symptoms in the lymphogram and the histological findings. However, histological verification of the diagnosis cannot be omitted in differentiating both the various lymphomas and the various subgroups of Hodgkin's disease.

Lymphography is today a routine method in the diagnosis of malignant lymphomas. It is particularly valuable in the evaluation of the retroperitoneal lymph-node system, which cannot be studied by other non-surgical diagnostic procedures unless there is already gross lymph-node involvement.

The main reasons for lymphography in malignant lymphoma are

1. *Staging* in histologically proven cases.
2. *Monitoring* of response to therapy.
3. *Study* of the spread of the disease.
4. *Examination* of the retroperitoneal lymph-node system in cases where clinical findings indicate suspicion of malignant lymphoma without the diagnosis being established.

Retroperitoneal lymph-node examination and the value of lymphography for staging purposes will now be discussed in more detail.

Lymphographic Differential Diagnosis

Lymphographic differential diagnosis requires precise analysis of all structures in the lymphogram. In the filling phase ("lymphangiogram"), pathologic changes of lymph vessels can be recognized.

In the storage phase ("lymphadenogram"), the shape, number, and size of lymph nodes and the distribution pattern of contrast material are studied.

Localization of pathological lymph nodes and disturbances of normal storage patterns are the most important reasons for differential diagnosis.

In the *lymphangiogram*, the number, position, course, lumen diameter and condition of valves of the lymph vessels can be used for differential diagnosis. Lymphatic block is a very conspicuous lymphographic finding. Collateral vessels and delayed drainage of lymph vessels indicate hindrance of lymph flow (Table 1).

In the differential diagnosis of malignant lymphomas, the lymphadenogram is of more importance than the filling phase. Both the number of opacified lymph nodes, their size, shape and storage pattern and the localization of pathological lymph nodes within the lymphatic system are significant (Table 2).

Table 1. Diagnostic criteria: Lymph vessels

1. Number (decreased — normal — increased)
2. Position (normal — displacement — distortion)
3. Course (normal — stretched — twisted)
4. Lumen width (narrow — normal — dilated)
5. Condition of the valves
6. Blockage of lymph flow
7. Contrast medium extravasation
8. Collateral vessels
9. Delayed drainage of contrast medium
10. Localization of the pathological process

Table 2. Diagnostic criteria: Lymph nodes

1. Number (non-opacified — decreased — normal — increased)
2. Size (max. cross section of normal oval lymph nodes: 2.5×1.0 cm; round lymph nodes 1.5 cm; FFD: 110 cm)
3. Shape (round — oval — deformed — conglomerate)
4. Storage pattern (decreased — increased)
5. Localization of the pathological process

Changes in the *storage pattern* involve the concentration and the distribution of contrast material. Changes in the concentration pattern include spotted, streaky, lumpy, and mesh-like structures. The distribution of the contrast material can be regular or irregular (Table 3).

Storage defects vary in size, form and localization within the lymph node. They can be round, oval or irregularly shaped ("lacunar") with clear or blurred contours. They can be located marginally, when they include the peripheral sinus of the lymph

Table 3. Diagnostic criteria: Storage pattern of the lymph nodes

A: Type of storage pattern
1. Spotted (small — medium — large)
2. Lumpy
3. Streaked (usually in horizontal lines)
4. Reticular (fine mesh, large mesh)
B: Type of contrast medium distribution
1. Regular
2. Irregular

Table 4. Diagnostic criteria: Storage pattern of the lymph nodes

C: Shape of the storage defects
1. Round
2. Irregular
D: Localization of the storage defects
1. Marginal
2. Central
3. Diffuse

node; they can be located centrally, or they can be evenly distributed throughout the lymph node (Table 4). Examples of different storage patterns and various localizations of storage defects are given in Figs. 1—3.

What is the significance of these symptoms in the lymphangiogram and lymphadenogram for differential diagnosis of malignant lymphoma? Analysis of the storage pattern in the lymphogram can never replace histological diagnosis. Comparative lymphographic-histological studies in benign and malignant lymph-node diseases have

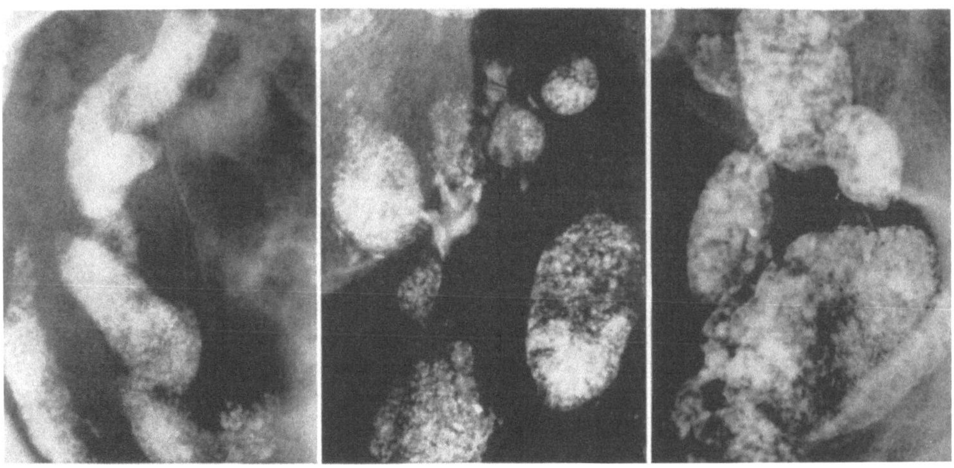

a b c

Fig. 1 a—c. Storage pattern of the lymph nodes, a Small spotted, b Medium spotted, c Large spotted

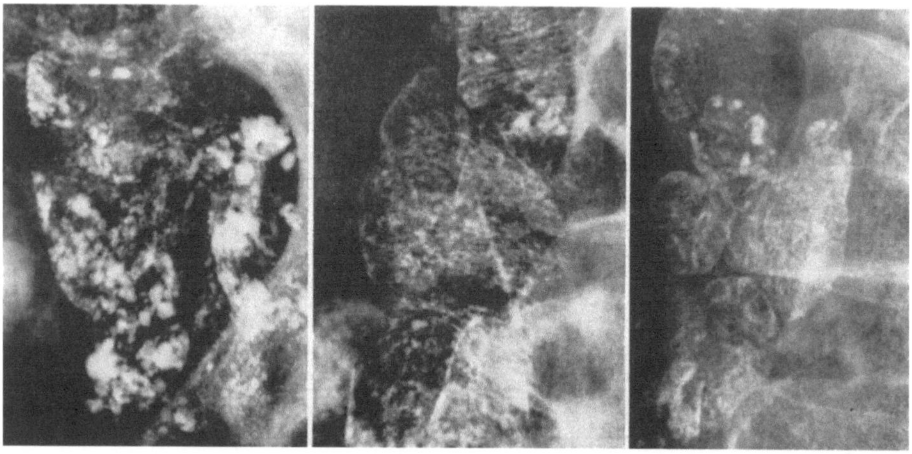

a b c

Fig. 2 a—c. Storage pattern of the lymph nodes, a Lumpy, b Streaked, c Reticular

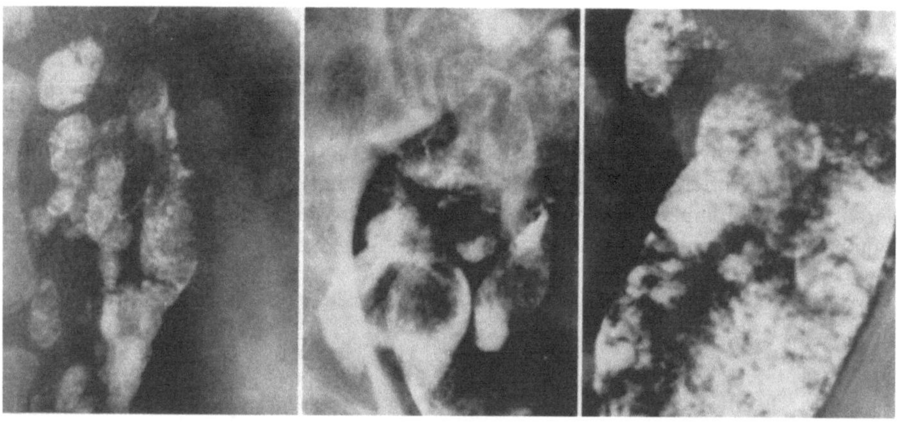

a b c

Fig. 3 a—c. Localization and shape of storage defects of the lymph nodes, a Marginal and regular, b Central and regular, c Diffusely distributed and irregular

shown that there is no single specific symptom correlated with a certain disease. The sum of several lymphographic symptoms, however, often leads to differential conclusions, particularly in late-stage disease with generalized involvement of lymph nodes [1, 4, 8, 10, 11].

The most characteristic lymphographic findings in the malignant lymphoma group are seen in Hodgkin's disease (HD). In early stages the lymph nodes are of normal size or slightly enlarged and reveal a coarsened storage pattern with central and marginal storage defects which tend to be confluent.

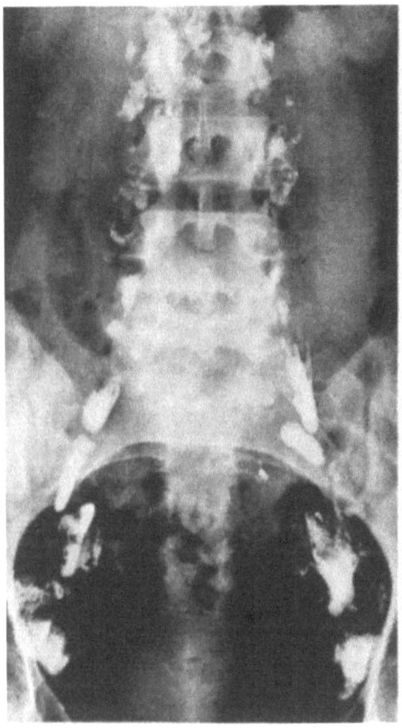

Fig. 4

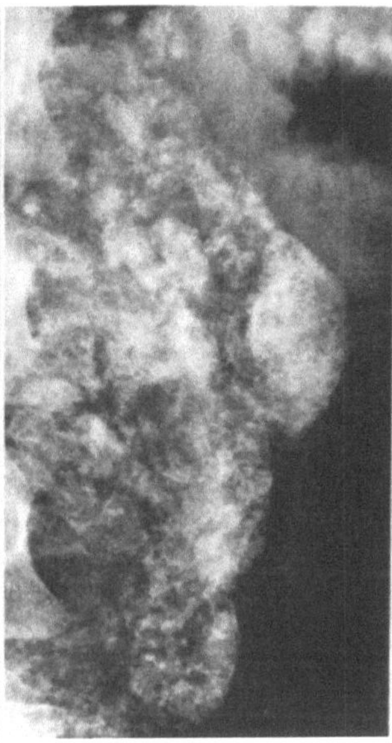

Fig. 5

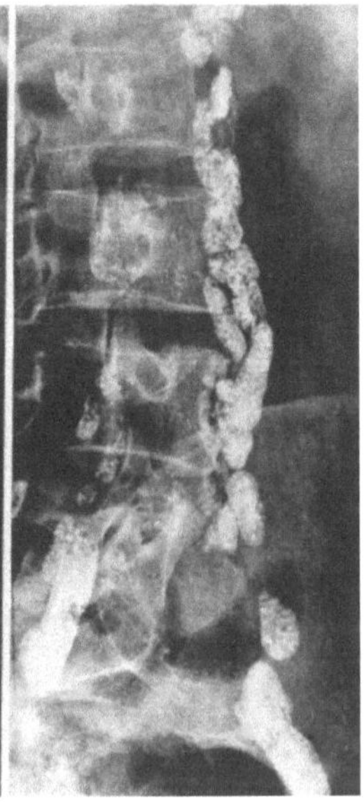

Fig. 6

Fig. 4. Hodgkin's disease: Normal and pathological lymph nodes
Fig. 5. Hodgkin's disease: Generalized lymph-node involvement with enlargement
Fig. 6. Sarcoidosis: Generalized lymph-node involvement without marginal defects

In early-stage HD normal and pathological lymph nodes are often found simultaneously (Fig. 4). As a rule, HD first involves the para-aortic lymph nodes, often only unilaterally. In late-stage disease there is generalized lymph node involvement with significant enlargement of nodes and subsequent delayed drainage of lymph; a characteristic blurred storage pattern is seen (Fig. 5).

Retroperitoneal lymph-node involvement in *sarcoidosis* can be readily differentiated from HD [5]. In sarcoidosis, lymph nodes are markedly enlarged even in the early stages, with a mesh-like diffuse storage pattern and several round, sharply delineated areas of defective storage. Interruptions of marginal contours are rarely seen (Fig. 6).

The non-caseous form of *lymph-node tuberculosis* is mostly restricted to a few nodes. These show moderate enlargement with loosening of storage structure similar to the findings in unspecific lymphadenitis. The caseous form, however, reveals relatively large central and marginal storage defects. It is difficult to differentiate this form from HD (Fig. 7).

Early *lymph-node metastasis* cannot be separated lymphographically from early-stage HD, since both show scattered small storage defects. Advanced cases of lymph-node metastasis can still be diagnosed with a high degree of certainty because of their generally unilateral involvement of single lymph nodes. The diseased nodes are enlarged. They are characterized by peripheral storage defects of moth-eaten appearance, while the storage pattern is otherwise normal. Delayed drainage of the contrast material or total blockage of lymph flow are further signs of advanced lymph-node metastasis.

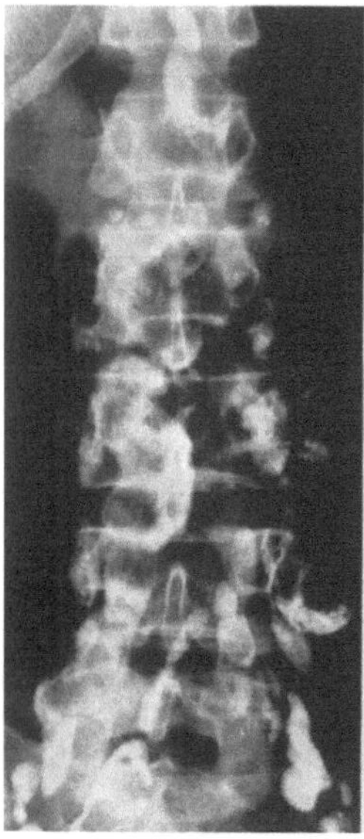

Fig. 7

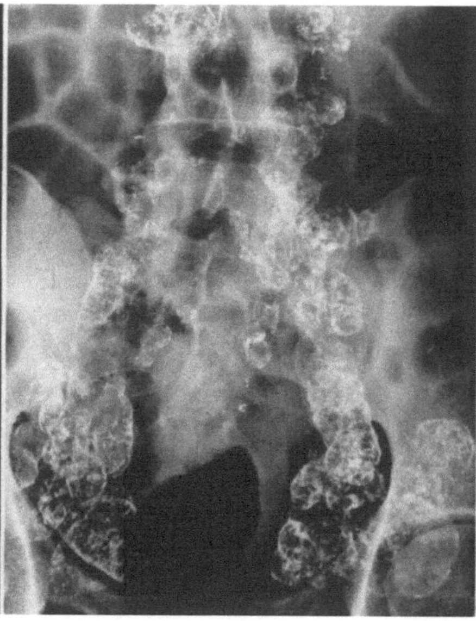

Fig. 8

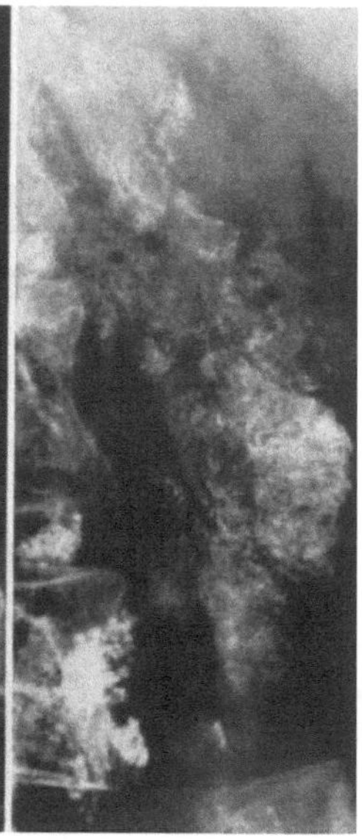

Fig. 9

Fig. 7. Caseous lymph-node tuberculosis: Central and marginal storage defects
Fig. 8. Lymphosarcomatosis: Generalized lymph-node involvement, foamy storage pattern with diffusely distributed defects
Fig. 9. Lymphosarcomatosis: Generalized lymph-node involvement with streaked storage pattern

In *lymphosarcomatosis* the lymph nodes are grossly enlarged. The storage pattern has a foamy-blistery appearance and numerous nodes are almost entirely destroyed. Storage defects varying in form and size are distributed over the lymph nodes, the contours of which are irregular (Fig. 8). Occasionally one sees horizontal streaks (Figs. 8 and 9).

Reticulum-cell sarcoma is also characterized by generalized lymph-node involvement and cannot be differentiated lymphographically from lymphosarcoma. Horizontal streaks are not found in reticulum-cell sarcoma, however (Fig. 10).

Very similar lymphographic patterns to those in lympho- and reticulum-cell sarcoma are observed in *Brill-Symmers giant follicular lymphoblastoma* (Fig. 11).

Generalized retroperitoneal lymph-node involvement in *Waldenström's disease (macroglobulinemia)* also reveals a similar lymphographic picture (Fig. 12).

Horizontal streaks as demonstrated in lymphosarcoma can also occur in *chronic lymphatic leukemia* (Fig. 13).

The differential diagnostic possibilities of lymphography are illustrated schematically in Table 5. According to this scheme, lymphosarcoma, reticulum-cell sarcoma, chronic lymphatic leukemia and Brill-Symmer's disease cannot be differentiated lymphographically [9], while HD shows a fairly characteristic combination of lymphographic symptoms. The main difficulties in diagnosis of HD arise in the very early stages, where it has to be differentiated from fibrolipomatosis, nonspecific lymphadenitis, tuberculosis, and early lymph-node metastasis.

Table 5. The possibilities for differential diagnosis in various lymph node diseases (simplified)

	Fibro-lipomatosis	Unspecified lymphadenitis	Tuberculosis	Sarcoidosis	Hodgkin's disease	Chronic lymphatic leukaemia	Lympho-sarcomatosis	Lymph node metastases
Fibrolipomatosis	—	++	caseated: (+) T. B. lymph-adenitis: ++	++	initial: + later: ++	++	++	initial: (+) later: +
Unspecified lymphadenitis	++	—	caseated: ++ T. B. lymph-adenitis ∅	++	initial: (+) later: ++	++	++	initial: (+) later: ++
Tuberculosis	caseated: (+) T. B. lymph-adenitis: ++	caseated: (+) T. B. lymph-adenitis: ∅	—	caseated: + T. B. lymph-adenitis: ++	caseated: (+) T. B. lymph-adenitis: ++	++	++	caseated: (+) T. B. lymph-adenitis: ++
Sarcoidosis	++	++	caseated: + T. B. lymph-adenitis: ++	—	++	++	++	++
Hodgkin's disease	initial: + later: ++	initial: (+) later: ++	caseated: (+) T. B. lymph-adenitis: ++	++	—	++	++	initial: (+) later: ++
Chronic lymphatic leukaemia	++	++	++	++	++	—	∅	++
Lymphosarcomatosis Lymphoreticulo-sarcomatosis and others	++	++	++	++	++	∅	—	++
Lymph node metastases	initial: (+) later: +	initial: (+) later: +	caseated: (+) T. B. lymph-adenitis: ++	++	initial: (+) later: ++	++	++	—

∅ = differentiation not possible, (+) = differentiation in individual cases, + = frequent differentiation, ++ = differentiation usually possible.

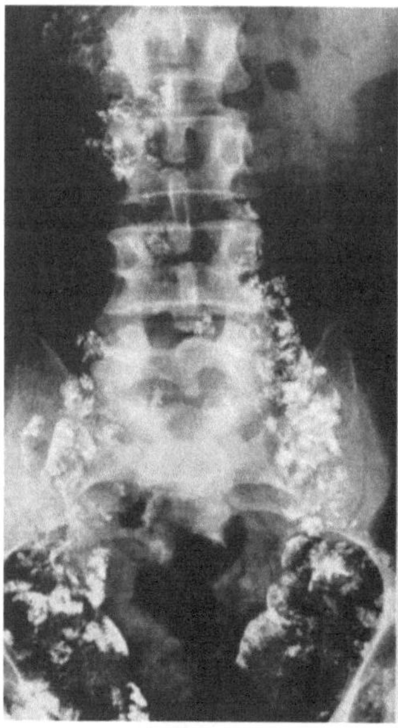

Fig. 10

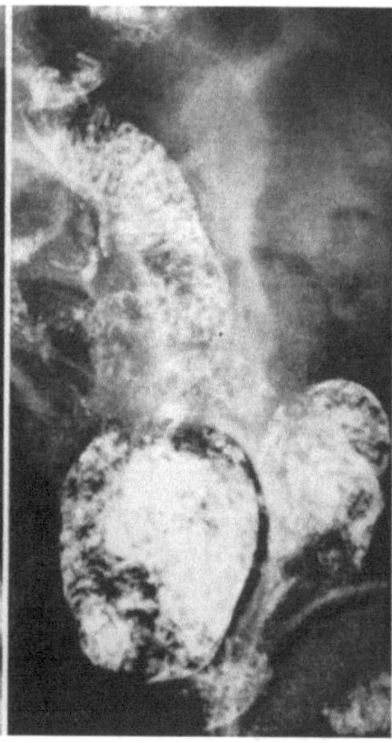

Fig. 11

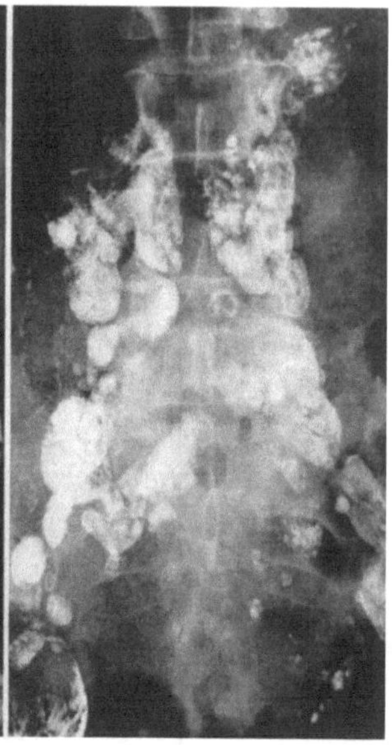

Fig. 12

Fig. 10. Reticulum cell sarcoma: Generalized lymph-node involvement
Fig. 11. Giant follicular Brill-Symmers lymphoblastoma: Generalized lymph-node involvement
Fig. 12. Waldenström's disease: Generalized lymph-node involvement

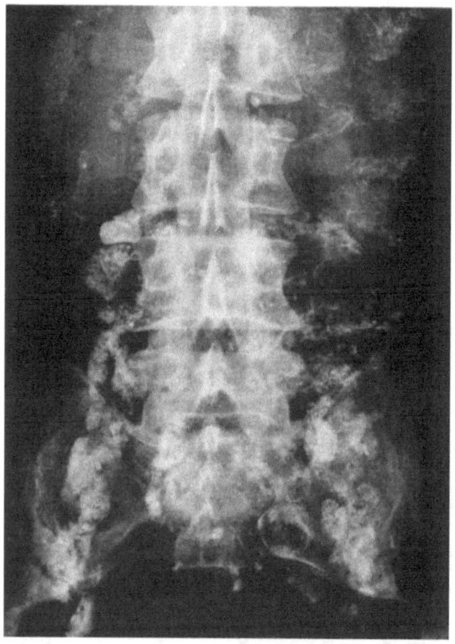

Fig. 13. Chronic lymphatic leukemia: Generalized lymph-node involvement with streaked storage pattern

Correlation of Lymphographic Symptoms with Histological Subgroups of Hodgkin's Disease (Luke's Classification)

The correlation of lymphographic symptoms with histological subgroups of HD (Luke's classification [3]) was painted out for the first time by [2]. Our own study in this field, presented at the meeting of the International Society of Lymphology in Brussels in 1970 [7], reported on a computer analysis of 121 lymphograms (Table 6). The majority of our patients were untreated at the time of lymphography. 61 cases (50.4%) showed an unequivocal pathologic lymphogram, 49 cases had normal lymphographic findings, and 11 cases were undetermined. Histologically, most cases fell into the categories of nodular sclerosis and mixed cellularity.

Table 6. Hodgkin's disease. Histological subtype and lymphographic diagnosis in 121 lymphograms

Histological subtype LUKES and BUTLER 1966	No. of lymphograms				
	Total n	%	Abnormal n	Normal n	Equivocal n
L+H, nodular	4	3	0	4	0
L+H, diffuse	12	10	6	5	1
Nodular sclerosis	50	41	19	24	7
Mixed cellularity	30	25	19	11	0
Diffuse fibrosis	13	11	7	4	2
Reticular	12	10	10	1	1
Total	121	100	61	49	11

There were 4 cases of the lymphohistiocytic form of the nodular type, none of which showed involvement of the subdiaphragmatic lymph nodes. The percentage of retroperitoneal lymph-node involvement was higher in subgroups with poor cellularity. All 10 patients with the reticular type of HD had a pathologic lymphogram.

Generally, all types of disturbance of the storage structure, i. e. coarsening, streaky, foamy, reticular or blurred patterns, were seen in all histological subgroups. Often the lymphographic appearance was not uniform and several different storage patterns were found simultaneously. In most cases, however, certain symptoms or a combination of symptoms were predominant in the lymphogram. Coarsening of the storage structure, for instance, was the dominant symptom in about 40 to 50% of the cases with nodular sclerosis, mixed cellularity and the diffuse form of the lymphohistiocytic type. In subgroups with poor cellularity, the coarsened storage pattern was seen less frequently. In the reticular type it could be found in only 10% of the cases (Table 7).

Here, in the reticular type, a blurred mesh-like storage structure dominated. Streaky, foamy and mesh-like patterns were relatively often connected with the diffuse form of the lymphohistiocytic type, while they were seldom seen in cases with nodular sclerosis or mixed cellularity.

Table 7. Hodgkin's disease. Histological subtype and changes in storage pattern of contrast medium in 61 abnormal lymphograms

Histological subtype LUKES and BUTLER 1966	Storage pattern of lymphographic contrast medium				
	Coarse-grained %	Streaked %	Bullous %	Net-like %	Blurred %
L+H, nodular	0	0	0	0	0
L+H, diffuse	50	17	17	17	0
Nodular sclerosis	39	6	6	6	6
Mixed cellularity	56	5	0	5	17
Diffuse fibrosis	30	0	0	17	33
Reticular	10	20	20	50	40

Taking all lymphographic criteria — not only those relating to the storage structure — into consideration, the correlation of lymphographic findings with the different histological subgroups of HD gave the following results:

Nodular sclerosis and mixed cellularity show lymphographically the well-known features of HD, such as lymph-node enlargement of varying degrees with coarsened storage pattern and central and marginal filling defects. The number of diseased lymph nodes depends on the duration of illness (Fig. 14).

Diffuse fibrous and reticular types are characterized lymphographically by mesh-like, blurred storage structures with marginal storage defects. Generalized lymph-node involvement is already present in early stages of the disease. The lymph nodes are diffusely interspersed with malignant tissue (Fig. 15).

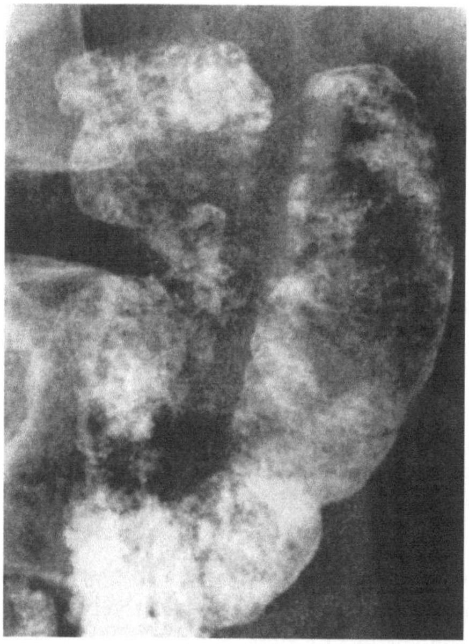

Fig. 14. Hodgkin's disease: Nodular sclerosis subtype

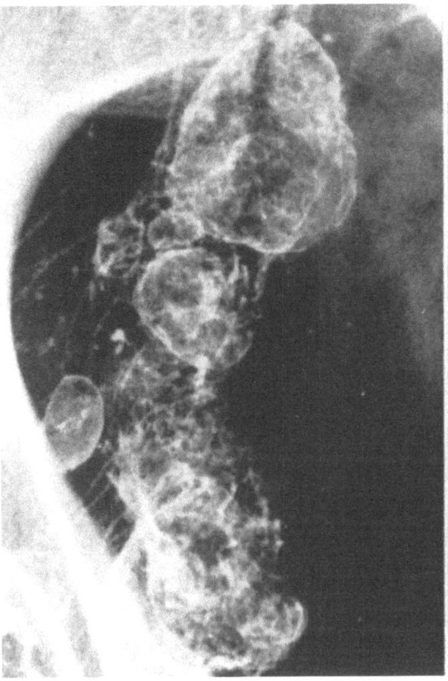

Fig. 15

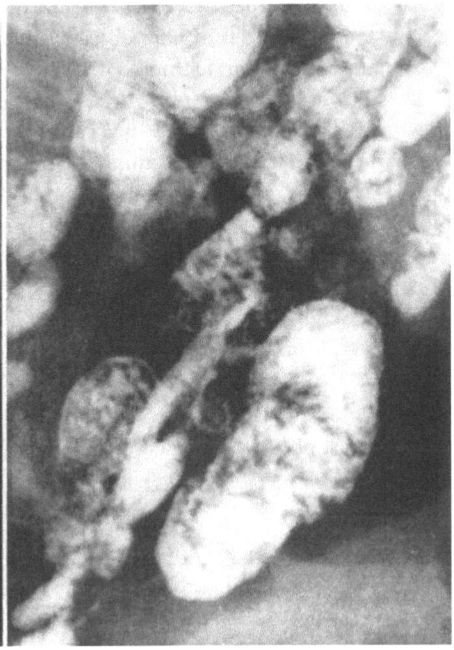

Fig. 16

Fig. 15. Hodgkin's disease: Reticular subtype
Fig. 16. Hodgkin's disease: Diffuse form of the lymphohistiocytic subtype

The dominant symptom in the *diffuse form of the lymphohistiocytic type* is coarsening of the storage structure. Occasionally, foamy and streaky structures are found in diffusely interspersed lymph nodes. In contrast to forms with poor cellularity, marginal filling defects are typically absent. Only single lymph nodes are involved. Lymphographically, this picture resembles that of sarcoidosis (Fig. 16).

In conclusion, differential diagnosis of malignant lymphomas by means of lymphography is possible, but only to a limited extent. It does not replace histological diagnosis. In most cases the lymph-node involvement in malignant lymphoma starts above the diaphragm. Biopsy for histological verification can easily be performed. At Freiburg, primary affection of abdominal lymph nodes was found in only 3% of all cases with HD [6]. Similar percentages are reported for other malignant lymphomas.

Staging by Lymphography

Differential diagnostic consideration may be interesting and challenging, but lymphography for staging purposes is much more significant. Only precise knowledge of the stage of the disease can allow us to assess the prognosis and to initiate optimal therapy. Knowledge of the typical lymphographic symptoms makes it easier to decide whether there is retroperitoneal lymph-node involvement in a given case of histologically proved malignant lymphoma. Differentiation between an early stage of the disease and inflammatory or degenerative changes is extremely difficult.

About 8% of the 121 cases remained "undetermined" at the time of lymphography. Final diagnosis was established by radiographic monitoring of the opacified lymph nodes at short time intervals.

The role of lymphography for staging purposes in 205 patients with histologically proved HD is demonstrated in Table 8. Lymphography placed 45.3% of these patients in another stage. A similar figure was obtained in early cases where the time interval between establishing the diagnosis histologically and performing lymphography was less than 6 months. Here the stage had to be changed in 41.9% of the cases after lymphography [6].

The recently recommended procedure of laparotomy with open lymph-node biopsy for staging purposes will give reliable data on the accuracy of lymphography in early lymph-node disease.

Table 8. Hodgkin's disease: Stage changing as result of lymphography in 205 cases with a time interval of less than 6 months between histological diagnosis and lymphography

Stage I, II, $IV_{p.c.}$ → III, $IV_{p.c.}$ + abdominal involvement					
Interval histology → lymphography				Total	
< 6 Months		> 6 Months			
n	%	n	%	n	%
39	41,9	54	48,3	93	45,3
(93)		(112)		(205)	

References

1. Fuchs, W. A., Davidson, J. W., Fischer, H. W.: Lymphography in cancer, p. 179. Berlin-Heidelberg-New York: Springer 1965.
2. Fuchs, W. A., Härtel, M. P.: Die Prognose des M. Hodgkin auf Grund der Lymphknotenstruktur im Lymphogramm. Fortschr. Röntgenstr. **109**, 553 (1968).
3. Lukes, R. J., Butler, JJ., Hicks, F. B.: The natural history of Hodgkin's disease as related to its pathologic picture. Cancer (Philad.) **19**, 317 (1966).
4. Rüttimann, A., del Buono, M. S.: Die Lymphographie. In: Schinz, Glauner, Rüttimann: Ergebnisse der med. Strahlenforschung. N. F. I, 248. Stuttgart: Thieme 1964.
5. Strickstrock, K.-H., Weissleder, H.: Lymphografische Diagnose und Differentialdiagnose bei der Sarkoidose. Fortschr. Röntgenstr. **108**, 576 (1968).
6. Strickstrock, K. H., Musshoff, K., Weissleder, H., Boutis, L., Bauer, S., Propping, D.: Der abdominelle Morbus Hodgkin. 49. Röntgen-Kongress, Hamburg 1968, Strahlentherapie **131** Suppl.: Maligne Lymphome. München: Urban & Schwarzenberg 1969.
7. Strickstrock, K.-H., Weissleder, H., Schmiedel, E.: Computer analysis of lymphographic and histological examination results in cases of Hodgkin's disease. p. 110. 3rd Congress of the International Society of Lymphology. Brüssel: Abstracts 1970.
8. Weissleder, H.: Die Lymphographie. Ergebn. inn. Med. Kinderheilk. **23**, 297 (1965).
9. Weissleder, H., Peters, P. E.: Lymphografische Differentialdiagnose bei Lymphknotenerkrankungen. Fortschr. Röntgenstr. **114**, 517 (1971).
10. Welin, S., Johansson, S.: Lymphography. In: Diethelm, L. (Ed.): Handbuch der Medizinischen Radiologie, Vol. VIII, p. 179. Berlin-Heidelberg-New York: Springer 1968.
11. Wiljasalo, M.: Lymphographic differential diagnosis of neoplastic diseases. Acta radiol. (Stockh.) Suppl. 247 (1965).

Lymphography in Clinical Stage III Hodgkin's Disease

W. A. FUCHS, I. TRILLER, and M. HAERTEL

Summary

35 patients with CS III Hodgkin's disease at first presentation were subdivided by lymphography into two groups: CS III_{1N} presenting only the aortic lymph nodes involved and CS III_{2N} with additional involvement of the iliac (inguinal) lymph nodes. The 3-year survival rate of CS III_{1N} was 70%, of CS III_{2N} 8% and of CS III as a whole 55%.

Lymphography is a routine procedure for the clinical staging of Hodgkin's disease [15]. The accurate delineation of the portal fields in radiation therapy and the control of the results of radiotherapy and chemotherapy are other important reasons for routinely performing this method. Our present study, like our previous preliminary reports [4, 5], indicates that lymphography offers additional information in patients with CS III disease.

Material and Methods

35 consecutive patients with CS III at first presentation were investigated between 1961 and 1972. 10 patients were women and 25 were men. The age of the adult subjects ranged at onset from 17 to 74 years (mean: 37,3 years).

The clinical staging was done according to the report of the Committee on Hodgkin's disease staging procedures (*Ann Arbor* 1971) [3].

The histopathology of the lymph node disease was classified according to the Rye modification [11] of the classification of LUKES and BUTLER [10].

All cases had been subjected to a rigorous *clinical study*. This included history and physical examination, with careful mapping and measurement of clinically involved lymph nodes, spleen, liver and other palpable disease; complete blood counts, erythrocyte sedimentation rate, liver function tests (alkaline phosphatase, bilirubin serum, glutamic oxalic and glutamic pyruvic transaminases) supplemented by isotope scanning and needle biopsy of the liver in cases with hepatic enlargement or abnormal tests. Radiographic examination of the chest and skeleton and bilateral lymphography with inferior cavography and urography were done in all patients.

Strict criteria of *lymphographic interpretation* were applied. Positive lymphograms were classified into two groups: 1. moderately enlarged lymph nodes with solitary or contiguous lacunar filling defects of varying size (Fig. 1) and 2. markedly enlarged lymph nodes with cystic pattern characterized by a delicate net-like structure (Fig. 2). Enlargement of lymph nodes alone without a pathological lymphographic pattern was not judged to be abnormal.

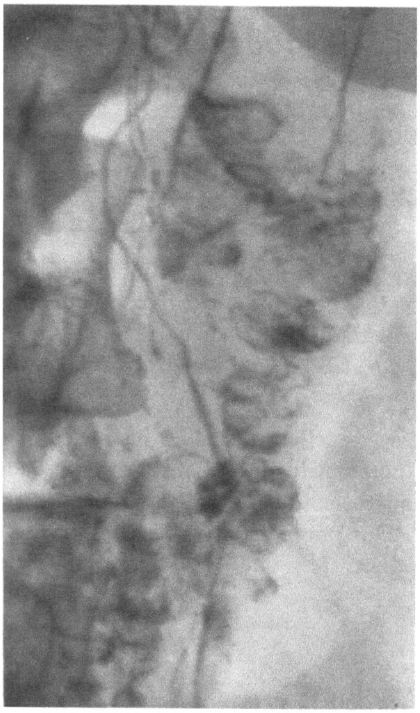

Fig. 1

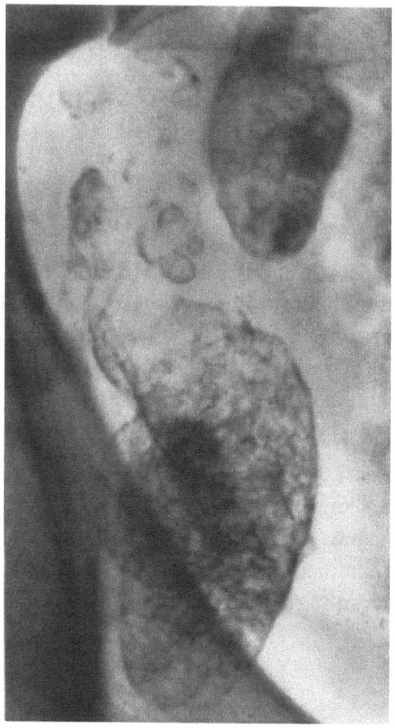

Fig. 2

Fig. 1. Contiguous lacunar filling defects in moderately enlarged aortic lymph nodes
Fig. 2. Cystic pattern of enlarged aortic lymph nodes

The aortic, iliac left and right, inguinal left and right lymph nodes were each considered to represent one region.

The *radiotherapeutic program* consisted in a modification of the extended-field radical megavoltage therapy program proposed by Kaplan and Rosenberg [9]. The portal fields routinely included the supraclavicular, mediastinal, aortic and iliac areas. Doses in the range of 4000 rads, given at the rate of about 1000 rads/week, were administered. The cervical, axillary and inguinal regions were irradiated with similar doses only in the presence of disease or when adjacent to an involved area. 17 patients were treated by radiotherapy alone, 5 patients underwent a combined radiotherapy-chemotherapy treatment, 13 patients had only chemotherapy.

Chemotherapy was done with a cyclic program utilizing nitrogen mustard, vincristine, procarbazine and prednisone in 9 more recent cases. The other 9 earlier patients received high dose procarbazine, chlorambucil, nitrogen mustard, vincristine, cyclophosphamide and vinblastine.

The survival of these patients has been analyzed by the actuarial method of Berkson and Gage [2], without correction for natural attrition.

Results

In 16 patients only a single region, the aortic lymph nodes, was involved (CS III_{1N}). 19 patients showed involvement of two or more contiguous regions, e.g. the aortic and iliac (inguinal) regions (CS III_{2N}).

The 3-year survival rate of all patients in CS III was 55%, with 5 out of 35 patients living after 5 years (Fig. 3). Comparison of the actuarial survival rates of the patients according to the number of infradiaphragmatic lymph node regions involved results in a 3-year survival rate of 70%, with 5 patients living after 5 years for patients of group CS III_{1N}. In CS III_{2N} the 3-year survival rate was only 8%; none of the patients of this group survived the 5-year limit. Consequently, the lymphographic findings subdivided the CS III into two groups of patients with an entirely different prognostic outlook.

25 patients had an abnormal lymphogram consisting exclusively of lymph nodes with lacunar filling defects. 10 patients showed a cystic lymphographic storage pattern in one or several pathological lymph nodes. The cystic storage pattern was predominantly found in patients of CS III_{2N} (9 out of 15 patients). 17 patients were classified as CS III A and 18 patients as CS III B. In CS III A, 9 out of 17 patients

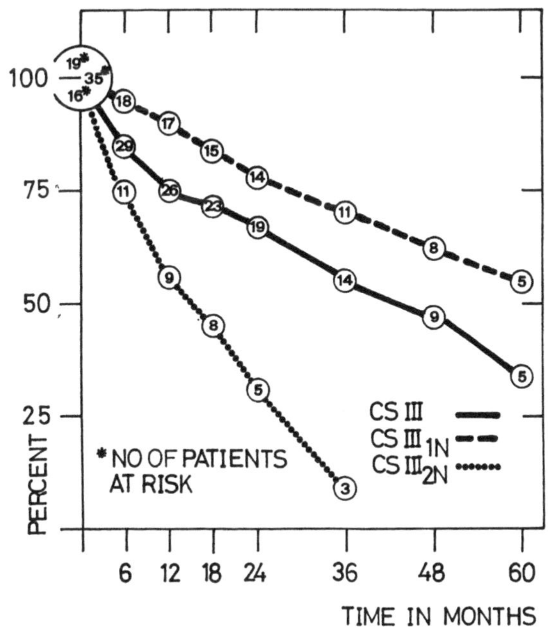

Fig. 3. Actuarial survival (Berkson-Gage) for patients with Hodgkin's disease CS III according to the number of infradiaphragmatic lymph node regions involved. CS III_{1N} = involvement of a single region, CS III_{2N} involvement of two or more contiguous regions

showed involvement of only a single lymph node region. Two or more contiguous lymph node regions were affected by the disease in 11 out of the 18 cases of CS III B disease. Consequently, no correlation seems to exist between A and B staging and the number of infradiaphragmatic lymph node regions involved.

No difference — topographical or structural — was noted in the site of involvement of the supradiaphragmatic lymph nodes in the two patient groups CS III_{1N} and CS III_{2N}. The histological subtypes did not show any predilection for one particular group. Although no statistical analysis was possible due to the limited number of cases, there seems to be no difference in survival rates between patients treated with radiotherapy and chemotherapy respectively in the two subgroups as judged by the survival time in each particular case.

Discussion

The main concern for a more refined classification of Hodgkin's disease CS III has been focused on the diagnosis of a possible involvement of the spleen and abdominal lymph node groups not visualized by lymphography. For this reason exploratory laparotomy, including splenectomy, is performed on a prospective basis in many centers [1, 6, 7, 8, 13, 16]. In CS I and CS II Hodgkin's disease, the number of lymph node regions involved and the specific key sites of involvement are considered to be important prognostic factors [12]. It is, therefore, reasonable to assume that CS III disease may also be further subdivided according to the number of infradiaphragmatic lymph node regions involved. The results of the present investigation indicate that CS III Hodgkin's disease can be subdivided according to lymphographic findings into two patient groups: 1. CS III_{1N} presenting only the aortic lymph nodes involved and 2. CS III_{2N} with additional involvement of the unilateral or bilateral iliac and in some cases inguinal lymph nodes. The 3-year survival rate of 70% for the patients with CS III_{1N} compared to 8% of the patients with CS III_{2N} is considerable and is in contrast to the 55% for the entire CS III group. Marked lymph node enlargement and the cystic lymphographic node pattern also indicate advanced disease, since these were found mainly in the CS III_{2N} group. These results confirm our findings described previously in preliminary reports [4, 5].

The limited number of patients did not allow us to group our case material according to different patterns of presentation. This could have been of particular interest, since more detailed long-term predictions are made in CS I and CS II according to the pattern of presentations within the supradiaphragmatic lymph node groups [12].

Certain reservations concerning the survival rate of the two subgroups must be made, since the therapeutic program for our case material was not standardized. Furthermore, the presence or absence of liver disease was only evaluated by conventional means and not by peritoneoscopy or laparotomy with liver biopsy. However, by applying strict selection criteria to eliminate questionable cases it is unlikely that an appreciable number of stage IV patients were included in this case material. Taking into account these limitations, caution has to be applied when reaching conclusions.

Nonetheless, the present study seems to indicate that lymphography may subdivide CS III Hodgkin's disease according to the number of infradiaphragmatic lymph node regions involved, and thereby furnish important information concerning the prognostic outlook of this patient group.

The Departments of Therapeutic Radiology (Prof. A. ZUPPINGER), Chemotherapy (Docent K. BRUNNER) and Pathology (Prof. H. COTTIER) are gratefully acknowledged.

References

1. AMIEL, J. L., LACOUR, J., GERARDAAMARCHANT, R., GENIN, J., LE MERLE, M., PARAMENTIER, C., SCHLIENGER, M., POUILLART, P., NETTER, G., TUBIANA, M., MATHÉ, G.: 135 laparotomies and splenectomies for Hodgkin's disease. Bull. Cancer (Paris) **58**, 167 (1971).
2. BERKSON, J., GAGE, R. P.: Calculation of survival rates for cancer. Proc. Mayo Clin. **25**, 270 (1950).
3. CARBONE, P. P., KAPLAN, H. S., MUSSHOFF, K., SMITHERS, D. W., TUBIANA, M.: Report of the committee on Hodgkin's disease staging Classification. Cancer Res. **31**, 1860 (1971).
4. FUCHS, W. A., HAERTEL, M.: Prognosis of Hodgkin's disease according to the radiographic pattern of lymphnodes. In: Progress in lymphology II, pp. 279—281. Ed. Stuttgart: Thieme 1970.
5. FUCHS, W. A., HAERTEL, M. P.: Die Prognose des Morbus Hodgkin auf Grund der Lymphknotenstruktur im Lymphogramm. Fortschr. Röntgenstr. **109**, 553 (1968).
6. GLATSTEIN, E., GUERNSEY, J. M., ROSENBERG, S. A., KAPLAN, H. S.: The value of laparotomy and splenectomy in the staging of Hodgkin's disease. Cancer (Philad.) **24**, 709 (1969).
7. GLATSTEIN, E., TRUEBLOOD, H. W., ENRIGHT, L. P., ROSENBERG, S. A., KAPLAN, H. S.: Surgical staging of abdominal involvement in unselected patients with Hodgkin's disease. Radiology **97**, 425 (1970).
8. KADIN, M. E., GLATSTEIN, E., DORFMAN, R. F.: Clinicopathologic studies of 117 untreated patients subjected to laparotomy for the staging of Hodgkin's disease. Cancer (Philad.) **27**, 1277 (1971).
9. KAPLAN, H. S., ROSENBERG, S. A.: Extended-field radical radiotherapy in advanced Hodgkin's disease: Short-term results of 2 randomized clinical trials. Cancer Res. **26** Part 1, 1268 (1966).
10. LUKES, R. J., BUTLER, J. J.: The pathology and nomenclature of Hodgkin's disease. Cancer Res. **26** Part 1, 1063 (1966).
11. LUKES, R. J., CRAVER, L. F., HALL, T. C., RAPPAPORT, H., RUBIN, P.: Report of the nomenclature committee. Cancer Res. **26** Part 1, 1311 (1966).
12. PETERS, M. V.: The need for a new clinical classification in Hodgkin's disease: Keynote address. Cancer Res. **31**, 1713 (1971).
13. PROSNITZ, L. R., FISCHER, J. J., VERA, R., KLIGERMAN, M. M.: Hodgkin's disease treated with radiation therapy — follow-up data and the value of laparotomy. Amer. J. Roentgenol. **114**, 583 (1972).
14. ROSENBERG, S. A.: A critique of the value of laparotomy and splenectomy in the evaluation of patients with Hodgkin's disease. Cancer Res. **31**, 1737 (1971).
15. ROSENBERG, S. A., BOIRON, M., DE VITA, V. T., Jr., JOHNSON, R. E., LEE, B. J., ULTMANN, J. E., VIAMONTE, M., Jr.: Report of the committee on Hodgkin's disease staging procedures. Cancer Res. **31**, 1862 (1971).
16. SMITHERS, D.: Indications for investigation in Hodgkin's disease. Proc. roy. Soc. Med. **65**, 61 (1972).

Alterations in Pulmonary Diffusion Capacity after Lymphangiography

K. Kröpelin, L. Baumeister, D. Frey, and W. Wanner *

Summary

Lymphangiography produces marked abnormalities of lung function, especially of gas diffusion, due to oil embolism. For this reason, patients with lung diseases affecting gas diffusion should be excluded from this diagnostic procedure. On the other hand, patients with normal lung function, but insufficient oxygen supply for cardiac or cerebral reasons, should be selected very carefully before lymphography. Patients suffering from chronic cor pulmonale should not undergo lymphography because of the additional stress to the lung circulation.

In X-ray examinations utilizing contrast media, lymphangiography is accompanied by a relatively large number of side-effects. In 20 to 30% of patients so examined, transitory reactions such as fever, nausea and vomiting, lymphangitis, and urticaria occurred [6, 11, 17]. Serious complications with cardiopulmonary symptoms are rare, but can be fatal [2, 4, 5, 6, 9, 10, 11, 16, 18, 20, 22].

Embolism of contrast medium into the lung can often be proved by the radiologist [2, 3, 7, 11, 13, 14, 23], and abnormalities in lung function show that contrast medium probably passes into the lung in all patients [7, 9, 12].

We examined the effect of lymphangiography on pulmonary gas exchange in 9 patients. The carbon monoxide diffusing capacity in steady state [1] and the arterio-venous oxygen and carbon dioxide tension were measured before and after lymphangiography (apparatus from Eschweiler, Kiel).

The general and physical data on the patients are shown in Table 1. Patient 6 was suffering from pseudo lupus erythematosus (pseudoLE) affecting the pleura and lungs. No other patients exhibited lung disease. Patient 5 received a therapeutic injection of 8 ml of Lipiodol-^{131}I for malignant melanoma.

Only in Patient 6 was oil embolism indicated by contrast-medium deposits in the lung on the X-ray film. Analysis of vital capacity, functional residual capacity, and airway resistance revealed a 37% deficit in the vital capacity of Patient 6. These parameters were within the normal range in all the other patients.

Table 2 gives the carbon monoxide-diffusing capacity and the oxygen tension readings before lymphangiography and at 5 and 30 h after lymphangiography. Carbon dioxide tension not listed in Table 2 was unchanged from initial values. This

* Supported by grants of VW-Stiftung.

Table 1. General and physical data on patients

Patients	Age	Diagnosis	Amount of Lipiodol ml	Embolism in X-ray film of the chest	Clinical symptoms
1	29	LGR [a]	14	—	dyspnea
2	21	LGR	14	—	—
3	36	LGR	10	—	fever
4	60	LGR	14	—	fever
5	42	Malignant melanoma	8 [b]	—	—
6	45	Pseudo LE	14	+	—
7	22	LGR	7	—	—
8	44	Seminoma	14	—	—
9	51	Lympho-sarcomatosis	14	—	—

[a] = Lymphogranulomatosis.
[b] = Lipiodol-^{131}J.

may indicate normal ventilation. Significant abnormalities of carbon monoxide-diffusing capacity were found only in Patients 5 and 6. Fig. 1 shows the relatively severe decrease of diffusing capacity in these patients. Oxygen tension fell by more than 5 Torr at least once in every patient (Table 2; Fig. 2).

There was no uniform relationship between oxygen tension and carbon monoxide-diffusing capacity. From these results one may conclude that measurement of oxygen tension, which is less time consuming and cheaper, is a more sensitive method than measuring the carbon-monoxide diffusing capacity. Fabel *et al.* [7] found lowered oxygen tension in nearly all cases. These findings are confirmed by our measurements. However, the significant reduction of carbon monoxide-diffusing capacity, seen by

Table 2. Diffusing capacity of the lung for carbon monoxide and arterial oxygen tension before and after lymphangiography

Patient	$D_L CO_{SS}$ ml/min/mm Hg			PaO_2 mm Hg			ΔPaO_2 mm Hg	
	before	after 5 h	30 h	before	after 5 h	30 h	after 5 h	30 h
1	24.3		24.9	74.6	60.6	74.5	−14.0	− 0.1
2	20.8	19.3	20.2	92.2	93.6	84.5	+ 1.3	− 0.7
3	34.7		33.4	81.6	70.6	75.6	−11.0	− 6.0
4	20.3		21.2	74.0	71.3	64.2	− 2.7	− 9.8
5	21.9	12.7	14.1	84.2	75.8		− 8.4	
6	9.6	6.8	7.4	86.5	68.2	68.5	−18.3	−18.0
7	30.1	29.3	27.1					
8	25.2	22.7	22.7	80.5	70.5		−10.0	
9	17.2	16.6	15.9					
Average	22.7	17.9	20.8	81.9	72.9	73.5	− 9.0	− 8.3
n	9	6	9	7	7	5	7	5

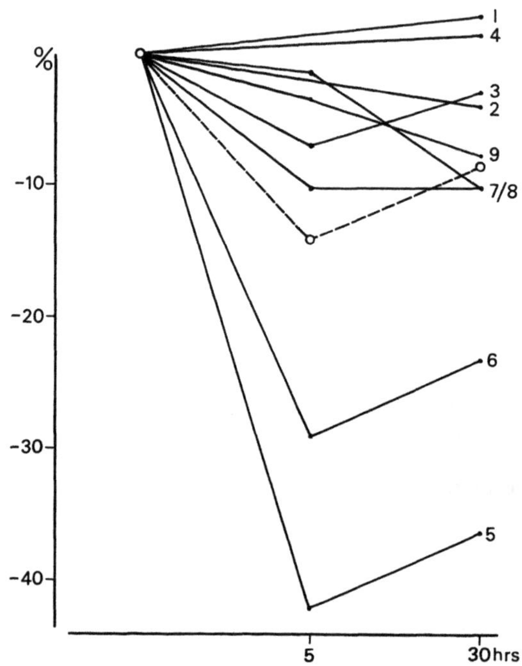

Fig. 1. Time course of changes in diffusing capacity in nine patients (dotted line = average)

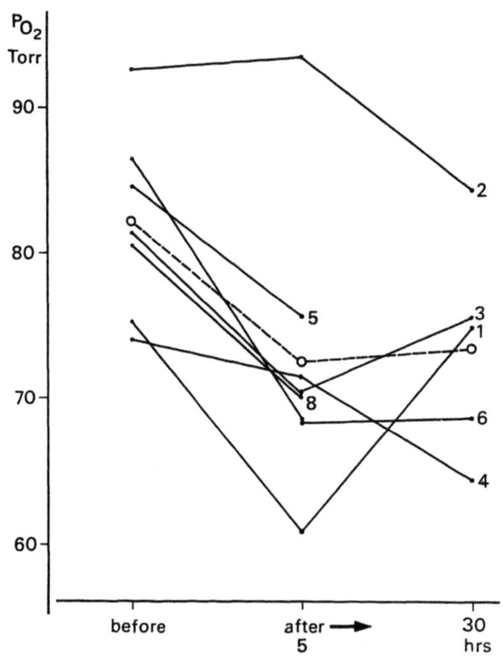

Fig. 2. Time course of changes in PaO_2 (dotted line = average)

FRAIMOW *et al.* [9] and GOLD *et al.* [12] in nearly all their patients, was found in only two of our patients.

The disturbances of oxygen uptake by the blood are caused by the oil emboli in the lung, as mentioned above [7, 8, 9, 12]. These disturbances are caused, at least in the first phase, not only by alveolar capillary block but predominantly by a diminution of vascular blood flow. In the later phase the disturbances are due to the swelling of the alveolar capillary membrane caused by migration of the contrast medium in the interstitial tissue. The pathogenesis of this process was determined by histological studies [2, 8, 12, 13, 15, 19]. The histological changes were reversible. In patients with coronary disease, however, these circulatory abnormalities can lead to sudden acute right ventricular failure [7, 9].

A correlation between the amount of injected contrast medium, size of total emboli and cardiopulmonary abnormalities was impressively shown by FABEL *et al.* [7].

In this context the analyses conducted after therapeutic lymphangiography need further discussion. Although we had injected no more than 8.0 ml of Lipiodol-^{131}I, we found a very marked decrease in diffusion capacity. This may lead to the conclusion that the radiation effect (a dose of 800 rad was calculated for the lungs) causes more damage to the pulmonary capillaries and of the interstitial tissues than the lymph-angiographic agent itself. As was shown in earlier experiments, chronic injury to lung tissue should not occur after application of radionuclides in lymphographic examinations of patients without lung disease [21]. However, there may be different results with higher dosages.

References

1. BATES, D. V., BOUCOT, N. G., DORMER, A. E.: The pulmonary diffusing capacity in normal subjects. J. Physiol. (Lond.) **129**, 237 (1955).
2. BRON, K. M., BAUM, S., ABRAMS, H. L.: Oil embolism in Lymphography. Radiology **80**, 194 (1963).
3. CLOSE, M. E., HALLGRIMSSON, J., WENDLAND, D. E.: Complications following lymphography with particular reference to pulmonary oil embolization. Amer. J. Roentgenol. **96**, 972 (1966).
4. DARGENT, M., CHASSARD, J. L., POMMATEAU, E., SAMIM, F.: Echecs et complications de la lymphographie au Lipiodol ultra-fluide. Lyon chir. **58**, 870 (1962).
5. DEPREZ-CURELY, J. P., BISMUTH, V., LAUGIER, A., DESCAMPS, J.: Accidents et incidents de la lymphographie. Ann. Radiol **5**, 577 (1962).
6. DOLAN, P. A.: Lymphography. Complications encountered in 522 examinations. Radiology **86**, 876 (1966).
7. FABEL, H., KUNITSCH, G., STENDER, H. ST.: Störungen der Lungenfunktion nach Lymphographie. Fortschr. Röntgenstr. **107**, 609 (1967).
8. FABEL, H., KUNITSCH, G., STENDER, H. ST.: Tierexperimentelle Untersuchungen zur Pathogenese der kardiopulmonalen Komplikationen nach Lymphographie. Z. ges. exp. Med. **147**, 143 (1968).
9. FRAIMOW, W. S., WALLACE, S., LEWIS, P., GREENING, R. R., CATHCART, R. T.: Changes in pulmonary function due to lymphangiography. Radiology **85**, 231 (1965).
10. FUCHS, W. A.: Complications in lymphography with contrastmedia. Acta radiol. (Stockh.) **57**, 427 (1962).
11. GERTEIS, W., GREUEL, H.: Kontrastmittelembolie der Lunge bei Lymphographie. Fortschr. Röntgenstr. **106**, 361 (1967).
12. GOLD, W. M., YOUKER, J., ANDERSON, S., NADEL, J. A.: Pulmonary function abnormalities after lymphangiography. New Engl. J. Med. **273**, 519 (1965).

13. Goldberg, M. E., Feinberg, S. B.: Pulmonary infarction following lymphography in dogs, its implications in human studies. Radiology **81**, 479 (1963).
14. Gough, J. H., Gough, M. M., Thomas, M. L.: Pulmonary complications following lymphography. Brit. J. Radiol. **37**, 416 (1964).
15. Guiney, E. J., Gough, M. H., Kinmonth, J. B.: Lymphography with fat-soluble contrast media. Studies of their effects in *Lepus* and *cuniculus*. J. cardiovasc. Surg. (Torino) **5**, 346 (1964).
16. Howett, M., Elmendorf, E. A.: Pelvic lymphangiography in normal and pathologic states. Obstet. and Gynec. **26**, 34 (1965).
17. Jackson, R. J. A.: Complications of lymphography. Brit. med. J. **1966 I**, 1203.
18. Jackson, L., Wallace, S., Schaffer, B., Gould, J., Kramer, S., Weiss, A.: The diagnostic value of lymphangiography. Ann. intern. Med. **54**, 870 (1961).
19. Kaufmann, E.: Experimentelle Lungenembolie mit jodhaltigem Kontrastmittel bei der Ratte. Z. ges. exp. Med. **152**, 201 (1970).
20. Koehler, P. R., Wohl, G. T., Schaffer, B.: Lymphangiography — a survey of its current status. Amer. J. Roentgenol. **91**, 1216 (1964).
21. Kröpelin, K., Doll, E.: Die Auswirkung einer therapeutischen Röntgenbestrahlung, einer heißen Lymphangiographie und einer Kombination beider auf die Lungenfunktion. Beitr. Klin. Tuberk. **141**, 177 (1969).
22. Lee, B. T., Nelson, J. H., Schwarz, G.: Evaluation of lymphangiography in clinical staging and management of Hodgkin's disease and lymphosarcoma. New Engl. J. Med. **271**, 327 (1964).
23. Schaffer, B., Koehler, P. R., Daniel, C. R., Wohl, G. T., Rivera, E., Meyers, W. A., Skelley, J. F.: A critical evaluation of lymphangiography. Radiology **80**, 917 (1963).

The Diagnostic Significance of Laparoscopy in Hodgkin's Disease

W. DISCHLER and G. KRIEGER

Summary

Laparoscopy was performed on patients with Hodgkin's disease. The value of this procedure in the diagnosis and staging of Hodgkin's disease by evaluation of the involvement of liver and spleen is documented. In 29 of 72 cases in stages I—III, staging had to be changed on the basis of laparoscopic findings. In 4 patients in whom Hodgkin's disease was unknown or uncertain, it was diagnosed with the aid of visually controlled hepatic biopsy. The figures show different pictures of liver and spleen involvement. Laparoscopy is also very useful in the evaluation of therapy.

Material

In this paper the data of 105 patients are referred to. The stage of Hodgkin's disease in the tables is not the primary stage of these patients but the secondary staging before or after laparoscopy. Only for the lesser part of this material were laparoscopies done for primary staging procedure, but for most of the cases it was done in the further onset of the disease, sometimes many years after primary diagnosis and therapy. That means that the results are not representative for the primary extension of the disease.

Results

The significance of clinical staging for the assessment of prognosis and therapy in Hodgkin's disease has been stressed by other authors. In this context we wish to emphasize the importance of hepatic involvement, which can be diagnosed by laparoscopy. We have done laparoscopies in about 150 patients with Hodgkin's disease, and the first 105 cases have been statistically analyzed.

Table 1 shows that in 21 out of 72 cases in stages 0—III [10] hepatic involvement was found and the stage at the time of investigation therefore had to be changed. Out of 5 cases in which diagnosis was uncertain, 4 were diagnosed as Hodgkin's disease by means of hepatic biopsy. Out of 33 cases in stage IV with known involvement of other organs, 16 had additional foci in the liver.

As Table 2 shows, not all cases in which foci were macroscopically visible exhibited typical granulomatous lesions on microscopical examination of forceps biopsies taken during laparoscopy. This problem is discussed below. Where there was no macroscopic evidence of Hodgkin's disease, the histological findings of biopsies done with the Silverman needle were always negative.

Table 3 summarizes the findings in 70 cases classified according to the criteria of [6] on the basis of the histology of the lymph nodes [4]. It is clear that the liver is less frequently involved in the lymphocytic predominance form. There is, however, no obvious relationship between histological type and type or intensity of hepatic involvement, except that in the mixed cellularity type the liver is more frequently involved than other organs.

Table 1. Detection of liver involvement by laparoscopy (Primary and secondary laparoscopy)

	Unknown Hodgkin's disease	Clinical stage previous to laparoscopy				Total
		I	II	III	IV	
Laparoscopies	5	3	11	53	33	105
Liver involvement confirmed by laparoscopy	4	1	4	12	16	37

Table 2. Accuracy of laparoscopic findings and biopsy

Laparoscopic findings	Ratio laparoscopy/biopsy	
	Liver	Spleen
Positive	37/26	25/18
Negative	68/68	63/56
Total	105	88 (17 without biopsy)

Table 3. Liver involvement in 70 patients classified according to the histological type of the lymph nodes

Histologic types	Clinical stage IV at the time of investigation				
			Involvement		Ratio
	Number	%	Liver %	Other organs only %	Liver/other organs
Lymphocytic predominance	9	33	33	66	1 : 2
Nodular sclerosis	30	50	74	26	3 : 1
Mixed cellularity	17	41	86	14	6 : 1
Lymphocytic depletion	14	72	60	40	1,5 : 1

Laparoscopic Pictures

We shall now present different laparoscopic pictures of liver and spleen involvement in Hodgkin's disease [2].

In Hodgkin's disease, as [7, 8] reported, there is nearly always a mesenchymal reaction in the liver with a general activation of the RES, a diffuse multiplication of Kupffer stellate cells and of lymphocytic and histiocytic cells, as well as the formation of loose aggregates of cells. This histological picture is that of an unspecific reactive hepatitis according to [11]. The macroscopic picture clearly shows the lobulated structure of the liver, with increased formation of lymphatic fluid and dilatation of lymphatic vessels in the liver capsule. This capsule of Glisson can show fibrous thickening along the lymphatic vessels. The blood capillaries of the liver capsule can also be enlarged and there may be an increase in their number (Figs. 1 and 2).

Another particular finding is peliosis of the liver, that is, dilatation of the sinusoids with stasis and extravasation of blood in the parenchyma. This results in the formation of blood pools, which present a bluish appearance at laparoscopy (Fig. 2). Peliosis has been found in Hodgkin's disease and in haemoblastosis.

In some cases we observed conspicuous scars in the liver, even in untreated cases. When these scars were compared with the appearance of the liver after therapy (Fig. 7), it was concluded that they must be the remains of spontaneously healed Hodgkin's granulomas in the liver. In some cases we found nothing except organized fibrous tissue in such lesions, which would support this hypothesis.

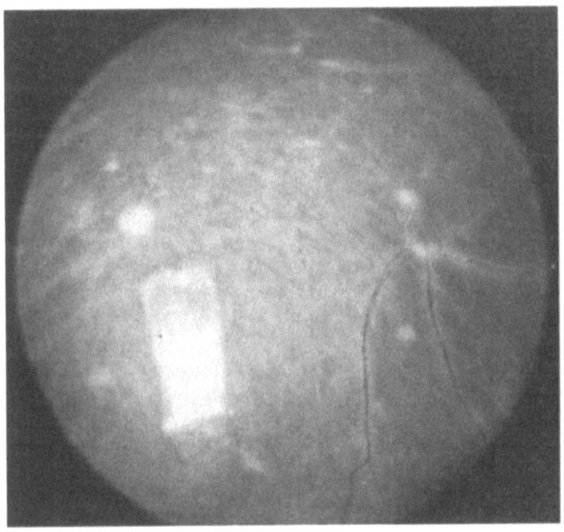

Fig. 1

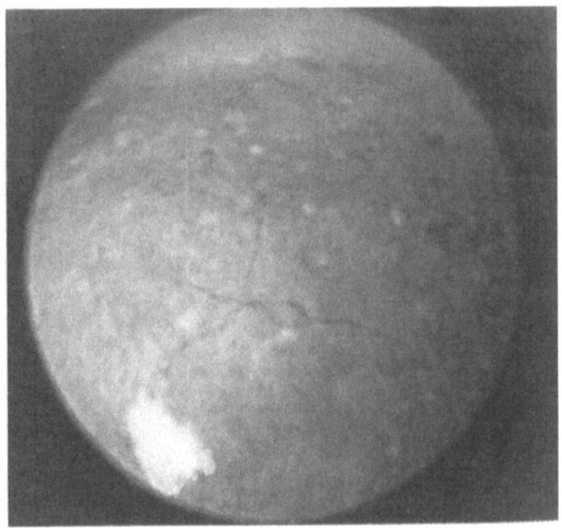

Fig. 2

Fig. 1. Capsular reaction and solitary Hodgkin's infiltrates: In this close-up view of the capsular surface of the liver dilatation of blood vessels and lymph vessels, typical of the mesenchymal reaction, can be demonstrated. Fibrinous changes of the capsule always occur along the lymphatic channels. These changes persist even if the disease is no longer active. — Several circular white Hodgkin's infiltrations of 1—2 mm in diameter can be seen. The light rectangular shape on the left is a reflection of the photographic flash

Fig. 2. Miliary type of Hodgkin's infiltrates and peliosis: White miliary infiltrates are disseminated. Dilatation of blood and lymph vessels. In the right upper part of the picture some dark irregular dots are visible

The significance of laparoscopy for the positive proof of Hodgkin's disease in the liver is also demonstrated in Fig. 1. Some small yellowish foci on the lateral edge of the right lobe of the liver removed by biopsy forceps were found on microscopic examination to be foci of Hodgkin's granuloma.

Sometimes little foci with indistinct outlines are recognizable laparoscopically; this foci can be caused by Hodgkin's infiltrates as well as by an unspecific mesenchymal reaction. The decision is made on the histological examination of the excised biopsy materials.

The different types of hepatic involvement in Hodgkin's disease are:

I. Miliary Type. Disseminated miliary foci are fairly often found, and may differ in size (Figs. 1 and 2). Macroscopically this looks like a miliary type of sarcoidosis or miliary tuberculosis of the liver. Biopsy and histological examination are therefore necessary in all cases.

II. Aggregated Type. In the most common type of Hodgkin's disease of the liver, white or yellow foci are aggregated in groups of different sizes, which are more or less prominent on the surface of the liver (Fig. 3). This picture is typical of Hodgkin's disease, but as it is sometimes imitated by tuberculosis or echinococcus alveolaris, biopsy is required.

III. Nodular Type. The type with huge nodules of various sizes is less frequent. Nodules may sometimes protrude from the surface of the liver capsule (Fig. 6) and can resemble a nodular sarcoidosis of the liver. Single large nodes may look like

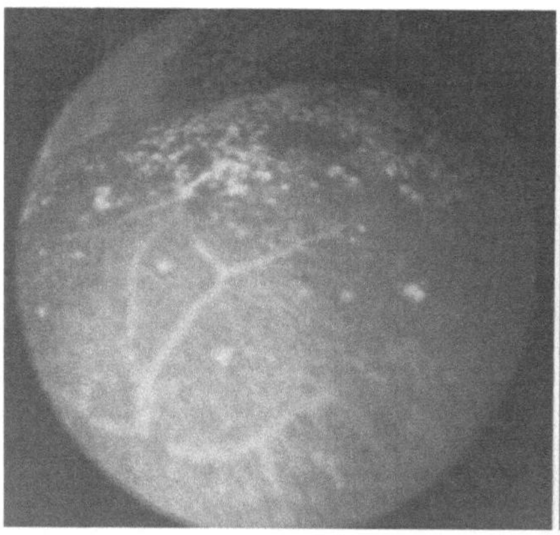

Fig. 3

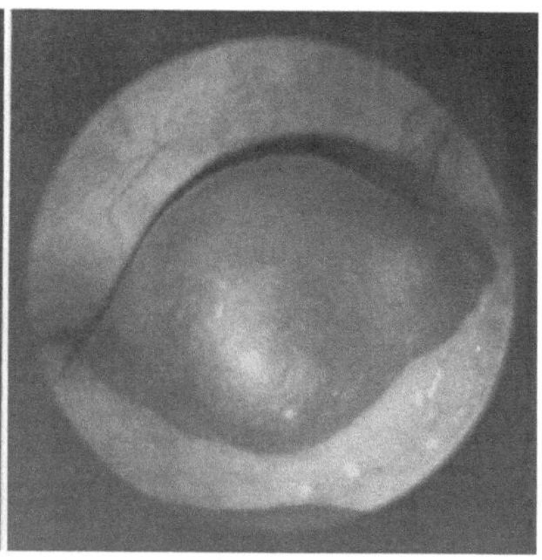

Fig. 4

Fig. 3. Aggregates of Hodgkin's infiltrates: This picture, looking towards the right hemidiaphragm, shows the larger part of the left liver lobe. In the foreground we see some round Hodgkin's foci between dilated lymph channels which present as white ramifications. In the background one sees a group of Hodgkin's foci of various sizes, more or less densely grouped together. These changes on the diaphragmatic surface of the liver could not be seen at laparotomy

Fig. 4. Enlarged spleen with Hodgkin's nodes: One looks towards the left hemidiaphragm. The spleen, which is enlarged and thickened, shows nodular and spherical protuberances. One of these reflects the photographic flash. — In a biopsy taken with the Menghini needle Hodgkin's infiltrates could be found

Table 4. Size of the spleen in "false negative" cases. Laparoscopy: No foci or nodes recognizable. Biopsy: Histologic involvement of the spleen

Enlargement of the spleen	Untreated patients	Radiation of the spleen and/or chemotherapy
Slight	0	1
Moderate	1	7
Considerable	0	0
Total	9	

metastases of a carcinoma and may even show the characteristic central indentation of carcinomatous nodules.

IV. Diffuse Type. Diffuse infiltrations of the liver by Hodgkin's disease, in our opinion, represent an especially fast progressing form. The picture resembles generalized metastases.

With manifestations of Hodgkin's disease in the spleen, as in the liver, we find in most cases an unspecific capsular reaction with small white dots or streaks of connective tissue. Enlargement of the spleen is shown by a crenellated edge. Splenic enlargement is present when the lower pole descends below the phrenico-colic ligament (Fig. 4).

Biopsy of the spleen with the Menghini needle involves no risk, as bleeding from the biopsy site can be controlled. This means that biopsy is possible, even with platelet counts as low as 40,000 per mm^3.

In some cases we found, to our surprise, typical Hodgkin granulomas in the needle biopsy although the surface of the spleen was normal (see Table 2). Table 4 shows, in addition, that in 9 cases with histologically confirmed involvement in which the splenic surface showed no evidence of Hodgkin's disease, the spleen was moderately enlarged.

As we pointed out above, splenic size can be estimated satisfactorily at laparoscopy (Fig. 4). When we correlate splenic size and the finding of typical Hodgkin

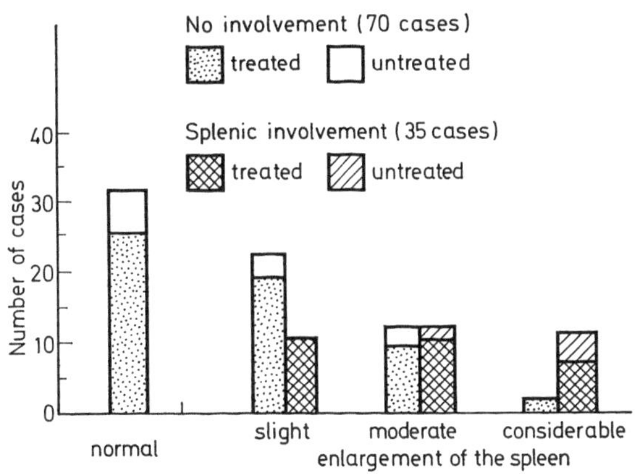

Fig. 5. Laparoscopic evaluation of the size of the spleen

granulomas on needle biopsy we find that with increasing size of spleen there is increased incidence of granulomas (Fig. 5). [3] obtained similar results when they examined spleens which had been removed surgically.

Typical Hodgkin nodules are also found in the spleen; in most cases they protrude above the level of the splenic capsule (Fig. 4). As in the liver, we sometimes find old scars beside fresh nodules in the spleen. As long as the platelet count ist not below 50,000 per mm³, forceps biopsy under direct vision is not dangerous.

Additional Findings

In addition to the assessment of hepatic and splenic manifestations, laparoscopy in Hodgkin's disease provides other important information. For instance, congested lymph vessels in the intestinal serosa or chylous ascites indicate severe disturbance of lymphatic drainage due to the involvement of mesenteric lymph nodes. Rarely, para-aortic lymph nodes become sufficiently enlarged to push the left lobe of the liver forward. In 2 cases Hodgkin infiltrations were found in the falciform ligament and diaphragm respectively, thus indicating peritoneal involvement.

Laparoscopy not only possesses great diagnostic significance but is also important in assessing the effects of therapy. In one case steroid therapy had caused severe fatty cirrhosis of the liver. A control laparoscopy carried out later showed the fatty induration to have been fully reversible, although the increased fibrous tissue remained.

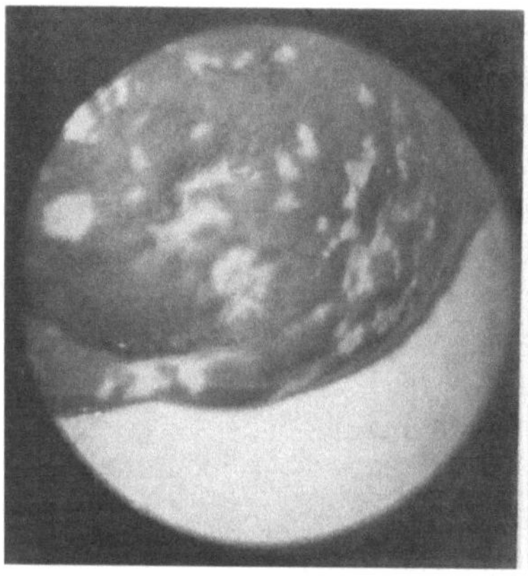

Fig. 6

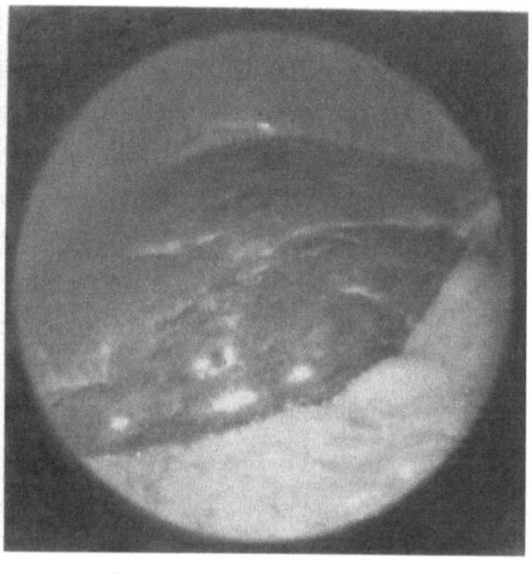

Fig. 7

Fig. 6. Nodular Hodgkin's infiltrates (before treatment): This picture shows a large part of the left lobe of the liver which covers part of the stomach (bottom in the picture). There are irregular white Hodgkin's infiltrates which are reminiscent of carcinoma metastases. Near the hepatic edge a linear scar can be seen

Fig. 7. Control laparoscopy after 2 years of combined chemotherapy: (Same patient as in Fig. 6.) The left lobe of the liver is visible up to the diaphragm. All Hodgkin infiltrates have disappeared and funnel-shaped and linear scars can be seen. The light spots at the edge of the liver are reflexions of the photographic flash

We regret that reproduction of the original color photographs was not possible as the black-and-white copies are much less informative

Occasionally part of the liver falls within an irradiated area; this results in destruction of the parenchyma or radiation fibrosis of the hepatic capsule. Because of the fibrous thickening of Glisson's capsule, the liver appears grey. It is gratifying when laparoscopy shows that therapy has been successful. In one case, infiltrations disappeared completely after 2 years of intermittent chemotherapy (Figs. 6 and 7). Deep scars remained, a feature we sometimes found in untreated cases, as mentioned above.

Indications for Laparoscopy

Are there systemic symptoms that indicate splenic or hepatic involvement so that the indication for laparoscopy could be limited to these cases? As Table 5 shows, this is unfortunately not the case. Therefore, laparoscopy must be done in all cases of Hodgkin's disease, sometimes several times.

A comparison of our figures with those of GLATSTEIN *et al.* [3] shows that these authors cite a lower incidence of hepatic involvement. This is not astonishing because these authors' figures are the results of primary staging procedures. This can give misleading results, as is shown by one of our cases. The patient had undergone splenec-

Table 5. Frequency of liver and spleen involvement in Hodgkin's disease

	Systemic symptoms		Total
	No	Yes	
Liver only involved	6	11	17
Spleen only involved	6	9	15
Liver and spleen both involved	9	11	20
Neither involved	36	17	53
	57	48	105

Table 6. The value of laparoscopy for the detection of liver involvement in different systemic diseases

	Total	Laparoscopy negative for liver involvement	Confirmed by histology n (%)	Histology discordant n (%)
Hodgkin's disease	105	68	68 (100)	0 (0)
Reticulosis	29	20	6 (30)	14 (70)
Chronic lymphatic leukemia	4	2	0 (0)	2 (100)
Lymphosarcoma	5	5	5 (100)	0 (0)
Chronic myelocytic leukemia	5	4	1 (25)	3 (75)
Multiple myeloma	4	4	2 (50)	2 (50)
Sarcoidosis	33	27	3 (11)	24 (89)

tomy 3 weeks prior to laparoscopy and the surgeon had considered the liver to be entirely normal. This is because the state of the liver was assessed during splenectomy, looking from the left side of the abdomen. At laparoscopy, however, we found extensive Hodgkin infiltrations in the subdiaphragmatic area (as in Fig. 3); these were invisible to the surgeon from the left side of the abdomen.

Table 6 shows that the assessment of hepatic involvement in Hodgkin's disease, as compared with other systemic diseases, is very accurate. This may be due to the fact that the Hodgkin infiltrates are connected to the lymphatic channels and are therefore most extensive in the liver capsule. The liver capsule is very rich in lymphatic vessels which drain along the falciform ligament. In the spleen, on the other hand, the lymphatic vessels are subcapsular. Therefore only larger nodes can be seen at laparoscopy.

Conclusions

Laparoscopy should be carried out in all patients with Hodgkin's disease [2]. This procedure involves less stress for the patient than a lymphography, which is nevertheless necessary. Depending on the actual stage of the disease, laparoscopy shows hepatic involvement in up to 50% of cases and infiltrates in the spleen in up to 35% of cases.

Patients in whom hepatic or splenic involvement cannot be proved by forceps or needle biopsy [1] but who have negative bone marrow findings should be considered for a more radical diagnostic approach, i. e. splenectomy, if warranted by the circumstances [5, 9].

References

1. Bagley, Ch. M., Jr., Roth, J. A., Thomas, L. B., Devita, V. T., Jr.: Liver biopsy in Hodgkin's disease. Ann. intern. Med. **76**, 219 (1972).
2. Beck, K., Dischler, W., Helms, M., Kiani, B., Sickinger, K., Tenner, R.: Color atlas of laparoscopy. Arranged H. J. Schaefer. Stuttgart-New York: F. K. Schattauer 1970.
3. Glatstein, E., Guernsey, J. M., Rosenberg, S. A., Kaplan, H. S.: The value of laparotomy and splenectomy in the staging of Hodgkin's disease. Cancer (Philad.) **24**, 709 (1969).
4. Hamann, W., Oehlert, W., Musshoff, K., Nuss, A., Schnellbacher, B.: Histologische Einteilung dés Lymphoma malignum Hodgkin und seine Bedeutung für die Prognose. Dtsch. med. Wschr. **95**, 112 (1970).
5. Hanks, G. E., Terry, L. N., Bryan, J. A., Newsome, J. F.: Contribution of diagnostic laparotomy to staging non-Hodgkin's lymphoma. Cancer (Philad.) **29**, 41 (1972).
6. Lukes, R. J., Craver, L. F., Hall, Th. C., Rapaport, H., Ruben, P.: Report of the nomenclature comittee. Cancer Res. **26**, 1311 (1966).
7. Oehlert, W., Dischler, W.: Unspezifische Mesenchymreaktion und Parenchymschäden der Leber bei Patienten mit Morbus Hodgkin. Dtsch. med. Wschr. **97**, 323 (1972).
8. Oehlert, W., Musshoff, K., Wunsch, B., Willmann, H., Beck, K.: Unspezifische Mesenchymreaktion der Leber bei Patienten mit Morbus Hodgkin. Klin. Wschr. **48**, 126 (1970).
9. Prosnitz, L. R., Nuland, S. B., Kligerman, M. M.: Role of laparotomy and splenectomy in the management of Hodgkin's disease. Cancer (Philad.) **29**, 44 (1972).
10. Schmidt, C. G.: Diagnostik und Stadieneinteilung der Lymphogranulomatose (M. Hodgkin). Dtsch. med. Wschr. **98**, 836 (1973).
11. Thaler, H.: Leberbiopsie — Ein klinischer Atlas der Histopathologie. Berlin-Heidelberg-New York: Springer 1969.

Splenectomy

Indications, Techniques, Complications, Intraoperative Diagnostic Methods

I. STAIB, D. KAISER, and K. MUSSHOFF

Summary

After considering the risk of splenectomy in general, we report on our technique of this procedure, marking the place of removed lymph nodes and liver biopsy.

The low overall incidence of complications is demonstrated and analysed in the 61 cases under discussion.

Values are given on thrombocytosis, hospital stay, and drainage of the splenic bed. The diagnostic value of the whole procedure is discussed.

1. Introduction

1.1. Splenectomy in patients with proven Hodgkin's disease (HD) has so far met with reservations or criticism in the German medical press [1]. On the basis of KAPLAN's reports [2] and the results of a retrospective study [3], one of us (K. M.) instituted a controlled trial of splenectomy on HD patients in his care. We took this opportunity to monitor the diagnostic success of the radiologist by surgical means in the hope of increasing therapeutic success (the later is discussed below by Dr. PAULI-BEISEL).

1.2. Before any operation, indications and risks must be carefully assessed. Previous indications for splenectomy were traumatic rupture of the spleen, hematological disorders, malignant disease of adjacent organs or of the spleen itself, portal hypertension in which bleeding causes an emergency situation, or splenorenal anastomosis [4, 5]. Hodgkin's disease constitutes a third large group of indications; out of a total of 162 splenectomies performed in the period between January 1969 and the end of June 1972, 69 were for HD, 43 for trauma, and the rest miscellaneous.

1.3. The factors to be considered in assessing the risk of the operation are:

a) Severity of the disease. We have staged our patients on the basis of the Freiburg modification of the Freiburg Classification, or the Ann Arbor Classification. Only patients in stages I—IV p.c. of the Rye Classification, or in stages I—III of the Ann Arbor Classification were operated upon [6, 7].

b) Age of the patients. The ages of our patients ranged from 11 to 59 years.

c) Concomitant disease, particularly that affecting lungs, liver, or kidney.

d) Obesity.

e) Severity of the operation. According to MOORE's Classification [8] splenectomy is an operation of medium severity. As late as 1970, HODAN reported an operative mortality of 12%. However, in his series, various diseases provided the indication for splenectomy [9].

f) In HD, splenectomy is not absolutely indicated, and optimal postoperative care must be guaranted.

Of particular importance are reliable blood clotting estimates (Dr. BÖTTCHER reports on this in detail [10]).

2. Technique

2.1. We use an incision along the left costal margin to luxate the whole spleen from behind to the anterior abdominal wall. This approach has the advantage that the splenic hilus can easily be inspected and dissected. Stomach and liver can be inspected as well as small intestine, transverse colon, mesenteries and greater omentum. The patient experiences little postoperative respiratory distress such as is seen after a

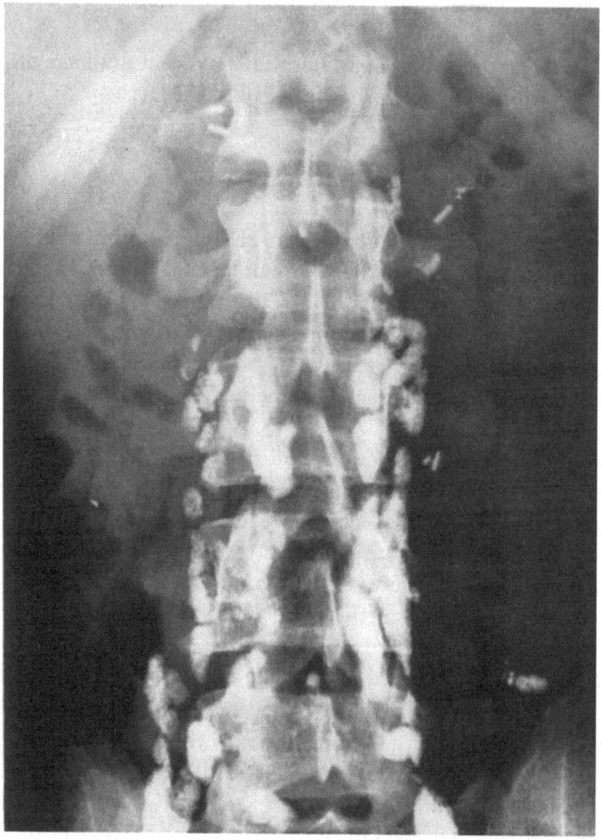

Fig. 1. Postoperative X-ray with silver clips inserted at operation. 4 clips — liver hilus, 3 clips — lesser omentum, 2 clips — para-aortal lymph nodes, 1 clip — splenic hilus

median upper abdominal incision. The disadvantage of this approach is that the retroperitoneal space, particularly below the aortic bifurcation, is difficult to reach. The incision is closed with an intracutaneous suture so that only a fine line remains. We consider this aspect to be of some importance, especially in female patients. After removal, the spleen is weighed to allow an objective assessment of its size.

2.2. As in laparotomy, we systematically examine the abdomen to obtain diagnostic information about the spread of the disease. The hili of spleen and liver, the lesser curvature of the stomach, head and body of the pancreas, mesentery, greater omentum and aortic bifurcation are inspected. We remove as many lymph nodes as possible even if they do not appear to be enlarged and mark the sites of removal with silver clips (Fig. 1). We use a protocol to record the numbers so that after histological examination we can apply radiotherapy in a differentiated manner. The protocol also allows a comparison with the preoperative findings.

2.3. Next, a liver biopsy is taken. Three different techniques were used:

a) A biopsy from the liver margin. This did not prove a good site for histological examination, as only fibrosis was found in most cases.

b) Biopsy with the Vlim-Silbermann needle. This method did not provide sufficient material for adequate histological investigation.

c) We now use the Menghini needle, which removes a tissue core 4 cm in length. However, this usually necessitates hemostasis by stitch-ligature of vessels supplying the local liver parenchyma.

2.4. The operation allows us to discuss whether radiotherapy produces adhesions. Adhesions were found in 33 cases; 20 of these patients had received no infradiaphragmatic radiotherapy and 13 had been irradiated. In 28 laparotomies, no adhesions were found; of these patients, 6 had received radiotherapy. On the basis of these findings, no major effect of radiotherapy can be demonstrated.

3. Intra- and Postoperative Complications

Among the unselected results of 61 cases in our series, there were 9 complications, only one of which was really dangerous.

3.1. There were no per- or postoperative hemorrhages (this being the most dangerous potential acute complication). None of our patients needed blood transfusion. Hemodynamic changes after splenectomy are expected only in cases of extreme splenomegaly with splenic perfusion of more than 1000 ml. None of our patients had a spleen of this size.

3.2. Wound healing problems may occur because of the increased susceptibility to infection frequently postulated for HD patients. Two patients had healing by second intention. In 2 further cases, accumulations of non-infected serous fluid had to be drained. In one case, the drain had to be extracted under an anesthetic. There was no overall increase in incidence of wound infection.

3.3. Two patients had pulmonary complications. In one case we found atelectasis of the right lower lobe, which disappeared after bronchoscopic aspiration; the other had a pleural effusion in the left lower lung field, resection of the right upper lobe having been done 2 years before. The effusion was tapped and removed. This patient (stage IV p.c.) also had one of the 2 wound infections. Postoperatively his platelet count went up to 1.2 million. Heparin treatment was started, but the patient suffered a thrombosis of the brachial artery which had to be treated by embolectomy.

3.4. The low overall incidence of complications is reflected in the short hospital stay (average 10 days). Most patients were discharged on day 7 to 12 after operation. The shortest stay (4 days) was due to transfer to another department after satisfactory surgical progress. The longest stay (23 days) was necessary in the case of the patient with multiple complications mentioned above. The number of complications is too small to allow correlation with the stage of the disease.

3.5. Particularly dangerous post-splenectomy complications, such as atonia of the bowel or splenic fever, did not occur in this series. There were 3 cases of cystitis, and in one patient, a small intestinal obstruction occurred in the 8th postoperative day. We reopened the abdomen, and the further postoperative course was uneventful.

3.6. Drainage of the splenic bed was not carried out in 8 patients in whom we found the surroundings of the spleen to be absolutely free of excess fluid. When the operating surgeon considers a drain necessary, it serves to monitor the bleeding and is, as a rule, removed after 3 to 4 days (in our series the time varied from 1 to 10 days). Most authors do not recommend drainage of the splenic bed [11, 12]. However, introduction of infection through the drain is not observed unless it is kept in the wound for more than 7 days.

4. The Diagnostic Value of Splenectomy

4.1. In order to assess the diagnostic value of splenectomy, it is necessary to correlate macroscopic and microscopic findings. Of spleens with suspected involvement, 45% showed histological evidence of HD. Of spleens which had been described as unaffected on macroscopic examination, 20% were histological positive.

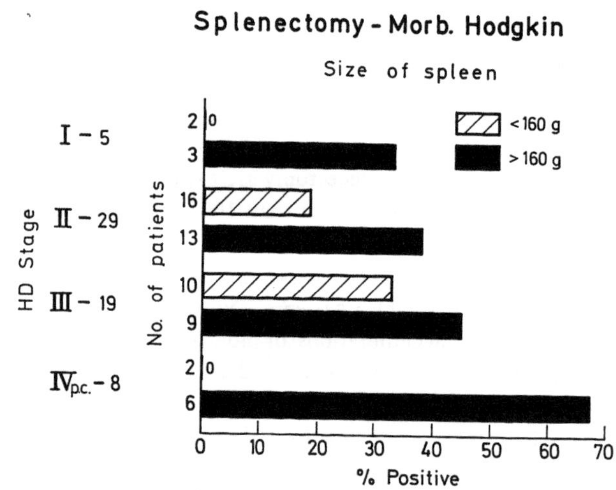

Fig. 2. Relation of positive histological findings to spleen size at the different stages of Hodgkin's disease

A special serial technique was used for histological examination (described by OEHLERT [13]). In 30 HD cases, lymph-node involvement was suspected; in 21% this was histologically confirmed. Few liver biopsies have been satisfactory from the technical point of view (for technique see § 2.3.c).

4.2. We tried to correlate the stage of the disease with splenic size and histological diagnosis (Fig. 2). Spleens weighing more than 160 g were defined as enlarged and showed a markedly higher incidence of lymphogranulomatosis than spleens of "normal" size. However, the latter were by no means free of lymphogranulomatous infiltrates.

4.3. Dr. PAULI-BEISEL discusses changes made in preoperative staging on the basis of operative findings [14].

Conclusions

The value of splenectomy for the diagnosis of Hodgkin's disease, in particular for staging and infradiaphragmatic spread, cannot be doubted. We can fully support the recommendations of American authors to perform splenectomy in Hodgkin's disease. Operative risk can be kept low by a critical selection of patients, impeccable operative technique, and cooperation with a hematologist in postoperative care. Our observations allow no assessment of the therapeutic value of splenectomy.

References

1. KABOTH, W., BEGEMANN, H.: Neuere Aspekte zur Prognose der Lymphogranulomatose. Lebensversicher.-Med. **24**, 73 (1972).

2 a. SALZMAN, J. R., KAPLAN, H. S.: Effect of prior splenectomy on hematologic tolerance during total lymphoid radiotherapy of patients with Hodgkin's disease. Cancer. (Philad.) **27**, 471 (1971).

2 b. WAGENKNECHT, L., ALBERTO, P., MAURICE, P. A.: The place of laparotomy-splenectomy in the therapeutic management of Hodgkin's disease. Schweiz. med. Wschr. **100**, 1999 (1970).

3. MUSSHOFF, K.: Grundlagen der Strahlentherapie des Morbus Hodgkin, Indikation und Ergebnisse. (11. Wissenschaftl. Tagung der deutschen Krebsgesellschaft.) Z. Krebsforsch. **78**, 162 (1972).

4. MAPPES, G., FISCHER, J.: Erfahrung mit der Splenektomie bei Blutkrankheiten. Dtsch. med. Wschr. **94**, 584 (1969).

5. WEINREICH, J.: Die Indikation zur Milzexstirpation bei haematol. Erkrankungen. Dtsch. med. Wschr. **95**, 348 (1970).

6. CARBONE, P. P., KAPLAN, H. S., MUSSHOFF, K., SMITHERS, D. W., TUBIANA, M.: Report of the Hodgkin's disease staging classification committee. Conference on staging in Hodgkin's disease. Ann Arbor, April 26—28, 1971. Cancer Res. **31**, 1860 (1971).

7. MUSSHOFF, K.: Therapy and prognosis of two different forms of organ involvement in cases of malignant lymphoma. (Hodgkin's disease, Reticulum cell sarcoma, Lymphosarcoma) as well as a report about stage division in these diseases. XIIth International Congress of Radiology, Tokyo Oct. 1969. Klin. Wschr. **48**, 673 (1970).

8. MOORE, F. D.: Metabolic care of the surgical Patient. Philadelphia and London: Saunders Company 1959.

9. HODAN, R. P.: The risk of splenectomy a review of 310 cases. Amer. J. Surg. **119**, 709 (1970).

10. BÖTTCHER, D., BLÜMEL, I., STAIB, I.: Changes in blood clotting after splenectomy. In: K. MUSSHOFF (Ed.). Diagnosis and therapy of malignant lymphomas. Recent Results in Cancer Research Vol. 46. Berlin-Heidelberg: Springer 1974 in press.
11. SLATE, R. W., GETZEN, L. G., LANING, R. C.: One hundred cases of traumatic rupture of the spleen. Arch. Surg. 99, 498 (1969).
12. OLSON, W. R., BEAUDOIN, D. E.: Wunddrainage nach Splenektomie. Amer. J. Surg. 117, 615 (1969).
13. OEHLERT, W.: personal communication.
14. PAULI-BEISEL, CH., MUSSHOFF, K., OEHLERT, W.: Preliminary results of laparotomy with splenectomy in patients previously treated for Hodgkin's disease. In: K. MUSSHOFF (Ed.). Diagnosis and Therapy of Malignant Lymphomas. Recent Results in Cancer Research, Vol. 46, p. 123—127. Berlin-Heidelberg: Springer 1974.

Changes in Blood Coagulation after Splenectomy

D. Böttcher, J. Blümel, and I. Staib

Summary

The changes in blood clotting characteristics after splenectomy affect mainly the platelet system. The changes are quantitative as well as qualitative. The changes in plasmatic coagulation on the other side are comparable to those after surgical operations of similar severity. It is remarkable that a marked rise in Factor VIII activity, which lasts several days, occurs after splenectomy. This makes a major influence of the spleen on Factor VIII synthesis appear very unlikely.

Postoperative thromboembolic episodes are among the rarer but particularly dangerous complications of splenectomy. In a series of 70 patients, the majority of whom had diagnostic laparotomy with splenectomy for Hodgkin's disease, severe thromboembolic complications occurred in 2 patients. One patient had repeated embolic incidents, including pulmonary embolism and peripheral vascular occlusion.

These complications are ascribed to the special relationship between spleen and blood platelets. We know from experiments with labeled platelets that the spleen influences platelet turnover by two different mechanisms operating at different stages. One mechanism is the initially reversible storage of functioning platelets, the other is destruction. The normal splenic pool of platelets is estimated to be about 40% of the total platelet mass. Free interchange can occur with circulating platelets. The platelets are destroyed, mainly in the spleen, after a life span of 8 to 11 days [2, 4, 9].

After splenectomy, the platelet count rises by 2 to 6 times the initial value, reaching a maximum around the 10th postoperative day (Fig. 1). Within 3 months of splenectomy the platelet count returns to the initial value. This is a much larger increase in platelets than the usual rise of 30—50% after surgical procedures.

It cannot be explained solely by removal of the splenic pool. A change in the life span of the platelets after removal of the major site of their destruction is also unlikely to be the causative factor, for the life span is usually found to be normal [7]. The cause of this post-splenectomy thrombocytosis is perhaps an increased rate of platelet production. Animal experiments indicate that this could occur in the absence of a humoral regulator substance normally produced in the spleen. Reimplantation of the spleen, even in a semipermeable chamber, was shown to prevent post-splenectomy thrombocytosis [14]. The absolute rise in platelet numbers, however, cannot be regarded as the sole reason for thromboembolic complications. Changes of platelet function must be discussed as additional factor. Hirsch *et al.* [6] observed an increase in platelet stickiness. We observed an increase in platelet aggregation and adhesiveness

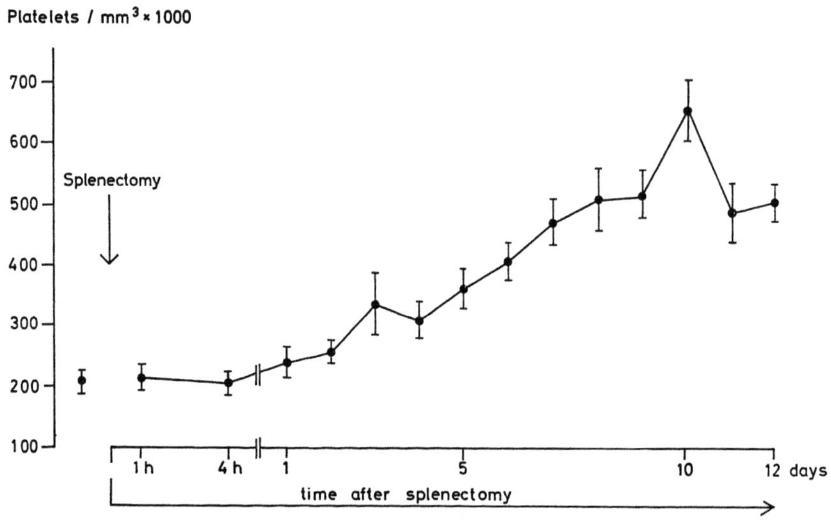

Fig. 1. Changes in platelet count after splenectomy (mean values and standard deviations for 30 patients)

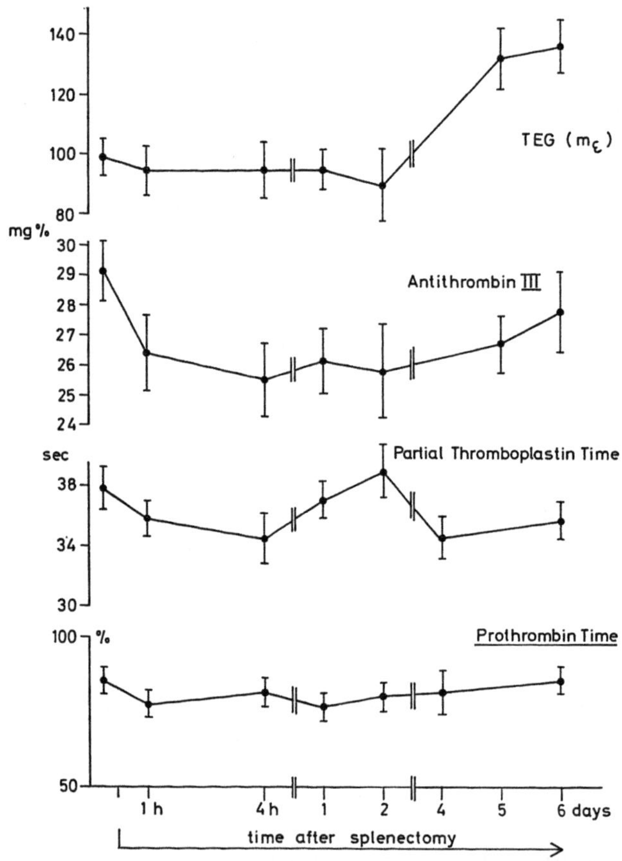

Fig. 2. Coagulation studies of 30 patients after splenectomy for Hodgkin's disease (mean values and mean standard deviations)

in a patient who had a pulmonary embolism after splenectomy. Treatment with acetyl-salicylic acid prevented further embolism, in spite of a further rise in platelet count to more than a million. When the drug was stopped because of gastric disturbance, a second embolic accident occurred.

The changes in plasmatic coagulation, on the other hand, are very similar to those occurring postoperatively after comparable surgical procedures. As Fig. 2 shows, in 30 patients there was a transitory fall in fibrinogen and an increase in prothrombin time, neither statistically significant, immediately after operation. A moderate fall in partial thromboplastin time and a significant fall in antithrombin III occurred in the first 5 days after operation. At about the 5th postoperative day the thrombelastogram showed a significant increase of the maximum amplitude which was correlated with the rise in platelets.

Factor VIII activity after splenectomy gave interesting results. We observed a significant rise from preoperative values during the first 6 postoperative days. One-stage and two-stage Factor VIII assays were used (Fig. 3). There was no correlation between Factor VIII activity and platelet count (Fig. 4).

A postoperative rise in Factor VIII activity has been described in humans as well as laboratory animals [1]. It is considered to be due to the effects of circulating catecholamines, and the mechanism appears to be the same that causes the Factor VIII rise after physical exercise, adrenaline injection and stimulation of hypothalamic centres, with resulting activation of the adrenal medulla [8, 10, 13]. The theory that this Factor VIII rise may be triggered by hemodynamic changes is supported by its being blocked by β-adrenergic blockers [8]. This adrenaline-dependent effect does not occur in the splenectomized person, nor can a postoperative rise of Factor VIII activity be

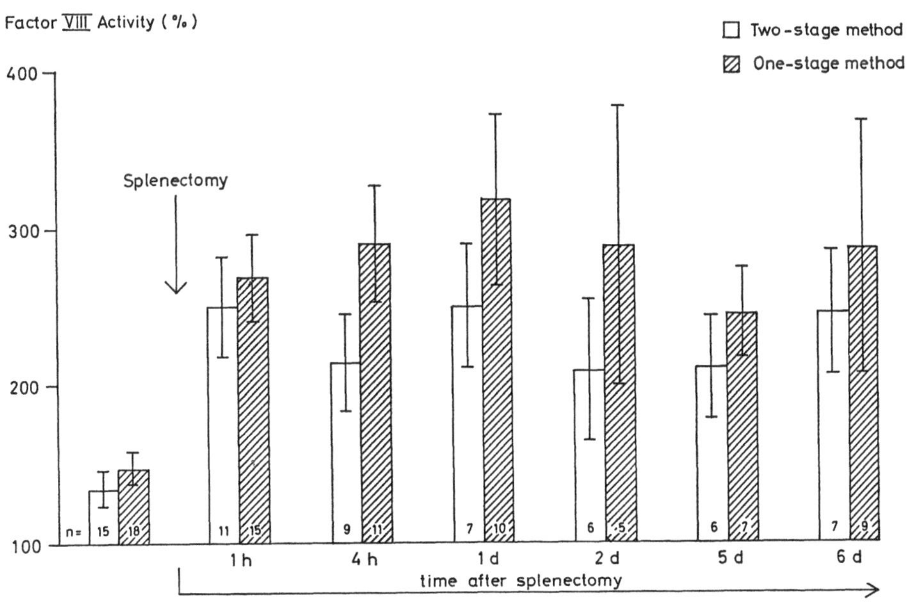

Fig. 3. Factor VIII activity following splenectomy in Hodgkin's disease (mean values and mean standard deviations). Factor VIII assays by the one-stage method of Geiger *et al.* [5] and the two-stage method of Pitney [12]

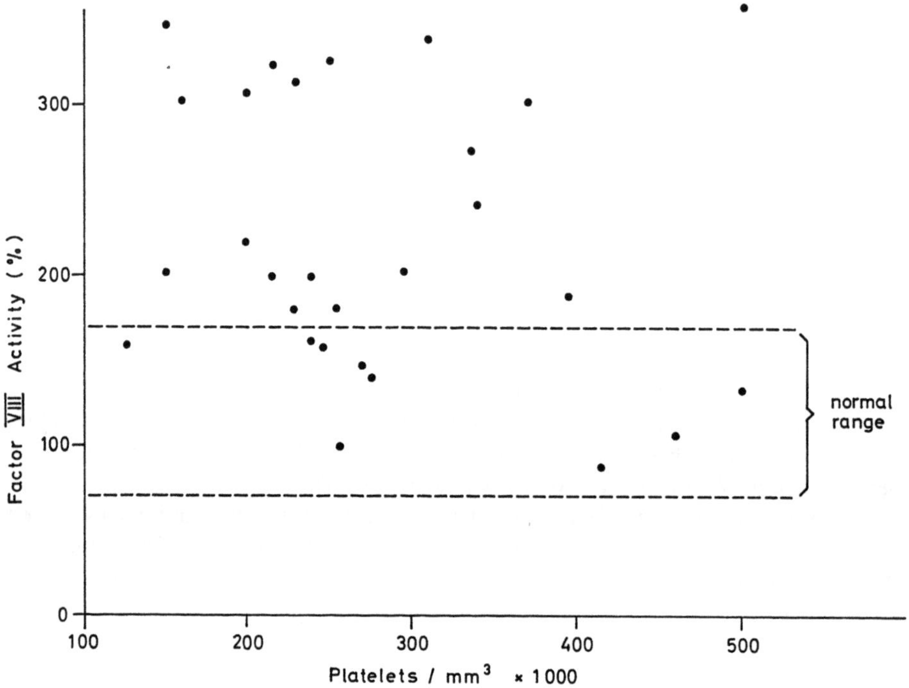

Fig. 4. Factor VIII activity and corresponding platelet counts in 22 patients after splenectomy for Hodgkin's disease. (Factor VIII assay according to Pitney [12])

observed in splenectomized laboratory animals [10, 11]. Because of these findings and of spleen perfusion experiments in which an increase in Factor VIII was found in the perfusion fluid [15], the spleen is thought to play a decisive role in the synthesis and storage of Factor VIII. However, McKee *et al.* [11] excluded the spleen as a site for synthesis of Factor VIII. Our findings of a sustained rise in Factor VIII activity after splenectomy could be interpreted in the same way. Storage of Factor VIII by the spleen will have to be discussed further, especially in view of the absence of a rise in Factor VIII activity after adrenaline injection in post-splenectomy patients.

If thrombosis after splenectomy is to be prevented, the changes in the platelet system will require particular attention. In addition to anticoagulants of the heparin and dicoumarol types, drugs, like acetylsalicylic acid, should be used, since these have an immediate effect on platelet function.

References

1. Amundsen, M. A., Spittell, J. A., Jr., Thompson, J. H., Owen, C. A. J.: Hypercoagulalability associated with malignant disease and with the postoperative state. Evidence for elevated levels of antihemophilic globulin. Ann. intern. Med. **58**, 608 (1963).
2. Aster, R. H.: Pooling of platelets in the spleen: role in the pathogenesis of "hypersplenic thrombocytopenia". J. clin. Invest. **45**, 645 (1966).

3. Breslow, A., Kaufman, R. M., Lawsky, A. R.: The effect of surgery on the concentration of circulating megakaryocytes and platelets. Blood **32**, 393 (1968).
4. Gehrmann, G.: Milz und normaler Thrombocytenhaushalt. In: Die Milz (Lemert, K., Harms, D., Eds.), p. 276. Berlin-Heidelberg-New York: Springer 1970.
5. Geiger, M. T., Duckert, F., Koller, F.: Quantitative Bestimmungen von Faktor VIII (Antihämophiles Globulin) und Faktor IX (Christmas-Factor, PTC) bei Blutersippen. 5th congr. Europ. Soc. Hemat., p. 413. Berlin-Göttingen-Heidelberg: Springer 1956.
6. Hirsch, J., McBride, J. A., Dacie, J. V.: Thrombo-embolism and increased platelet adhesiveness in post-splenectomy thrombocytosis. Aust. Ann. Med. **15**, 122 (1966).
7. Hjort, P. F., Paputchis, H.: Platelet life span in normal, splenectomized and hypersplenic rats. Blood **15**, 45 (1960).
8. Ingram, G. I. C. (Discussion): In: The Haemophilias, International Symposium, Washington, D. C. (Brinkhous, K. H., Ed.), p. 243. Chapel Hill: Univ. of North Carolina Press 1964.
9. Kotilainen, H.: Platelet kinetics in normal subjects and in haematological disorders. Scand. J. Haemat. Suppl. 5 (1969).
10. Libre, E. P., Gowan, D. H., Watkins, D. H. C., Jr., Shulman, N. R.: Relationship between spleen, platelets and Factor VIII levels. Blood **31**, 358 (1968).
11. McKee, P. A., Cousson, R. T., Buchner, R. G., Williams, G. R., Hampton, J. W.: Effect of the spleen on canine Factor VIII levels. J. Lab. clin. Med. **75**, 391 (1970).
12. Pitney, W. R.: The assay of antihaemophilic globulin (AHG) in Plasma. Brit. J. Haemat. **2**, 250 (1956).
13. Rizza, G. R., Eipe, J.: Exercise, Factor VIII and the spleen. Brit. J. Haemat. **20**, 629 (1971).
14. Tarnuzi, A., Smiley, R. K.: Hematologic effect of splenic implants. Blood **29**, 373 (1967).
15. Webster, W. P., Reddick, R. L., Roberts, H. R., Penick, G. D.: Release of Factor VIII (antihaemophilic factor) from perfused organs and tissues. Nature (Lond.) **213**, 1146 (1967).

Staging Laparotomy and Splenectomy in Hodgkin's Disease

Analysis of Indications and Patterns of Involvement in 285 Consecutive Unselected Cases

H. S. KAPLAN, R. F. DORFMAN, T. S. NELSEN, and S. A. ROSENBERG

Summary

The frequency of subdiaphragmatic involvement in a series of 285 consecutive, unselected, previously untreated patients with Hodgkin's disease, of whom 272 underwent staging laparotomy with splenectomy, is analyzed with respect to the influence of age, sex, histopathological type, preoperative sites of anatomical involvement, constitutional symptoms, lymphangiographic findings, and other factors. From these data, low- and high-yield groups may be identified, providing a basis for the selection of Hodgkin's disease patients in whom staging laparotomy is indicated. Diagnostic information made available by laparotomy with splenectomy and biopsy resulted in a change of stage in 18% and influenced treatment decisions in 35% of all cases.

Editor's Note

Since Dr. DORFMAN was not able to attend the convention to report on the results obtained by the Stanford group, Dr. KAPLAN was kind enough to place at my disposal the tables that he showed at the International Hodgkin Symposium in Stanford on May 22—24, 1972.

The contributed material will appear in detailed form in the National Cancer Institute Monograph 36. I have, with permission of the authors, compiled for the Freiburg convention a shortened selection which concisely and convincingly states the aims and tasks of staging laparotomy.

Comments on Table 1. The distribution of histological types in the Stanford collective shows a conspicuously high percentage (71%) of nodular sclerosis and low percentage (1%) of lymphocyte depletion. Nodular sclerosis totaled 74% of 185 patients, which DORFMAN [1] reported in Ann Arbor in 1971; lymphocyte depletion was 2%.

Published results show the following values for the proportion of nodular sclerosis (proportion of lymphocyte depletion in parentheses): LUKES and BUTLER [8]: 40% (18%); FRANSSILA *et al.* [2]: 47% (11%); KELLER *et al.* [6]: 52% (6%); LANDBERG and LARSSON [7]: 21% (13%); HAMANN *et al.* [5]: 46% (21%); GOUGH [4]: 15% (36%); FULLER *et al.* [3]: 53% (4%) and MUSSHOFF *et al.* [9]: 34% (16%).

The particular histological distribution of the Stanford collective must be taken into account in evaluation of the results.

One third of these Hodgkin's disease patients had a positive abdominal lymph node or spleen involvement or both at the time of diagnosis.

Table 1. Hodgkin's disease. Histopathologic type vs. frequency of para-aortic and splenic involvement in 272 cases given staging laparotomy

Histopathological Type	Cases [a]		Para-aortic nodes positive	Spleen positive
	No.	%	%	%
Lymphocyte Predominance	26	9.6	19	12
Nodular Sclerosis	194	71.3	34	34
Mixed Cellularity	48	17.6	44	56
Lymphocyte Depletion	3	1.1	67	67
Unclassified	1	0.4	—	—
Total	272	100.0	34	36

[a] No. of cases of each type submitted to laparotomy and splenectomy (percent of total series).

Table 2. Hodgkin's disease stage distribution

<table>
<tr><th>Stage (Ann Arbor Classification) [a]</th><th>No.</th><th>%</th><th>No.</th><th>%</th><th>No.</th><th>%</th></tr>
<tr><td>I A</td><td>29</td><td>10</td><td rowspan="2">32</td><td rowspan="2">11</td><td rowspan="2">32</td><td rowspan="2">11</td></tr>
<tr><td>B</td><td>3</td><td>1</td></tr>
<tr><td>II A</td><td>64</td><td>22</td><td rowspan="2">103</td><td rowspan="2">36</td><td rowspan="3">129</td><td rowspan="3">45</td></tr>
<tr><td>B</td><td>39</td><td>14</td></tr>
<tr><td>IIII_E (A+B)</td><td>26</td><td>9</td><td>26</td><td>9</td></tr>
<tr><td>III A</td><td>10</td><td>3.5</td><td rowspan="2">11</td><td rowspan="2">4</td><td rowspan="6">91</td><td rowspan="6">32</td></tr>
<tr><td>B</td><td>1</td><td>0.5</td></tr>
<tr><td>III_E (A+B)</td><td>4</td><td>1</td><td rowspan="4">80</td><td rowspan="4">28</td></tr>
<tr><td>III_S A</td><td>42</td><td>15</td></tr>
<tr><td>B</td><td>26</td><td>9</td></tr>
<tr><td>III_{ES} (A+B)</td><td>8</td><td>3</td></tr>
<tr><td>IV A</td><td>5</td><td>2</td><td rowspan="2">33</td><td rowspan="2">12</td><td rowspan="2">33</td><td rowspan="2">12</td></tr>
<tr><td>B</td><td>28</td><td>10</td></tr>
<tr><td></td><td>285</td><td>100</td><td>285</td><td>100</td><td>285</td><td>100</td></tr>
</table>

[a] The stage was based on laparotomy findings (272 cases).

Comments on Table 2. In the Ann Arbor Stage II group, 26 (20%) of a total of 129 patients had localized extranodular organ involvement of subcategory type E. In Ann Arbor Stage III, the proportion of localized extranodular organ involvement, including involvement of the spleen, amounted to 80 (88%) of 91 patients; therefore, involvement is limited to the lymph nodes in only 12% of all patients in Stage III.

At the time of diagnosis, the signs of generalization corresponding to Ann Arbor Stage IV were found in only 33 (12%) of 285 patients.

Table 3. Hodgkin's disease influence of laparotomy findings of final stage

Initial clinical stage (Ann Arbor)	Total No. of cases	Postlaparotomy pathologic stage in-creased	de-creased	Change of stage	
	No.	No.	No.	No.	%
I A	36	8	—	8	22
I B	3	0	—	0	
II A II_E A	99	21	0	21	21
II B II_E B	57	11	0	11	19
III A III_E A [a]	33	1	1	2	6
III B III_E B [a]	36	7	1	8	22
IV A	2	—	0	0	
IV B	6	—	0	0	
	272 [b]	48	2	50	18.2

[a] Laparotomy revealed spleen involvement in 22/33 CS IIIA and in 25/36 CS IIIB cases. When these cases, reclassified within Stage III as $PSIII_SA$ and $PSIII_SB$, respectively, are combined with those in which a change of stage was documented, laparotomy is seen to have yielded significant additional information in a total of 97/272 cases (35%).

[b] Laparotomies were not performed in 12 other cases (11 Stage IV, 1 geriatric case).

Comments on Table 3. Results of laparotomy with splenectomy caused the clinical stage to be altered in 50 patients (18.2%). If the change from negative to positive spleen involvement (Stage III to Stage III_S) is taken into account, then the percentage change in evaluation is 35%. The spleen is additionally involved in 22 of 33 patients = 67% in Stage III A, and in 25 of 36 patients = 69% in Stage III B.

Comments on Table 4. According to the laparotomy results presented here, the following conclusions can be drawn from the pre-operative lymph node pattern as to the effect of the disease:

1. An infradiaphragmatic involvement of lymph nodes and spleen has until now not been seen together with a primary involvement of the mediastinum or of an axilla in Stage I. It can be concluded, therefore, that direct dissemination of the disease from the mediastinum and the axillae to the abdomen does not occur, or if so, only rarely.

2. With primary involvement of the cervical-supraclavicular nodes and the para-aortic nodes, the spleen and the splenic hilar nodes are involved in an average of one

Table 4. Hodgkin's disease. Association of subdiaphragmatic involvement at laparotomy with various preoperative patterns of lymphadenopathy [a]

Preoperative sites of involvement	Total No. of cases	Laparotomy findings	
		Para-aortic and/or splenic hilar nodes positive	Spleen positive
		%	%
1. a) Mediastinal nodes only	11	0	0
b) Unilateral axillary nodes only	5	0	0
2. a) Cervical-supraclavicular nodes only:			
Left	26	38	35
Right	13	8	23
Bilateral	13	46	38
b) Cervical-supraclavicular and mediastinal nodes only:			
Left	24	25	29
Right	15	13	13
Bilateral	42	38	40
c) Cervical-supraclavicular nodes alone or with other supradiaphragmatic sites:			
Left	68	32	35
Right	44	18	20
Bilateral	126	45	47
3. Inguinal, femoral, iliac nodes alone or in combination	16	50	31

[a] 285 consecutive previously untreated cases, of which 272 were submitted to staging laparotomy.

third of cases. The percentage of abdominal involvement is greater in combination with involvement of the neck and supraclavicular nodes of the left side than in combination with those of the right side, and is greatest when both sides are involved.

When the mediastinal nodes are involved in addition to the cervical-supraclavicular nodes, the percentage of abdominal findings not only does not increase, but actually decreases. Even when all remaining supradiaphragmatic regions involved are combined with the cervical-supraclavicular nodes, the infradiaphragmatic inclusion does not increase, or if so, only insignificantly.

These findings indicate that the disease spreads from the cervical and supraclavicular regions, which are the most frequently involved primary body areas, in caudal direction into the abdomen, proceeding, however, not over the mediastinum, but via the ductus thoracicus.

Table 5. Hodgkin's disease. Association of liver and bone marrow involvement with spleen and para-aortic nodes involvement [a]

	Total No. of cases	Laparotomy findings		
		No. with laparotomy	Spleen positive	Para-aortic nodes positive
Liver biopsy positive	10	9	9	8
Bone marrow biopsy positive	9	6	6	6

[a] All cases with positive liver or bone marrow biopsy among 285 consecutive, previously untreated patients are represented. Of the 3 patients with bone marrow involvement who did not have staging laparotomies, 2 had lymphangiograms, both of which were positive for para-aortic node involvement.

3. In Clinical Stages I and II with primary subdiaphragmatic involvement of the inguinal, femoral or iliac nodes, or both, the para-aortic nodes are additionally involved in half of the cases and the spleen in one third of the cases.

Comments on Table 5. In all cases in which the liver biopsy was positive, a positive spleen (in 9 of 9 cases) and, with one exception (in 8 of 9 cases), positive para-aortic nodes were found in the laparotomy.

With positive bone marrow findings, a positive spleen as well as positive para-aortic nodes were found in all cases in which laparotomy with splenectomy was performed.

References

1. DORFMAN, R. F.: Relationship of histology of site in Hodgkin's disease. Cancer Res. **31**, 1786 (1971).
2. FRANSSILA, K. O., KALIMA, T. V., VOUTILAINEN, A.: Histologic classification of Hodgkin's disease: A correlation of histopathology with survival. Int. J. Cancer **5**, 273 (1970).
3. FULLER, L. M., GAMBLE, J. F., FUTLER, J. J.: Influence of specific histology and clinical presentation on prognosis in localized Hodgkin's disease treated with intensive large volume radiotherapy. J. Radiol. **98**, 641 (1971).
4. GOUGH, J.: Hodgkin's disease: A correlation of histopathology with survival. Int. J. Cancer **5**, 273 (1970).
5. HAMANN, W., OEHLERT, W., MUSSHOFF, K., NUSS, A., SCHNELLBACHER, B.: Histologic classification of Hodgkin's disease and its relevance to prognosis. Dtsch. med. Mschr. **15**, 509 (1970).
6. KELLER, A. R., KAPLAN, H. S., LUKES, R. J., RAPPAPORT, H.: Correlation of histopathology with other prognostic indicators in Hodgkin's disease. Cancer (Philad.) **22**, 487 (1968).
7. LANDBERG, T., LARSSON, L.: Hodgkin's disease. Acta radiol. (Stockh.) **8**, 390 (1969).
8. LUKES, R. J., BUTLER, J. J.: The pathology and nomenclature of Hodgkin's disease. Cancer Res. **26**, 1063 (1966).
9. MUSSHOFF, K., HARTMANN, CH., NIKLAUS, B., RÖSSNER, R.: Results of therapy in Hodgkin's disease, Freiburg im Breisgau 1964—1971. This volume, p. 206—220.

Preliminary Results of Laparotomy with Splenectomy in Patients Previously Treated for Hodgkin's Disease

C. Pauli-Beisel, K. Musshoff, and W. Oehlert

Summary

Between October 1969 and July 1972 primary staging laparotomies with splenectomy were carried out in 29 patients with Hodgkin's disease. In 41 cases secondary laparotomy with splenectomy was performed 1—12 years after the initial treatment. At secondary laparotomy, 4 of 27 cases (=15%) in clinical stages I and II (Ann Arbor) and 8 of 14 cases in stage III (Ann Arbor) showed involvement of abdominal lymph nodes and/or the spleen, and two cases with hepatic involvement were observed. Secondary laparotomy with splenectomy is an appropriate method when initial treatment has not been completely successful and further therapeutic measures are necessary to correct this.

A retrospective analysis of our patient series from 1964—1969 showed:

a) that there were a large number of recurrences in Stages II and III in the lymph nodes and lymphatic organs of the abdomen;

b) that results were poorer in Stage III cases where the spleen had not been included in treatment.

From October 1969 onwards we therefore performed laparotomy with splenectomy (as discussed by Staib).

The series of 70 patients falls into two main groups. In the first group, laparotomy was carried out as part of the initial course of treatment as a primary staging method, i. e. before radiotherapy was started, between two courses of radiotherapy, or immediately after radiotherapy was finished. The second group consists of patients who had a laparotomy 2—12 years after the end of treatment. Most patients in this group were in full remission, some showed radiological evidence of splenomegaly and, in some patients, laboratory data indicated active disease.

Table 1 shows the staging on the basis of the Ann Arbor Classification. Group I (primary laparotomy) includes 29 patients and group II 41 patients. Of 36 patients in Stage II (both groups), 3 had localized extranodular manifestations (8.5%); of the 26 extranodular manifestations (23%), the overall percentage for the series being 14.5%.

As Table 2 shows, a very high incidence of abdominal manifestations occurred in the group of patients submitted to primary laparotomy. In Stages I and II, 47%, and in Stage III, 67% were found to have abdominal involvement. The spleen and lymph nodes were about equally affected, but no foci were found in the liver.

Table 1. Hodgkin's disease. Patients group with laparotomy (1969, X—1972, VII) Ann Arbor Classification

Stage		Laparotomy primary or in the course of first treatment	Laparotomy subsequent to first treatment	♂	♀	Total	
		No.	No.	No.	No.	No.	No.
I	A	1	7	4	4	8	8
	B						
II	A	12	17	12	17	29	36 [a]
	B	4	3	1	6	7	
III	A	10	11	8	13	21	26 [b]
	B	2	3	4	1	5	
		29	41	29	41	70	70

[a] 3/36 with Stage II_E
[b] 6/26 with Stage III_E

Table 2. Results of laparotomy made in the course of first treatment related to clinical stage

Stage		Hodgkin's disease positive in						
		abdominal lymph nodes		spleen		liver	total lymph nodes, spleen, liver	
	No.	No.	%	No.	%	No.	No./No. [a]	%
I	1	—		—		—	0/1	0
II	16	5	31	5	31	—	8/16	50
III	12	5	42	6	50	—	8/12	67
	29	10	34	11	38	—	16/29	55

[a] Number of patients with positive diagnosis of disease in lymph nodes, spleen and liver or both/number of patients at risk.

Table 3 shows that in the group of patients in whom laparotomy was performed at a later stage only 15% in Stages I and II were found to have abdominal manifestations. In Stage III, however, 57% of cases showed involvement of spleen, liver and lymph nodes, in spite of the previous therapy. Taking the two groups together, positive abdominal findings occur in 29% of all cases.

We would like to stress that in the second group (in which laparotomy was performed later) the liver was involved in 2 cases. One case was a female patient who had been given radiotherapy when she was in Stage II. After 4 years the disease progressed to the para-aortic region. A combination of radiotherapy and cytotoxic drugs

Table 3. Results of laparotomy subsequent to first treatment up to 12 years later, related to clinical stage

Stage		Hodgkin's disease positive in							
		abdominal lymph nodes		spleen		liver		total lymph nodes, spleen, liver	
	No.	No.	%	No.	%	No.	%	No./No. [a]	%
I	7	—		1	14	—		1/7	14
II	20	1	5	3	15	1	5	3/20	15
III	14	5	36	5	36	1	7	8/14	57
	41	6	15	9	22	2	5	12/41	29

[a] Number of patients with positive disease in lymph nodes, spleen, and liver or both/number of patients at risk.

induced a second full remission. Ten years after the first diagnosis and 5 years after the second course of treatment, laparotomy was performed and involvement of the liver and spleen was found.

The second case was a female patient who had been given supradiaphragmatic radiotherapy at another treatment centre. After a full clinical remission of one year, the patient again experienced symptoms of the disease. A lymphography was performed, and the patient was then given radiotherapy in the infradiaphragmatic region because of involvement of abdominal lymph nodes. After another 2 years, the patient returned to us. We performed a laparoscopy which showed no evidence of splenic or

Table 4. Results of laparotomy (all patients) related to clinical stage and symptoms A or B Ann Arbor Classification

Stage		Hodgkin's disease positive in							
		abdominal lymph nodes		spleen		liver		total lymph nodes, spleen, liver	
	No.	No.	%	No.	%	No.	%	No./No. [a]	%
I A	8	—		1	13	—		1/8	13
II B	0								
II A	29	3	10	6	21	—		8/29	28
II B	7	3	43	2	29	1	14	3/7	43
III A	21	9	43	8	38	1	5	13/21	62
III B	5	1	20	3	60	—		3/5	40
	70	16	23	20	29	2	3	28/70	40

[a] Number of patients with positive disease in lymph nodes, spleen, and liver or both/number of patients at risk.

hepatic involvement. A year later, laparotomy with splenectomy was performed, and involvement of both liver and spleen was found.

Table 4 shows the staging classification and the relation of the histological types A and B to the results in the two groups. It is evident that positive abdominal findings cannot be excluded in group A. In this series, which contains only a relatively small number of patients, the incidence of abdominal manifestations in group B (50%) is only slightly higher than in group A.

Table 5 shows the results of laparotomy related to the histological type for the whole patient series. It is important to realize that positive abdominal findings cannot be excluded in any of the histological types, not even in the lymphocytic predominance group, which has the most favorable prognosis.

Table 5. Results of laparotomy (all patients) related to histology

Histology		Hodgkin's disease positive in							
		abdominal lymph nodes		spleen		liver		total lymph nodes, spleen, liver	
	No.	No.	%	No.	%	No.	%	No./No. [a]	%
Lymphocytic Predominance	13	5	38	5	38	—		8/13	62
Nodular Sclerosis	32	8	25	11	34	2	6	15/32	47
Mixed Cellularity	14	3	21	4	29	—	—	5/14	36
Lymphocytic Depletion	8	—		—		—		0/8	0
Unclassified	3	—		—		—		0/3	0
	70	16	23	20	29	2	3	28/70	40

[a] Number of patients with positive disease in lymph nodes, spleen, and liver or both/ number of patients at risk.

The number of patients was small, but we found that the highest percentage of cases with abdominal manifestations occurred in the histological type with the best prognosis.

The two following figures give a synopsis of the time intervals in which abdominal manifestations of Hodgkin's disease were found.

Fig. 1 shows the results of laparotomy which had been carried out later in the course of the disease. The results are related to stage, clinical type and time. We see that in practically all stages (excluding in Stage I B in our series), abdominal manifestations were found up to 12 years after the time of first diagnosis.

Fig. 2 shows the results of laparotomy in Group 2, related to the histological type and to time. Both illustrations show clearly that the positive findings are distributed over the whole length of time up to 12 years, and that abdominal manifestations can be found even after intervals of several years.

When we summarize the results of our laparotomies, we see that involvement of abdominal lymph nodes, spleen and liver was found particularly often in the second

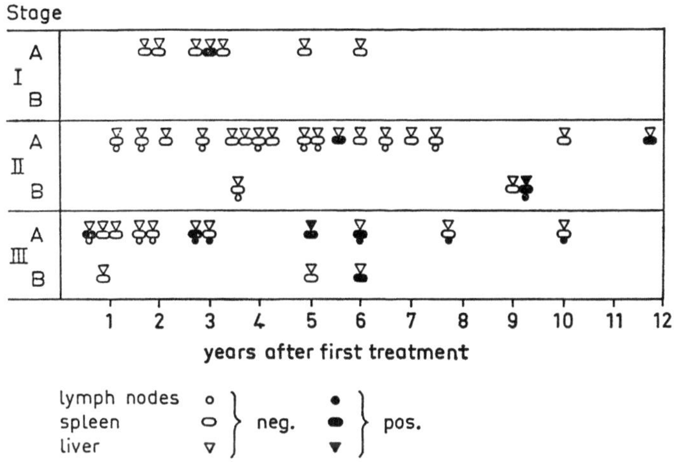

Fig. 1. Hodgkin's disease. Results of laparotomy from first treatment to 12 years. Stage (Ann Arbor Classification) and time interval

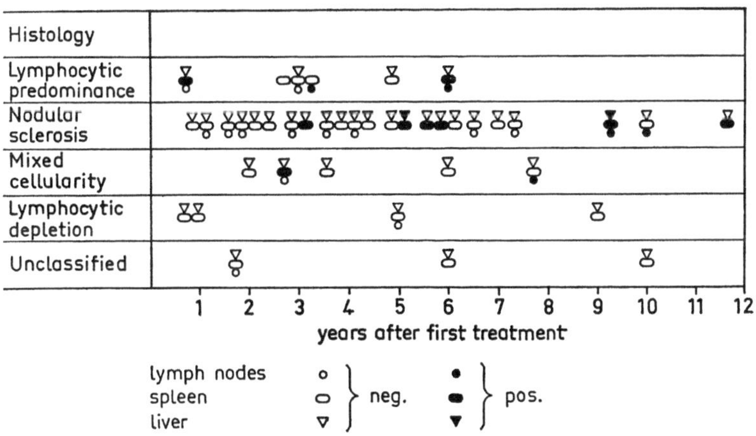

Fig. 2. Hodgkin's disease. Results of laparotomy from first treatment to 12 years. Histology and time interval

group of patients (in whom laparotomy was performed years after the first course of treatment). In such cases there may or may not be pathological clinical signs such as a marked or slight rise in erythrocyte sedimentation rate, alkaline phosphatase, or α-2 globulin.

On the basis of our findings we think that with patients who have not had primary treatment of the spleen, such treatment should be seriously considered later on. This could be radiotherapy or laparotomy with splenectomy. Indications for laparotomy should be considered in the context of the overall condition of individual patients.

Influence of Extensive Biopsy Sampling at Laparotomy on Planning of Radiotherapy in the Non-Hodgkin Lymphoma

R. E. Johnson, P. Chretien, and G. T. O'Conor

Summary

The natural history of the lymphoreticular lymphomas is ill-defined in comparison with Hodgkin's disease. In an effort to acquire information which would contribute to selection of more rational radiotherapeutic techniques, patients with non-Hodgkin's lymphoma have been subjected to surgical exploration of the abdomen. Lymph nodes suspected of involvement were removed for histologic study together with the spleen and wedge biopsies of the liver. Macroscopically normal lymph nodes also were generously sampled from the aortic-iliac chains, from the porta hepatis, and from the free portion of the mesentery. The findings support the general conclusion that non-Hodgkin's lymphomas display patterns of anatomical involvement which do not indicate the use of radiotherapy techniques generally employed for the treatment of Hodgkin's disease.

Introduction

The cornerstone of effective cancer therapeutics is an understanding of the developmental sequence of any given neoplasm and the ability to identify the relative position of each case within this sequence in order to plan rational treatment. During recent years, as more sophisticated diagnostic tools have become available, precision in defining the anatomical extent of disease and predicting the subsequent patterns of dissemination has greatly increased. The process often referred to as "staging" has been applied in particular to the malignant lymphomas and Hodgkin's disease. Recognition of the potential radiocurability of these tumors has accentuated the importance of accurate staging and led to the examination of exploratory laparotomy as a possible guide to decisions on therapy [1—3].

Knowledge of the lymphocytic and histiocytic lymphomas is much poorer than that of Hodgkin's disease. Deficient understanding of the patterns of involvement and dissemination has been reflected in the variety of radiotherapy techniques employed. In an effort to devise more rational approaches to treatment for the non-Hodgkin lymphomas, previously untreated patients have been subjected to surgical exploration of the abdomen following a routine comprehensive diagnostic evaluation. The influence of the laparotomy findings on the subsequent planning of radiation therapy is described in this report.

Clinic Material and Methods

Eighteen untreated patients with a histological diagnosis of malignant lymphoma other than Hodgkin's disease have been subjected to exploratory laparotomy when the routine diagnostic evaluation had failed to disclose evidence of extranodal dissemination. Ten of the 18 patients were male and the overall median age was 49 years (range 11 to 67). The diagnosis was poorly differentiated lymphocytic lymphoma (lymphosarcoma) in 10 cases, histiocytic lymphoma (reticulosarcoma) in 6 cases, and mixed lymphocytic-histiocytic lymphoma (reticulolymphosarcoma) in 2 cases.

The preoperative evaluation included a careful history and physical examination, radiographic studies (chest X-ray with tomography as indicated, metastatic skeletal survey, bipedal lymphography), liver studies (biochemical, radioisotopic scan, *and needle biopsy*), radioisotopic bone scan, hematology (complete and differential blood count and bone marrow biopsy), and such other tests as were considered to be indicated in individual patients. Patients with confirmed extranodal involvement prior to laparotomy were excluded from this review. Lymphographic evidence (positive suggestive) of retroperitoneal adenopathy was found in 11 of 18 patients; one of these patients had a palpable spleen tip and a second had a palpable retroperitoneal mass. Otherwise, there was no clinical or palpable evidence of abdominal disease in any of the sites biopsied at laparotomy.

The surgical approach to the abdomen was through an extended midline incision which permitted the inspection and systematic palpation of the entire peritoneal cavity. We sought an extensive representative sample of lymph nodes. Suspicious or clinically positive nodes were biopsied in addition to representative nodes from the aortic or iliac chains or both, and from the splenic pedicle. Splenectomy and liver biopsy (including a wedge from the right and left lobes) were performed. Lymph nodes of normal appearance were identified, often with difficulty, in the free portion of the mesentery and porta hepatics, and these were generously sampled. This procedure considerably extended the duration of the laparotomy as compared to Hodgkin's disease, the average operation for non-Hodgkin lymphomas requiring $2^1/_2$ to 3 hours.

Histopathological Findings and Influence on Treatment Planning

The cell type in all 10 of the lymphosarcoma patients was classified as poorly differentiated, and a nodular growth pattern was clearly present in 8 of the 10 cases. This nodular pattern usually persisted in some or all of the secondary sites found to be involved, particularly in the spleen and mesenteric lymph nodes. In the 2 cases classified as diffuse on the initial biopsy, a nodular pattern was found in the laparotomy specimens; in one instance, the tumor type was histiocytic.

Both lymphomas of the mixed lymphocytic-histiocytic type were nodular, and this nodular pattern persisted in the secondary sites although the cell type varied from pure lymphocytic to pure histiocytic in different specimens. Whereas only one of the 6 reticulosarcomas was classified as nodular on the initial biopsy, 2 of the 5 diffuse cases exhibited a nodular pattern in at least one secondary site biopsied at laparotomy. In the single reticulosarcoma patient with liver involvement the liver in-

Table 1. Histological findings with extensive biopsy sampling at laparotomy

Diagnosis and Case	Age	Sex	Histology on laparotomy biopsy specimens [a]				
			Liver	Spleen	Aorta	Porta	Mesentery
1. Lymphocytic lymphoma	11	M	–	–	(+)	–	–
2. Lymphocytic lymphoma	35	M	+	+	(+)	NE	NE
3. Lymphocytic lymphoma	56	F	+	+	(+)	+	–
4. Lymphocytic lymphoma	37	M	–	–	(+)	–	–
5. Lymphocytic lymphoma	60	M	–	–	–	+	–
6. Lymphocytic lymphoma	44	M	–	–	(+)	–	+
7. Lymphocytic lymphoma	54	F	–	+	+	+	+
8. Lymphocytic lymphoma	50	F	–	–	+	+	–
9. Lymphocytic lymphoma	65	M	–	–	(–)	–	–
10. Lymphocytic lymphoma	57	M	+	+	(+)	+	+
11. Lymphocytic-histiocytic lymphoma	28	F	+	(+)	(–)	+	+
12. Lymphocytic-histiocytic lymphoma	49	F	+	+	(+)	+	+
13. Histiocytic lymphoma	59	M	–	–	–	+	+
14. Histiocytic lymphoma	25	F	–	–	–	–	–
15. Histiocytic lymphoma	67	M	–	–	(+)	+	+
16. Histiocytic lymphoma	23	F	–	–	–	–	–
17. Histiocytic lymphoma	65	M	+	+	(+)	NE	NE
18. Histiocytic lymphoma	49	F	–	–	–	–	–

[a] Aorta, Porta, and Mesentery refer to lymph nodes from the aortic (or iliac) chain, porta hepatis region, and free mesentery respectively; the ( ) indicates sites preoperatively suspected of involvement; NE = Not Examined.

filtrate was composed predominantly of poorly differentiated lymphosarcoma cells. In addition, 2 other patients with reticulosarcoma had only nodular lymphosarcoma in the mesenteric nodes, while other abdominal nodes in the same patients contained diffuse histiocytic lymphoma.

The histological findings for the 18 extensively biopsied patients are summarized in Table 1. One third had confirmed liver involvement despite a negative (or non-diagnostic) preoperative assessment which included percutaneous liver biopsy and sometimes laparoscopy with multiple needle biopsies. In two thirds of the patients involvement of lymph nodes in the porta hepatis or free portion of the mesentery was proved by biopsy. No evidence of disease in these sites was clinically discernible

Table 2. Influence of laparotomy findings on the technique for radiation therapy

Histology	Number of patients	Tumor outside inverted-Y field		
		Nodes [a]	Liver	Combined
Lymphocytic lymphoma	10	6 (4)	3	7
Histiocytic lymphoma	8	5 (2)	3	5

[a] Mesenteric or porta-hepatis nodes or both; ( ) indicates the number with eccentric involvement in lymph nodes only.

prior to surgery, and in most cases the biopsied lymph nodes appeared normal and were often difficult to identify for excision.

The influence of these findings on the planning of radiation therapy is shown in Table 2. Two thirds of the patients had documented tumor involvement in sites which clearly rendered unsatisfactory the radiation technique utilized for Hodgkin's disease, the "inverted-Y" field. This high rate of involvement in locations unusual for Hodgkin's disease reflected the extensive sampling of "normal" nodes. This is illustrated by the following case:

Case 09-05-02: This 60-year-old male presented with cervical adenopathy which, on biopsy, was diagnosed as poorly differentiated lymphocytic lymphoma with a nodular pattern. Evaluation was unremarkable: it included a complete radiological workup of the gastrointestinal tract, liver function tests, needle biopsy of the liver, bipedal lymphography, and careful physical examination. At laparotomy, the usual specimens were obtained, including the spleen, liver wedge biopsies, representative lymph nodes of normal appearance obtained from the aortic chain (4 nodes), free portion of the mesentery (5 nodes), and the porta hepatis (4 nodes). All specimens were negative except for a single porta hepatis node, which was partially replaced with nodular lymphosarcoma.

Discussion

This experience is consistent with the few available descriptions [4, 5] of the laparotomy findings in non-Hodgkin lymphomas. It is evident from these combined reports that frequent diffuse abdominal involvement also mitigates against effective use of the radiotherapeutic techniques usually adopted for Hodgkin's disease. The routine technique for Hodgkin's disease is irradiation of the midline (para-aortic) lymph nodes in the upper abdomen; the porta hepatis and free mesentery are not encompassed in such a treatment field.

The frequency of unsuspected disease, particularly in the liver and non-axial abdominal nodes, is relatively high in our series and no doubt reflects the extensive random sampling of clinically normal tissues. In the case report, only a single lymph node of the total of 13 nodes examined was partially involved. The evident possibility of sampling error at laparotomy suggests that random biopsies are unreliable as a guide to treatment when the histological findings are negative.

All 3 reticulosarcoma cases with negative laparotomy findings had extranodal primary sites (two in the upper air passages and one in bone). One of these (Case 16) has already developed massive recurrence in the mesenteric lymph nodes within months of initial treatment, despite the negative laparotomy finding which had caused irradiation of the abdomen to be withheld. The 5 reticulosarcoma patients with primary lymph-node involvement all had confirmed involvement in the abdomen outside the area usually irradiated in Hodgkin's disease patients.

Two major questions are being prospectively examined and answers will shortly be available: "Is negative laparotomy reliable for decisions on treatment or should generalized abdominal involvement always be assumed?" and "Are the radiation doses that can be safely delivered to the entire abdomen sufficient to achieve frequent if not consistent control of disease in non-Hodgkin lymphomas?". The answers to these questions will further define the potential role of radiotherapy in the management of the lymphomas and provide a basis for the design of comparative clinical trials.

References

1. Glatstein, E., Guernsey, J. M., Rosenberg, S. A., Kaplan, H. S.: The value of laparotomy and splenectomy in the staging of Hodgkin's disease. Cancer (Philad.) **24**, 709 (1969).
2. Ultmann, J. E.: Current status: The management of lymphoma. Seminars Hemat. **7**, 441 (1970).
3. Johnson, R. E.: Is staging laparotomy routinely indicated in Hodgkin's disease? Ann. intern. Med. **75**, 459 (1971).
4. Hanks, G. E., Terry, L. N., Bryan, J. A., Newsome, J. F.: Contribution of diagnostic laparotomy to staging non-Hodgkin's lymphoma. Cancer (Philad.) **29**, 41 (1972).
5. Hass, A. C., Brunk, S. F., Gulesserian, H. P., Givler, R. L.: The value of exploratory laparotomy in malignant lymphoma. Radiology **101**, 157 (1971).

Bone Marrow Biopsy in Malignant Lymphoma

H. H. HENNEKEUSER *

Summary

Bone marrow biopsy detects involvement of bone marrow in Hodgkin's disease more often than aspiration does. Stage I and II patients very seldom show bone marrow involvement. In 10—50% of stage III patients, bone marrow involvement is found. These patients have to be reclassified in stage IV, where total nodular irradiation ist no longer possible. Lymphocytic depletion types are more often involved. In non-Hodgkin's lymphomas, biopsy delivers more information about bone marrow involvement than aspiration does. The difference is not as impressive as in Hodgkin's disease. Bone marrow involvement is found mostly in stage III and IV and in the lymphocytic types. A bone marrow biopsy should be performed in all patients with stage III malignant lymphomas before laparotomy staging procedures, and in stage I and II patients if systemic symptoms are present.

Exact staging of malignant lymphomas is of prognostic importance [1, 13, 19, 22, 24, 25]. It is of special importance to identify Stage IV cases, since in this stage the disease is generalized with extranodal tissue involvement and no curative X-ray treatment is possible [13, 19]. In addition to laparoscopy and diagnostic laparotomy, histological examination of bone marrow has a certain value as a diagnostic tool [24, 25, 27].

From June 1970 to June 1972 we examined 350 bone-marrow biopsies from patients of the University Medical Clinic, Freiburg i. Br. I report here the results from 98 cases of malignant lymphomas. We performed bone-marrow biopsy at the ventral upper iliac crest as an open biopsy with the myelotomy device by the method of BURKHARDT [3] under local anesthesia. Bone-marrow cores of 4 mm diameter and 10—20 mm length were obtained, treated by BURKHARDT's method [3], and embedded in methacrylate. The 3 µm-thick slices were stained with Gallamineblue-Giemsa, Ladewig, Gomori, and Turnbullblue [3]. In addition, esterase activity was demonstrated by the use of naphthol-AS-D-chloroacetate substrate; this served as a marker for neutrophil granulopoiesis and tissue mast cells [9]. Parallel to bone-marrow biopsy, cytological bone marrow examination by sternal or iliac crest aspiration was performed in all patients.

---

* Supported by a grant from the „Schutzkommission beim Bundesministerium des Inneren".

Histological classification of lymph nodes from all the Hodgkin's disease patients studied was performed by Professor OEHLERT, following the criteria of LUKES and BUTLER [17, 18].

Among the 60 HD patients we found bone-marrow metastasis in 11 cases (18%). Table 1 shows the variable degree of bone-marrow involvement reported in the literature: different investigators report between 2% and 29% [2, 4, 6, 7, 8, 13, 23, 25, 27]. All authors agree (Table 2) that bone-marrow biopsy is a better diagnostic tool than aspiration cytology for detecting tissue involvement [2, 3, 7, 13, 16, 23, 27]. Only the findings of GÜLLER *et al.* [8] are divergent; these should be reconsidered.

Table 1. Frequency of bone-marrow involvement in Hodgkin's disease

	All cases	Positive biopsy
BENNETT *et al.* (1968)	108	2%
KAPLAN (1971)	340	2%
GÜLLER *et al.* (1972)	42	4%
DORFMAN (1971)	185	4%
ROSENBERG (1971)	155	5%
HENNEKEUSER (1972)	60	18%
WEBB *et al.* (1970)	49	22%
GRANN *et al.* (1966)	42	26%
STUTZMAN (1971)	58	26%
DUHAMEL (1972)	100	29%

Table 2. Frequency of bone-marrow involvement in Hodgkin's lymphoma detected by biopsy and by aspiration

	All cases	% positive:	
		biopsy	aspiration
STUTZMAN (1971)	32	47	3
GRANN *et al.* (1966)	42	26	0
HENNEKEUSER (1972)	60	18	2
GÜLLER *et al.* (1972)	42	4	10

There is a positive correlation between the stage of disease and the frequency of bone-marrow involvement (Table 3): In HD Stages I and II tissue involvement is almost never observed (divergent findings have been reported by DUHAMEL [6]). Demonstration of bone-marrow involvement usually means infradiaphragmatic lymph-node involvement [1, 14, 23, 25, 27]. It is of special interest to study Stage III patients who show 10—50% bone-marrow involvement. In 5 patients with a positive bone-marrow biopsy during Stage III, no liver involvement had been found by laparoscopy and liver biopsy.

Most investigators report results on untreated patients who undergo biopsy during early phases of the disease, but some of the patients we studied had long-established HD. Tissue involvement may be expected rather frequently among these patients, and

Table 3. Clinical stage and bone-marrow involvement in Hodgkin's disease

Stage	Webb *et al.* 1970	Duhamel 1972	Rosenberg 1972	Stutzman 1971	Hennekeuser 1972
I	0/2 0%	8%	0/67 0%	0/12 0%	0/2 0%
II	0/8 0%	14%			0/8 0%
III	6/14 43%	50%	8/88 9%	5/20 25%	5/18 28%
IV	5/25 20%	58%		10/26 38%	6/32 19%
Total	11/49 22%	29/100 29%	8/155 5%	15/58 26%	11/60 18%

Table 4. Histological type and frequency of bone-marrow involvement detected by open iliac-crest biopsy in Hodgkin's disease in treated and untreated patients

Type	Biopsy in untreated patients	Biopsy after treatment	All cases
Lymphocytic Predominance	0/1	0/0	0/1
Nodular Sclerosis	2/8	0/9	2/17
Mixed Cellularity	2/12	1/11	3/23
Lymphocytic Depletion	3/11	3/8	6/19
Total	7/32	4/27	11/60

Table 5. Histological type and frequency of bone-marrow involvement detected by open iliac-crest biopsy in Hodgkin's disease

Type	Dorfman 1971	Hennekeuser 1972
Lymphocytic Predominance	0/13 0%	0/1 0%
Nodular Sclerosis	6/137 4%	2/17 12%
Mixed Cellularity	0/32 0%	3/23 13%
Lymphocytic Depletion	2/3 67%	6/19 32%
Total	8/185 4%	11/60 18%

Table 4 demonstrates its distribution in our patients. However, there was no difference between patients with early biopsy and those who had a later biopsy. Table 4 shows the correlation between the histological type of HD and the frequency of bone-marrow involvement: lymphocytic depletion types show more positive results than mixed cellularity and nodular sclerosis types. This agrees with the findings of Dorfman [4] (Table 5).

Histologically, bone-marrow metastasis in HD shows tumor-like expansive growth. The same histological pattern may be observed as in lymph-node histology. However, distinct reticulin-fiber formation is often found within HD foci [2, 4, 12, 17, 21]. In some remarkable cases (Fig. 1) a relatively cell-poor fibrosis of the marrow was observed without Sternberg-Reed cells. These fibrous alterations always suggest bone-marrow involvement [5, 12, 22, 26]. Two of our patients with such fibrosis showed positive results in repeat biopsies.

The importance of small non-caseating tubercle-like granulomas composed of epitheloid histiocytes but no Sternberg-Reed cells (Fig. 2) has not yet been elucidated. Such granulomas are occasionally found in liver, spleen, and in lymph nodes as well as in bone marrow [3, 11, 12, 15, 20, 21, 25]. Some of these granulomas are surrounded by a lymphocyte margin (Fig. 2). We found such granulomas in a sample from one patient, but this does not prove tissue involvement [11, 12, 21].

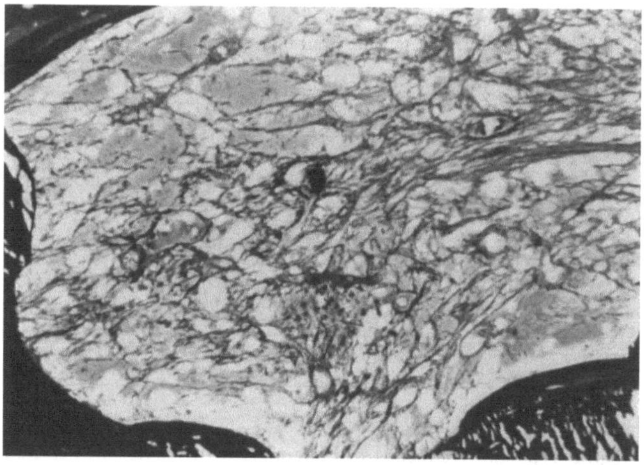

Fig. 1. Hodgkin's disease: Areas of fibrosis in hypoplastic bone marrow without Sternberg-Reed-cells. Gomori ×160

Other reactive marrow alterations have been observed frequently. About half the patients showed focal hyperplasia of eosinophilic granulocytes and about a third of all cases exhibited plasma-cell accumulation (mostly perivascular).

Among the patients with non-Hodgkin lymphomas (Table 6) we found bone-marrow involvement in 58%: 13 cases with diffuse and 9 cases with nodular involvement. As a possible explanation for the relatively high incidence of bone-marrow involvement in our cases (Table 7), the small number of patients investigated has to be considered. Among the non-Hodgkin lymphomas (Table 8) we can demonstrate once more that bone-marrow biopsy is superior to bone-marrow aspiration but the difference is less striking than with HD. This is probably due to the more localized changes and the distinct fibrosis in HD [1, 4, 7, 8, 10, 16]. The extensive studies of Jones *et al.* [10] also show a correlation in non-Hodgkin lymphomas between frequency of marrow involvement and histological type of the disease as well as clinical stage [10]. Lymphocytic types show bone-marrow involvement more frequently than histiocytic types (Table 9). Moreover, bone-marrow involvement during Stages I and II is rarely found, whereas nearly 25% of all Stage III and IV cases show bone-marrow involvement (Table 10).

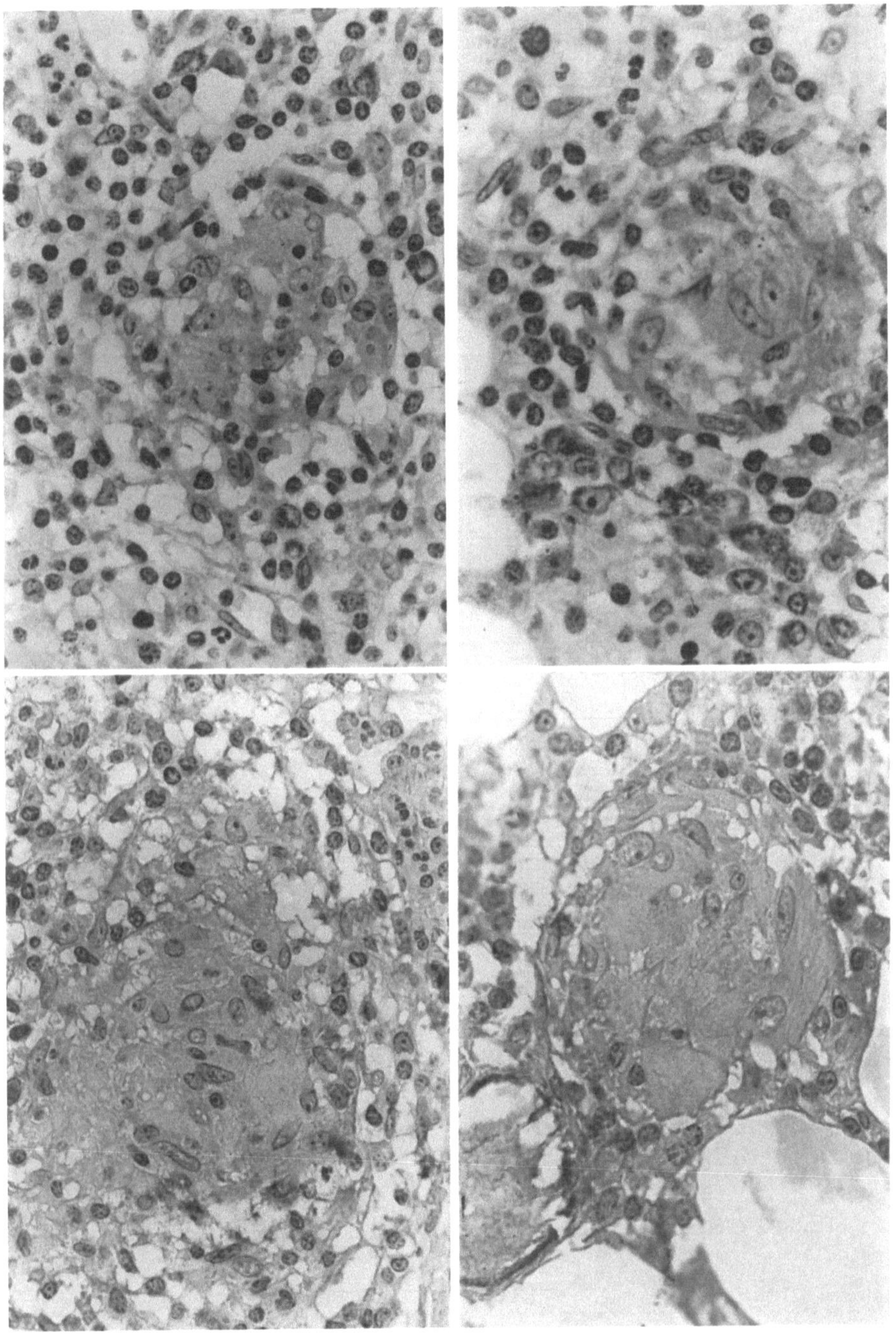

Fig. 2 a—d. Hodgkin's disease. Granulomas in the bone marrow. a and b Gallamine-Giemsa, c and d Hematoxylin. a and c ×800; b and d ×100

Table 6. Nodular and diffuse bone-marrow involvement in non-Hodgkin lymphomas

All cases	Bone-marrow involvement:		
	diffuse	nodular	total
38	13	9	22

Table 7. Frequency of bone-marrow involvement in non-Hodgkin lymphomas detected by biopsy and by aspiration

	All cases	% positive:	
		biopsy	aspiration
JONES *et al.* (1972)	218	18	6
GRANN *et al.* (1966)	39	33	33
GÜLLER *et al.* (1972)	23	38	34
HENNEKEUSER (1972)	38	58	29

Table 8. Frequency of bone-marrow involvement in non-Hodgkin lymphomas

	All cases	% positive
JONES *et al.* (1972)	218	18
GRANN *et al.* (1966)	39	33
GÜLLER *et al.* (1972)	35	39
HENNEKEUSER (1972)	38	58

Table 9. Bone-marrow involvement and histological type in non-Hodgkin lymphomas (JONES *et al.* 1972)

	All cases	% positive
Histiocytic	62	5
Mixed cellularity	85	18
Lymphocytic	68	26

Table 10. Clinical stage and bone-marrow involvement in non-Hodgkin lymphomas (JONES *et al.* 1972)

Stage	No. positive/ No. patients	%
I+II	2/78	3
III+IV	34/140	24

From the reported data we conclude that in all cases of malignant lymphoma in Stages III or IV, histological examination of the bone marrow should be performed when positive findings are followed by a change of the stage or therapy. During Stages I and II, increased alkaline phosphatase, unexplained anemia, granulocytopenia and thrombocytopenia, roentgenographic or scintigraphic evidence of bone disease as well as general symptoms (fever, night sweats, weight loss) are indications for bone-marrow biopsy [10, 23, 24, 25]. Moreover, a bone-marrow examination should be performed in all patients suffering relapse [23]. In HD positive results are more frequently observed with the lymphocyte depletion types and in non-Hodgkin lymphomas with the lymphocytic types (Tables 5 and 9). In 10—50% of patients in Stage III, generalization with extranodal tissue involvement is detected by histological examination of the bone marrow (Tables 3 and 10). The staging diagnosis is then changed to Stage IV. Bone-marrow biopsy, as the less dangerous procedure, should precede diagnostic laparotomy, since demonstration of marrow involvement is a sufficient criterion for Stage IV. Histological examination of the bone marrow also permits good determination of hematopoietic characteristics and is superior to aspiration for the detection of bone-marrow involvement in malignant lymphomas.

Acknowledgement

I would like to thank Mrs. A. H. LINDE for excellent technical assistance.

References

1. AISENBERG, A. C.: Primary management of Hodgkin's disease. New Engl. J. Med. **278**, 93 (1968).
2. BENNETT, J. M., GRALNICK, H. R., DE VITA, V. T.: Bone marrow biopsy in Hodgkin's disease. New Engl. J. Med. **278**, 1179 (1968).
3. BURKHARDT, R.: Farbatlas der klinischen Histopathologie von Knochenmark und Knochen. Berlin-Heidelberg-New York: Springer 1970.
4. DORFMAN, R. F.: Relationship of histology to site in Hodgkin's disease. Cancer Res. **31**, 1786 (1971).
5. DORFMAN, R. F.: Formal discussion of Robert J. Luke's paper "Criteria for involvement of lymph node, bone marrow, spleen, and liver in Hodgkin's disease". Cancer Res. **31**, 1768 (1971).
6. DUHAMEL, G.: Importance of the bone marrow biopsy for the staging of Hodgkin's disease. A study of 100 cases. XIV International Congress of Hematology, São Paulo 1972, Abstracts.
7. GRANN, V., POOL, J. L., MAYER, K.: Comparative study of bone marrow aspiration and biopsy in patients with neoplastic disease. Cancer (Philad.) **19**, 1898 (1966).
8. GÜLLER, R., SENN, H. J., NAGEL, G. A., GUDAT, F., GYR, K.: Die Bedeutung der Knochenmark- und Leberpunktion bei malignen Lymphomen. Schweiz. med. Wschr. **102**, 317 (1972).
9. HENNEKEUSER, H. H.: Histochemischer Nachweis von Naphthol-AS-D-Chloroacetat-Esterase an Methacrylat-Schnitten. Klin. Wschr. **50**, 213 (1972).
10. JONES, S. E., ROSENBERG, S. A., KAPLAN, H. S.: Non-Hodgkin's lymphomas. I. Bone marrow involvement. Cancer (Philad.) **29**, 954 (1972).
11. KADIN, M. E., DONALDSON, S. S., DORFMAN, R. F.: Isolated granulomas in Hodgkin's disease. New Engl. J. Med. **283**, 859 (1970).

12. KADIN, M. E., GLATSTEIN, E., DORFMAN, R. F.: Clinicopathologic studies of 117 untreated patients subjected to laparotomy for the staging of Hodgkin's disease. Cancer (Philad.) 27, 1277 (1971).
13. KAPLAN, H. S.: Clinical evaluation and radiotherapeutic management of Hodgkin's disease and the malignant lymphomas. New Engl. J. Med. **278**, 892 (1968).
14. KAPLAN, H. S.: Contiguity and progression in Hodgkin's disease. Cancer Res. **31**, 1811 (1971).
15. LENNERT, K., MESTDAGH, J.: Lymphogranulomatosen mit konstant hohem Epitheloidzellgehalt. Virchows Arch. Abt. A Path. **344**, 1 (1968).
16. LIAO, K. T.: The superiority of histologic sections of aspirated bone marrow in malignant lymphomas. Cancer (Philad.) **27**, 618 (1971).
17. LUKES, R. J.: Criteria for involvement of lymph node, bone marrow, spleen, and liver in Hodgkin's disease. Cancer Res. **31**, 1755 (1971).
18. LUKES, R. J., BUTLER, J. J.: The pathology and nomenclature of Hodgkin's disease. Cancer Res. **26**, 1063 (1966).
19. MUSSHOFF, K.: Grundlagen der Strahlentherapie des Morbus Hodgkin, Indikation und Ergebnisse. Z. Krebsforsch. **78**, 162 (1972).
20. OEHLERT, W., MUSSHOFF, K., WUNSCH, B., WILLMANN, H., BECK, K.: Unspezifische Mesenchymreaktionen und Parenchymschäden der Leber bei Patienten mit Morbus Hodgkin. Klin. Wschr. **48**, 126 (1970).
21. RAPPAPORT, H.: Atlas of Tumor Pathology, Section 3, Fascicle 8, Tumors of the hematopoietic system. Washington: Armed Forces Institute of Pathology 1966.
22. RAPPAPORT, H., BERARD, C. W., BUTLER, J. J., DORFMAN, R. F., LUKES, R. J., THOMAS, L. B.: Report of the committee on histopathological criteria contributing to staging of Hodgkin's disease. Cancer Res. **31**, 1864 (1971).
23. ROSENBERG, S. A.: Hodgkin's disease of the bone marrow. Cancer Res. **31**, 1733 (1971).
24. ROSENBERG, S. A., BOIRON, M., DE VITA, V. T., JOHNSON, R. E., LEE, B. J., ULTMANN, J. E., VIAMONTE, M.: Report of the committee on Hodgkin's disease staging procedures. Cancer Res. **31**, 1862 (1971).
25. TUBIANA, M.: Summary of informal discussion on staging procedures in Hodgkin's disease. Cancer Res. **31**, 1751 (1971).
26. UEHLINGER, E.: Über Knochenlymphogranulomatose. Virchows Arch. path. Anat. **288**, 36 (1933).
27. WEBB, D. J., UBOGY, G., SILVER, R. T.: Importance of bone marrow biopsy in the clinical staging of Hodgkin's disease. Cancer (Philad.) **26**, 313 (1970).

Radioisotope Investigations in Malignant Lymphoma

K. zum Winkel, B. K. Das, and U. Haubold

Summary

Radioisotopic investigations were performed in 145 patients with malignant lymphoma. A critical evaluation of the results was undertaken to assure the efficiency of different isotopic procedures. Liver and spleen scanning was successfully administered to verify involvement of the organs. Bone scanning rendered many positive results in cases of skeletal lesions. Comparative studies of lymphoscintigraphy and lymphography revealed a high percentage of conformity. Scintigraphy using 67 Gallium was successful in the localization of lesion particularly in the upper half of the body.

Introduction

Large-scale application of radioisotopic procedures in the diagnosis of the lymphoma group of neoplastic diseases is to be recommended for the following reasons:

1. The simple technique involves little inconvenience for the patient.
2. The low substance load and minimum radiation exposure results in minimal risk to the patient.
3. Lymphatic lesions are readily demonstrated.
4. Organ involvement outside the lymphatic system can be verified.

Several institutions have performed radioisotopic scanning of patients with malignant lymphoma [1, 2, 4, 5, 6, 7, 8, 10]. However, the efficiency of the different methods in systemic disease has been seldom reported. We have critically evaluated the results of various radioisotopic procedures in malignant lymphoma cases seen at our institute since 1969.

Method

Liver scans were performed with a multi-detector scanner (Dynapix) 30 min after i.v. injection of labeled colloids (Au-198, In-113m, Tc-99m). Anterior, posterior and lateral views of the liver were taken routinely.

Spleen scintigraphy was performed with a 5-in. scanner in the usual manner 30 min after injection of ^{197}Hg-BMHP. Anterior and lateral views of the spleen were routinely obtained.

This report deals with lymphoscintigraphic examination restricted to the retroperitoneal area and covering the inguinal, external and common iliac as well as the para-aortic lymph nodes. Twenty-four hours after the subcutaneous injection of 150 μCi colloidal ^{198}Au into the dorsum of each foot, scintigraphy was performed with a scintillation camera. Occasionally, a 5-in. scanner was used. Many of these patients (63 out of 89) had also undergone a lymphography, so the results of both methods could be compared.

Bone scans were performed 60 min after i.v. administration of ^{87m}Sr by means of a multi-detector scanner. Skeletal imaging was carried out at 3 levels: skull and neck to the middle of the thoracic vertebrae; from middle to the end of the lumbar vertebrae; pelvis including the proximal parts of the femora.

Scintigrams to localize the disease by means of ^{67}Ga were obtained 24 h after i.v. application of 1 to 2 mCi. ^{67}Ga citrate. The multi-detector scanner was used for this purpose.

Results

Table 1 summarizes results from our patients with Hodgkin's disease, retothelial sarcoma, lymphosarcoma and Brill-Symmers disease. All cases were histologically verified. Radioisotopic investigations have been carried out in 145 patients with malignant lymphoma over a period of 3$^1/_2$ years. The ratio of male to female patients was almost equal.

Table 1. Distribution of patients as determined by radioisotopic investigations

Histological diagnosis	Total number	Male	Female
Hodgkin's disease	83	42	41
Retothelial sarcoma	46	26	20
Lymphosarcoma	12	6	6
Brill-Symmers disease	4	1	3
Total	145	75	70

Hepatic scanning was performed in 120 patients. Follow-up examinations are not counted in addition to the first examination; only the latest finding in each case is evaluated. Various criteria such as size of liver, pattern of activity distribution and parenchymal defects are specially considered. Confluent inhomogeneity showing several cold areas is classified as multiple affection (Table 2).

Hepatomegaly was found in 39 cases (31%), whereas large parenchymal defects are rather rare (17 cases = 14%). Remarkably, all cases of Hodgkin's disease with confirmed cervical manifestation had a normal liver scan.

Spleen scans were carried out in 116 patients; 66 (57%) revealed a spleen of normal size though 5 had irregular uptake of radioactivity. The remaining 50 (43%) showed an enlarged spleen; large parenchymal defects were found in only 4 cases (Table 3).

Table 2. Results of liver scanning (120 patients)

Diagnosis	Normal size homogeneous distribution	Normal size nonhomogeneous distribution	Enlarged homogeneous distribution	Enlarged nonhomogeneous distribution	Multiple affections	Large defects
Hodgkin's disease (n=67)	24	3	12	13	6	9
Retothelial sarcoma (n=39)	15	5	5	5	3	6
Lymphosarcoma (n=10)	4	1	1	3	0	1
Brill-Symmers disease (n=4)	3	0	0	0	0	1

Table 3. Results of spleen scanning (116 patients)

Diagnosis	Normal size homogeneous distribution	Normal size nonhomogeneous distribution	Enlarged homogeneous distribution	Enlarged inhomogeneous distribution	Large defects
Hodgkin's disease (n=66)	35	3	21	5	2
Retothelial sarcoma (n=36)	18	1	13	3	1
Lymphosarcoma (n=10)	5	1	3	1	
Brill-Symmers (n=4)	3	0	0	0	1

Lymphoscintigraphy performed on 89 patients with malignant lymphoma showed a normal finding in the retroperitoneal area in only 9 cases. The remaining 80 cases reveal either generalized or localized involvement of iliac or para-aortic lymph nodes (Table 4). In this synopsis, only the primary findings of different investigators have been evaluated.

To compare lymphoscintigraphy with lymphography, we undertook a re-evaluation of the scintigraphic findings which differed partly (mainly in cases of "suspected affection") from the preliminary descriptions (Table 4). The radiological and scintigraphic results show a remarkable equivalence (Table 5). The divergent results in 13 cases are probably due to the long time interval between the two investigations. For example, in 4 cases with divergent results in lymphogranulomatosis, lymph-node scanning was conducted almost a year after lymphography. A further specification, however, was not made. It is interesting to note that affected lymph nodes with slight

Table 4. Results of retroperitoneal lymphoscintigraphy (89 patients)

Diagnosis	Normal	Generalized involvement	Localized involvement	Suspected affections
Hodgkin's disease (n=49)	5	21	20	3
Retothelial sarcoma (n=27)	3	14	7	3
Lymphosarcoma (n=9)	1	5	3	0
Brill-Symmers disease (n=4)	0	4	0	0
89	9	44	30	6

Table 5. Results of retroperitoneal lymphoscintigraphy compared with lymphography (63 patients)

Diagnosis	Normal	Suspected affections	Involvement	Conformity with lympho-graphy	No con-formity with lympho-graphy
Hodgkin's disease (n=34)	3	9	22	25	9
Retothelial sarcoma (n=20)	4	2	14	17	3
Lymphosarcoma (n=5)	0	1	4	4	1
Brill-Symmers disease (n=4)	0	0	4	4	0

enlargement and good uptake of Lipiodol in lymphography present an inconspicuous finding in lymphoscintigraphy. We observed this in 3 cases of Hodgkin's disease and in 2 cases of retothelial sarcoma.

Bone scanning was performed in 34 patients in various stages of malignant lymphoma. Only 10 had a normal finding, whereas 16 cases showed definite bone involvement. In the remaining 8 cases, only slightly increased localized ^{87m}Sr uptake was observed, and this could not be differentiated from benign bone conditions. We have recorded such cases as "suspected" bone lesions (Table 6).

The use of ^{67}Ga in tumor diagnosis has given interesting results in recent years. In our 35 patients with lymphoma who received gallium scintigraphy, significant localized concentration of radioactivity is found in Hodgkin's disease. Surprisingly, a high accumulation of ^{67}Ga is observed in sarcoidosis. No significant gallium concentration is seen in toxoplasmosis and syphilis nor in one patient with lymphogranulomatosis and one patient with lymphosarcoma (Table 7).

Of 14 patients who had already undergone treatment, positive localization was seen only in 2 cases, one being a case of Hodgkin's disease and the other of tuberculosis (Table 7).

Table 6. Results of bone scanning (34 patients)

Diagnosis	Normal	Bone lesions	Suspected bone lesions
Hodgkin's disease (n=17)	4	8	5
Retothelial sarcoma (n=12)	4	6	2
Lymphosarcoma (n=4)	1	2	1
Brill-Symmers disease (n=1)	1	0	0

Table 7. Accumulation of ^{67}Ga in lymphoma (35 patients)

	Untreated (21 patients)		Treated (14 patients)	
	+	∅	+	∅
Hodgkin's disease	11	1	1	6
Lymphosarcoma	1	1	—	—
Reticulosarcoma	—	—	∅	2
Brill-Symmers disease	—	—	∅	2
Boeck's disease	4	∅	∅	2
Toxoplasmosis	∅	2	—	—
Tuberculosis	—	—	1	—
Syphilis	∅	1	—	—

Table 8. Accumulation of ^{67}Ga and histological type in Hodgkin's disease (20 patients)

Histological type	Untreated		Treated	
	+	∅	+	∅
Lymphogranulomatosis without further classification	4	—	1	2
Reticulocellular	3	—	—	3
Lymphocytic	1 (+)	1	—	—
Mixed form	1	—	—	1
Sclerotic	1	—	1	—
Paragranuloma	1	—	—	—

Assuming that different histological types of Hodgkin's disease may have specific patterns of ^{67}Ga uptake, we undertook a further subdivision (Table 8). No ^{67}Ga accumulation was observed in an untreated case of the lymphocytic type, whereas significant concentration occurred even after treatment in a case of sclerotic type.

Discussion

Enlargement of the liver is easily diagnosed by means of liver scintigraphy. A diffuse involvement of the organ in the form of many small foci of diseases tissue cannot be distinguished from other benign affections and can only be described as inhomogeneous distribution of radioactivity. Multiple nodules showing large defects are rather seldom seen. Within these limitations, liver scintigraphy can be recommended as an useful diagnostic measure. Doubtful cases must be confirmed by means of celiac angiography or laparoscopy.

Similar results are obtained by scanning the spleen [3]. More than 40% of our patients had some enlargement; massive lesions were found only occasionally. Of course, no reference was made to the stage of the disease in the present study. Our series of patients is too small for subclassification. However, our experience leads us to recommend spleen scintigraphy of all patients in whom a malignant lymphoma has been found.

The retroperitoneal lymphatic system is a common site for manifestation of systemic disease. Lymphoscintigraphy is a simple diagnostic procedure for detecting involvement of retroperitoneal lymph nodes which are otherwise not easily accessible [14]. The affected lymph nodes are characterized by lack of uptake of radioactivity, localized or generalized reduction in concentration of radioactivity, and enlargement or dislocation of the uptake area [11]. Although a normal scintigraphic finding can almost rule out a lymphatic lesion, we observed a normal lymph node scan while the lymphograph showed an involvement in 3 cases of Hodgkin's disease and 2 cases of retothelial sarcoma. Lymphoscintigraphy allows selection of patients for endolymphatic therapy and should therefore be performed before a patient with malignant lymphoma is subjected to lymphography [15]. Another advantage of lymphoscintigraphy is that it can be repeated several times and is therefore suitable for therapeutic follow-up as well as in cases where the evacuation of lipiodol after lymphography has proceeded too far for evaluation.

Bone scanning is an unspecific procedure for localizing increased mineral metabolism. For determination of skeletal involvement, however, the method is eminently suitable; it demonstrates 80% [9, 13] of the total positive cases as opposed to 40% with radiological devices. Bone scintigraphy is therefore very important for localizing bone lesions in cases of malignant lymphoma. Another advantage is that of quick and accurate investigation of the whole skeletal system that can be repeated several times for follow-up studies after radiation therapy [12].

Our present experience indicates that ^{67}Ga scintigraphy is an excellent method for the localization of lesions, which are often found in unexpected areas. It is, however, difficult to distinguish lesions in the skeletal system from those in the vicinity of the gastrointestinal tract or in the liver, as ^{67}Ga is normally either accumulated or excreted in these regions. The procedure is particularly suitable for positive localization of lesions in the upper half of the body. Careful observation and further investigations of the pattern of ^{67}Ga uptake in different histological types are necessary, as this may afford prognostic predictions.

The results of this study have been presented in tabular form. Certain limitations, particularly in the comparison of lymphoscintigraphy and lymphography, could not be avoided. Both for diagnostic purposes and for the classification of patients with malignant lymphoma we consider all these radioisotopic procedures very valuable.

References

1. ALTENBRUNN, H.-J.: Die heutigen Möglichkeiten der positiven Tumorszintigraphie. In: Frontiers of Nuclear Medicine. (Ed.: W. Horst.) Berlin-Heidelberg-New York: Springer 1971.
2. FEINE, U., ZUM WINKEL, K.: Nuklearmedizin — Szintigraphische Diagnostik. Stuttgart: Thieme 1969.
3. FISCHER, J., LEON, A., WOLF, R.: Etat actuel de la scintigraphie splénique: résultats cliniques dans 4500 cas. In: Medical Radioisotope Scintigraphy, Vol. II, p. 381. Wien: IAEA 1969.
4. HAUBOLD, U.: Methoden und Ergebnisse der Leberszintigraphie. Dtsch. med. Wschr. **94**, 386 (1969).
5. KLEIN, U., HAUBOLD, U., HÖR, G., PAPST, H. W., SHEYBANI, M.: Die Szintigraphie in der Differentialdiagnose abdominaler Tumoren. In: Aktuelle Gastroenterologie. Stuttgart: Thieme 1968.
6. KLEIN, U., HAUBOLD, U., PAPST, H. W.: Die Lymphszintigraphie in der Verlaufskontrolle maligner Erkrankungen unter besonderer Berücksichtigung der Hämoblastosen. In: Maligne Lymphome. Strahlentherapie Suppl. 69 (1969).
7. LAHNHAMMER, H., GLAUBITT, G., GREBE, S. F., HAMPE, J. F., HAUBOLD, U., HÖR, G., KAUL, A., KOEPPE, P., KOPPENHAGEN, K., ROEDELER, H. D., VAN DER SCHOOT, J. B.: ^{67}Ga for tumor scanning. J. nucl. Med. **13**, 25 (1972).
8. MCAFEE, J. G., AUSE, R. G., WAGNER, H. N., Jr.: Diagnostic value of scintillation scanning of the liver. Arch. intern. Med. **116**, 95 (1965).
9. DE NARDO, G. L., VOLPE, J. A.: Detection of bone lesions with the strontium-85 scintiscan. J. nucl. Med. **7**, 219 (1966).
10. PAPST, H. W.: Nuklearmedizinische Möglichkeiten zur Diagnose und Lokalisation maligner Tumoren. Wien. med. Wschr. **120**, 788 (1970).
11. ZUM WINKEL, K.: Lymphologie mit Radionukliden. Berlin 1972.
12. ZUM WINKEL, K.: Determination of metastases in bone and lymph nodes. XII. Intern. Congr. Radiology, Tokyo, October 1969.
13. ZUM WINKEL, K., DREYER, H. J., HERB, R., HARBST, H., GEORGI, M., MAIER-BORST, W.: Szintigraphie von Knochen- und Gelenkaffektionen mit Fluor-18 im Vergleich zur Röntgendiagnostik. Deutscher Röntgenkongreß 1969, p. 23. Stuttgart: Thieme 1970.
14. ZUM WINKEL, K., VON KEISER, D.: Kombinierte Metastasensuche im Bauchraum mit der Szintigraphie des Lymphsystems und der Kavographie. Fortschr. Röntgenstr. **100**, 90 (1964).
15. ZUM WINKEL, K., BECKER, J., SCHEURLEN, H., GEORGI, M., JAHNS, E., HERZFELD, U.: Endolymphatische Therapie mit Radioisotopen. Therapiewoche **34**, 1170 (1967).

Diagnosis of Malignant Lymphoma with ^{67}Gallium

S. F. GREBE, H. G. SCHMIDT, F. DIETZEL, and M. RÖMER

Summary

^{67}Gallium shows a tendency to be accumulated in malignant tumors. However, the incorporation of this radioactive nuclide occurs also in acute or chronically inflammable processes (silicosis, tuberculosis). The critical organ is the liver. The absorbed dose in the liver is app. 1.3 rad. The accumulation in the tumor or lymphnodes can be measured optimally after 4—6 days, since by this time the interfering activity of the liver and intestine has worn off to a great extent. ^{67}Ga scans of malignant lymphoma in the abdomen are of considerably limited diagnostic value because of the superposition of the liver and intestinal activity. The mediastinum, however, which is not so easily accessible by X-ray, represents a suitable object for ^{67}Ga scans. This was shown in 20 cases of malignant lymphoma in the mediastinum; 16 of these cases showed a ^{67}Ga accumulation. In some cases the scan becomes positive prior to the radiograph.

The clinical use of ^{67}Ga in tumor scanning derives from the initial observation of EDWARDS and HAYES [3], that ^{67}Ga is concentrated in human neoplasms. These authors, while assessing the value of the ^{67}Ga as a bone-scanning agent, noted uptake in the enlarged cervical nodes of a patient with Hodgkin's disease. This affinity for carrier-free ^{67}Ga has been proved in a variety of human and animal malignant tumors by a number of authors [1, 2, 4—25]. We have also published a number of reports [8, 9, 15, 18, 23].

^{67}Ga is produced in a cyclotron (Philips). One ml of solution for injection contains 1 mCi ^{67}Ga, 1.6—2.6 mg sodium citrate and 9 mg benzyl alcohol in an isotonic solution of sodium chloride. The patients received the equivalent 2—3 mCi ^{67}Ga citrate intravenously. Scans were performed 2 and 3 days after injection with a 5-in. scanner (Friesecke or Siemens). For visualizing processes near to the surface, a fine-focus collimator was applied, and for deeply situated lesions, a coarse-focus collimator. In view of the technical limitations of the scanner, measurements were performed differentially (185—296 KeV) or integrally (lower window at 160 KeV).

The total body-radiation load is 506 mrad at doses of 2.5 mCi. The critical organ is the liver, in which the radiation dosage amounts to about 1.3 rad [8, 9, 15, 18].

One can detect and locate soft tissue scintigraphically and estimate its extent [1, 2, 4—25]. Superficial tumors can be demonstrated, if the diameter exceeds 0.8 cm, and for more deeply situated tumors if the diameter exceeds 2 cm [8, 9]. It is remarkable that dependence of ^{67}Ga accumulation on the histological type of tumor was not found [15, 18]. The uptake of ^{67}Ga in the cytoplasm of malignant cells is greater in non-necrotic than in necrotic tumors [6]. The mechanism of ^{67}Ga citrate uptake is unknown, but may be related to metabolic activity, protein synthesis or macrophage activity [22]. The affinity of ^{67}Ga for malignant tumors is not specific since non-malignant processes can also store ^{67}Ga. This was observed often in silicosis [23] and tuberculosis [15, 18, 23] but seldom in inflammatory lesions [20]. Concentration of

Fig. 1. ^{67}Ga accumulation in a peripheral bronchial carcinoma of the right lung and in a lymph node metastasis from the mediastinum. The physiological ^{67}Ga accumulation in the liver is visible at the base of the lung

^{67}Ga in tumors was found in untreated as well as in treated patients [14, 15, 18], but a negative scan was found more frequently in treated patients [15, 18]. Comparative control examinations before and after therapy are in progress.

Outside the abdominal area 80—90 percent of malignant diseases have a positive scan [8, 9, 15, 18]. Fig. 1 demonstrates a ^{67}Ga accumulation in a peripheral bronchial carcinoma on the right lung and in a lymph-node metastasis from the mediastinum. At the base of the lung one can see physiological ^{67}Ga enrichment of the liver. In the abdominal cavity, distinction of ^{67}Ga accumulation by a tumor from physiological ^{67}Ga concentration in the liver and colon may be difficult, though they are of different intensity. To separate pathological ^{67}Ga accumulation from colon and liver activity, we performed serial scannings on different days. Fig. 2 shows the same

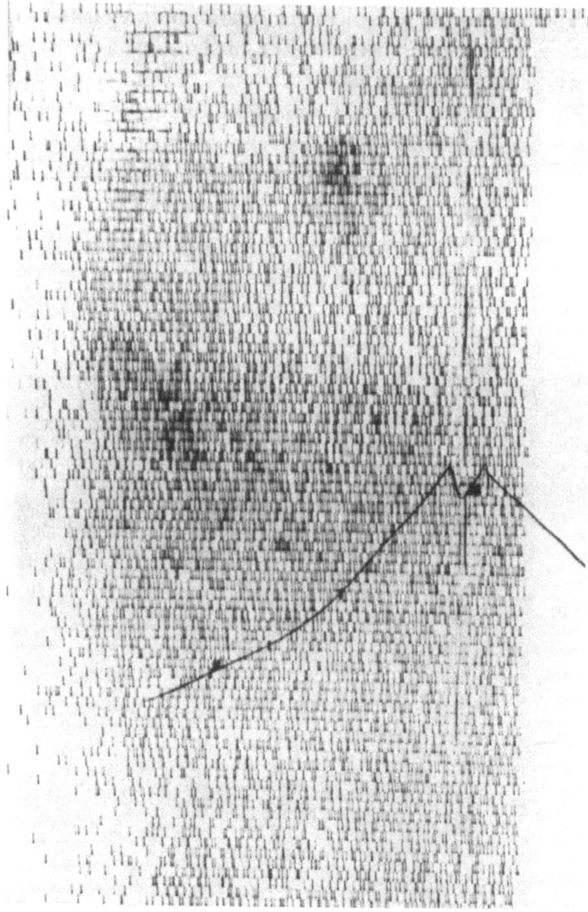

Fig. 2. The same patient as in Fig. 1. Scanned on the following day. ^{67}Ga has left the liver

patient as in Fig. 1; this scan was carried out on the following day. At this time ^{67}Ga has left the liver, and activity remains only in the peripheral bronchial carcinoma and in the lymph-node metastasis from the mediastinum. ^{67}Ga can often be removed from the colon by means of a purgative and the tumor can be demonstrated by scintigraphy between days 4 and 6 [9, 15, 18].

A large number of positive scans (70—90%) were found in local or generalized malignant disease of the reticulohistiocytic system [9, 15, 17, 18, 19, 22, 23, 24]. We obtained 16 positive scans in 20 cases. Among 16 patients with Hodgkin's disease, 14 showed ^{67}Ga accumulation in the pathological nodes.

One can often visualize a pathological area earlier with a ^{67}Ga scan than with other methods. The mediastinum is a particularly difficult area for assessment by conventional methods, and Fig. 3 is an example of the results obtained with ^{67}Ga. Hodgkin's disease was found histologically in the enlarged cervical nodes on the right. Some years before, this patient had tuberculosis, and a thoracoplasty was performed on the right side. The X-ray did not show any enlarged lymph nodes in the mediastinum.

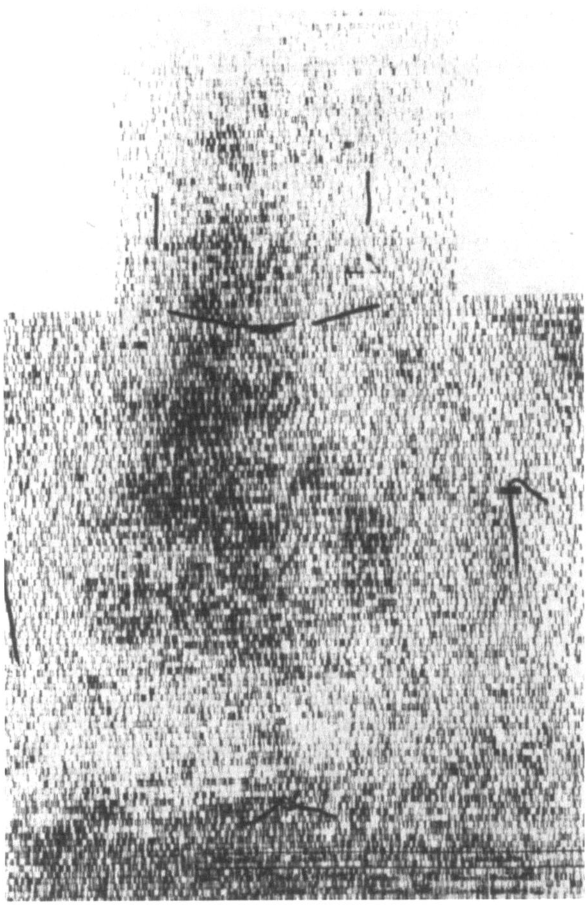

Fig. 3. ^{67}Ga accumulation in a chain of lymph nodes in the mediastinum

Although the uptake of ^{67}Ga is nonspecific, ^{67}Ga scanning is a helpful tool in the clinical diagnosis of malignant lymphoma or Hodgkin's disease when used in conjunction with clinical, laboratory, and radiological findings. There are still many problems to be resolved, for example:

Is there any change in ^{67}Ga accumulation before and after irradiation or chemotherapy? What ^{67}Ga accumulation is seen in the spleen when this organ is affected? What are the percentages of false-positive and false-negative results?

References

1. Ando, A., Hisada, K.: Affinity of Gallium-67 for malignant tumor. Radioisotopes **19**, 239 (1970).
2. Chaudri, M. A., Lavender, J. P., Barker, J. R., Lowe, J.: ^{67}Ga citrate for localization in neoplastic and inflammatory tissue. 8. Jahrestg. Ges. Nuclearmed. Hannover 1970. Stuttgart: Schattauer 1972.

3. Edwards, C. L., Hayes, R. L.: Tumor scanning with ^{67}Ga-citrate. J. nucl. Med. 10, 103 (1969).
4. Edwards, C. L., Hayes, R. L.: Scanning tumors of soft tissue and bone with ^{67}Ga-citrate. J. nucl. Med. **11**, 332 (1970).
5. Edwards, C. L., Hayes, R. L., Nelson, B. M., Tehranian, N.: Clinical investigation of ^{67}Ga for tumor scanning. J. nucl. Med. **11**, 316 (1970).
6. Edwards, C. L., Hayes, R. L.: Scanning malignant neoplasms with gallium 67. J. Amer. med. Ass. **212**, 1184 (1970).
7. Fehling, H., Würdinger, H.: Untersuchungen der Tumorspezifität von Gallium-67. 8. Jahrestg. Ges. Nuclearmed. Hannover 1970. Stuttgart: Schattauer 1972.
8. Grebe, S. F., Steckenmesser, R., Römer, M.: Radioaktives ^{67}Ga in der nuklearmedizinischen Tumordiagnostik. Münch. med. Wschr. **113**, 238 (1971).
9. Grebe, S. F., Schoen, H., Steckenmesser, R., Heger, N.: Die Möglichkeiten des Nachweises und der Lokalisation von malignen Tumoren mit der ^{67}Ga-Szintigraphie. Fortschr. Röntgenstr. **116**, 73 (1972).
10. Hayes, R. L., Burd, B. L., Carlton, J. E., Rafto, J. J.: Factors affecting the localization of ^{67}Ga in animal tumors. J. nucl. Med. **11**, 324 (1970).
11. Hayes, R. L., Nelson, B., Swartzendruber, D. C., Carlton, J. E., Byrd, B. L.: Gallium-67 localization in rat and mouse tumors. Science **167**, 289 (1970).
12. Higasi, T., Ikemoto, S., Nakayama, Y., Hisada, T.: Diagnosis of malignant tumor with ^{67}Ga-citrate. Jap. J. nucl. Med. **6**, 226 (1969).
13. Higasi, T., Hisada, T., Nakayama, Y., Kinosita, Y., Kawat, K., Sozuki, S., Kato, H., Murata, A., Sugiyama, M., Kawaguchi, R., Nakamura, I.: Diagnosis of malignant tumor with ^{67}Gallium-citrate (2nd report). Radioisotopes **19**, 311 (1970).
14. Hisada, T., Hiraki, T.: Limit and significance of ^{67}Ga for diagnosis of malignant tumors. Igaku No Ayumi 72 (1970).
15. Hör, G., Glaubitt, D., Grebe, S. F., Hampe, J., Haubold, U., Kaul, A., Koeppe, P., Koppenhagen, J., Langhammer, H., van der Schoot, J. B.: Tumorszintigraphie mit ^{67}Ga. 8. Jahrestg. Ges. f. Nuclearmed. Hannover 1970. Stuttgart: Schattauer 1972.
16. Hundeshagen, H., Brase, A., Dittmann, A.: Möglichkeiten der positiven Tumordarstellung mit ^{67}Gallium. 8. Jahrestg. Ges. f. Nuclearmed. Hannover 1970. Stuttgart: Schattauer 1972.
17. Kay, D. N., McCready, V. R.: Clinical isotope scanning using ^{67}Ga citrate in the management of Hodgkin's disease. Brit. J. Radiol. **45**, 437 (1972).
18. Langhammer, H., Glaubitt, D., Grebe, S. F., Hampe, J. F., Haubold, U., Hör, G., Kaul, A., Koeppe, P., Koppenhagen, J., Roedler, H. D., van der Schoot, J. B.: ^{67}Ga for tumor scanning. J. nucl. Med. **13**, 25 (1972).
19. Larson, St. M., Milder, M. S., Tretner, I. H., Johnston, G. S.: Interpretation of ^{67}Ga in lymphoma and Leukemia. J. nucl. Med. **13**, 448 (1972).
20. Lavender, J. P., Lowe, J., Barker, J. R., Burn, J. I., Chaudhri, M. A.: Gallium 67 scanning in neoplastic and inflammatory lesions. Brit. J. Radiol. **44**, 361 (1971).
21. Manfredi, O. L., Quinones, J., Bartok, St.: ^{67}Ga-citrate scanning for tumor localization with microradioaudiography correlation. J. nucl. Med. **13**, 452 (1972).
22. Schwarzendruber, D. C., Nelson, B., Hayes, R. L.: Gallium-67 localization in lysosomalike granules of leucaemic and non-leucaemic murine tissues. J. nat. Cancer Inst. **46**, 941 (1971).
23. Steckenmesser, R., Grebe, S. F., Wentz, D., Bayindir, S.: Nuclearmedizinische Diagnostik im Thoraxraum. Congressus radiologicus Cechoslovacus, Brno 1972.
24. Turner, D. A., Gottschalk, A., Hoffer, P. B., Ultmann, J. E., Harper, P. V.: ^{67}scanning in the staging of malignant lymphoma: successes and failures. J. nucl. Med. **13**, 474 (1972).
25. Winchell, H. S., Sanchez, P. D., Watanabe, C. K., Hollander, L., Anger, H. O., McRae, J., Hayes, R. L., Edwards, C. L.: Visualization of tumors in humans using ^{67}Ga-citrate and the Anger whole-body scanner, scintillation camera and tomographic scanner. J. nucl. Med. **11**, 459 (1970).

Primary Extent, Later Extension and Stage as Factors in Therapy of Malignant Lymphoma

Presentation and Progression of Hodgkin's Disease

T. LANDBERG

Summary

Hodgkin's disease is primarily a disease of the lymphatic system. It may be unicentric from the beginning and then spread at first locally in the lymphatic system. Spread via the blood-stream seems to be more frequent with advancing disease, but may occur early. Direct overgrowth to extranodal sites may occur early in the course of the disease.

Initial Symptoms

The first symptom usually noted by the patient with Hodgkin's disease is enlarged lymph nodes, most often in the neck (Table 1). In about 15% of the patients, fever, weight loss, or asthenia is the first symptom.

Table 1. Initial symptom reported by the patient. From WESTLING [31]

Lymphoma in the	%
neck	56
axilla	7
groin	6
Fever, weight loss, asthenia	15
Cough, dyspnea, congestion	6
Other symptoms e. g. pruritus, pain	8
No symptoms at all	2

Evaluation of the Extent of Disease

In evaluating the extent of the disease, the larger lymph-node clusters are often divided into different regions. Fig. 1 illustrates the location of these lymph nodes. The division into different regions is purely topographical and linked with the different methods used to investigate particular regions. No sharp delineations seem to exist between the regions.

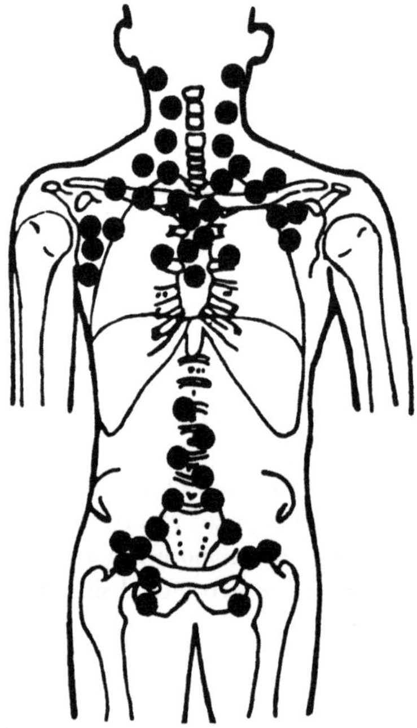

Fig. 1. Different lymph node regions (cervical, axillary, mediastinal, para-aortic, para-iliac and inguinal) frequently involved in Hodgkin's disease

When the extent of the disease is assessed without the aid of lymphography or staging laparotomy, the most common pathological finding is lymphomas in the neck, followed by the axilla, mediastinum and groin (Table 2; [14, 15]). Abdominal lymphomas, involvement of the lung tissue and of the spleen may also be detected in a considerable number of patients.

When first seen, most patients have involvement of the lymphatic tissue only. This applied to 71% of patients first seen during 1944—1965 (Fig. 2; [13, 14, 15, 16]), whereas the remaining 29% of the patients had extranodal disease and usually nodal disease in addition.

	Total 182 patients	
130/182=71% Involvement of lymph node groups only	← $p < 0.001$ →	52/182=29% Involvement of tissues outside the lymph node groups
91/130=70% Two or more groups involved		44/52=85% Two or more lymph node groups involved
72/91=79% All affected groups per continuitatem	← $p < 0.001$ →	19/44=43% All affected lymph node groups per continuitatem

Fig. 2. 182 patients with Hodgkin's disease grouped according to involvement before the beginning of treatment. Lund 1944—1965

Table 2. Clinical manifestations at the beginning of treatment in 149 patients with Hodgkin's disease evaluated without lymphography or laparotomy. Lund 1944—1960

	Number of sites involved
Lymphomas in the	
neck [a]	122
axilla [a]	73
mediastinum	57
groin [a]	40
cubital or popliteal Fossa	4
abdomen	16
Waldeyer's ring	1
Lung parenchyma	16
Liver	9
Spleen	10
Skeleton	3
Skin	9
Other tissues	7

[a] uni- or bilateral

Altogether, about 75% of the patients had involvement of at least two groups of lymph nodes, and all affected groups were contiguous in 72% of the patients with exclusively nodal disease, whereas this was the case in only 43% of patients who also had extranodal disease. These differences are highly significant. Thus, with the limited methods of evaluation used, the disease seemed to be mainly confined to the lymph nodes at the beginning of treatment, and then to affect mainly adjacent lymph-node regions. If extranodal sites were involved, the location of the disease at the beginning of treatment seemed to be more random.

The type of presentation is largely determined by the histological type of the disease [17]. It is well known that the lymphocyte predominance and nodular sclerosis types have a slower clinical course than the mixed cellularity or lymphocyte depletion types (Table 3). In patients with lymphocyte predominance or nodular sclerosis, involvement of two or more lymph-node groups was more often contiguous (Table 4) than in patients with mixed cellularity or lymphocyte depletion. The difference is highly significant.

The tendency for the nodular sclerosis type to affect mainly the mediastinum is well known, and in a group of 149 patients the frequency of mediastinal involvement was significantly higher for patients with nodular sclerosis than for patients with other histological types at the beginning of treatment, and almost significantly higher at the end of the follow-up (Table 5). PETERS [22] reported a better survival rate for patients with local disease if the mediastinum was affected, and stated that most patients who survived for 10 years had nodular sclerosis.

The histological type appears to affect both the location of disease and the speed of its spread.

In the patient groups mentioned so far, abdominal disease had been charted mainly by intravenous urography and liver function tests. The introduction of lymphography made it clear that these methods are highly unreliable in excluding abdominal disease.

Table 3. 146 patients with Hodgkin's disease grouped according to stage, histological type of lesion and duration of disease up to the beginning of treatment. Lund 1944—1960

	History (months)	Clinical stage according to JELLIFFE [8]	
Histological type		I or II	III
Lymphocyte predominance	< 6	6	1
	6—12	6	0
	> 12	4	0
Nodular sclerosis	< 6	14	6
	6—12	4	0
	> 12	2	5
Mixed cellularity	< 6	19	24
	6—12	4	12
	> 12	6	13
Lymphocyte depletion	< 6	3	10
	6—12	1	2
	> 12	0	4

Table 4. 135 patients with Hodgkin's disease in whom at least two lymph node groups were involved at the beginning of treatment. Lund 1944—1965

Histological type	All affected groups continuous	Affected groups discontinuous
Lymphocyte predominance or Nodular sclerosis	37 (=90%)	4 (=10%)
	↕ $p < 0.001$	
Mixed cellularity or Lymphocyte depletion	54 (=57%)	40 (=43%)

Table 5. Frequency of mediastinal involvement in 149 patients with Hodgkin's disease. Lund 1944—1960

Histological type	Mediastinal involvement At the beginning of treatment	At end of follow-up
Nodular sclerosis	65%	74%
Lymphocyte predominance Mixed cellularity Lymphocyte depletion	31%	49%
	38%	54%

Thus SCHWARZ [28] found that, prior to lymphography, 56% of the patients studied were placed in Stage I or II, whereas after lymphography 26% were transferred to Stage III. A further step towards the early detection of abdominal disease has been the introduction of staging laparotomy (Table 6). The inadequacy of staging without lymphography and laparotomy is thus apparent.

Table 6. Reports on findings at laparotomy in patients with Hodgkin's disease

	Number of patients	Positive findings at laparotomy (%)		
		10	Spleen	Abdominal lymph nodes
JELLIFFE *et al.* [9]	22	10	55	43
FARRER-BROWN *et al.* [5]	50	8	50	70
KADIN *et al.* [10]	117	26	38	32
HASS *et al.* [7]	50	0	50	35
PROSNITZ *et al.* [23]	40	11	38	50
	279	Liver	43	40

KAPLAN [11] illustrated the number of involved sites in 340 patients subjected to charting procedures that included lymphography and, in some instances, also laparotomy. The most common sites to be involved were the left side of the neck, the right side of the neck and the mediastinum; each site was involved in about 200 patients. The lumbar-para-aortic lymph nodes, the left axilla and, somewhat less often, the right axilla were involved in about 90 patients. The iliac or inguinal lymph nodes were involved in about 50 patients, the spleen in 44, lung parenchyma in 20 and the liver in 9 patients. If only one site was involved, as was the case in 54 patients, the location of disease was usually on one side of the neck or, more rarely, in the mediastinum, axilla, para-aortic or inguinal region.

Routes of Spread

There are three main routes of spread in Hodgkin's disease: via the lymphatics, via the blood stream [24], and by direct invasion [18]. The spread via the lymphatics may occur from one node to the next one, but the thoracic duct can act as a short cut between the abdomen and the left side of the neck ("mediastinal skip", [12]). The incidence of abdominal disease [3] was the same (54%) when the left or both sides of the neck were involved, but much lower (17%) when only the right side of the neck was involved. [4] have shown that Sternberg-Reed cells may be found in the thoracic duct lymph in patients with Hodgkin's disease, and if these cells are neoplastic, they may be of importance in the hematogenous spread of the disease. Such spread seems to be more common with advancing disease [30] and may explain some of the widespread manifestations seen in advanced disease. Even early in the disease, however, invasion of the blood stream may be detected [24], and invasion of veins in lymph-node biopsy material and spleens have been observed in up to 20% of the cases [25].

Such patients have a high frequency of extranodal involvement. It may be assumed that the spleen acts like a filter, removing some of circulating neoplastic cells from the blood stream. It has been suggested that the liver is usually involved via the portal system from the spleen [25].

Hodgkin's disease also has a tendency to spread locally, and it may invade neighbouring tissues directly from involved lymph nodes [18]. Such local overgrowth is most often seen in the lung, the chest wall and the skeleton. It does not worsen the prognosis [19].

Extension after the Initial Treatment

In a cluster of lymph nodes, the disease process may be more advanced than was expected from palpation. SLAUGHTER *et al.* [29] demonstrated in a neck dissection specimen that lymph nodes invaded by the pathological process in varying degrees merged with normal ones.

Radical radiotherapy should include not only the areas where the disease may be detected, but also areas with occult disease. For a long time it has been customary to irradiate only manifestly involved regions. Patients treated with such techniques often developed metastases. Fig. 3 illustrates how it may be impossible to catch up the progression of the disease in such a case.

The location of the first extension after the initial treatment has been reported by a number of authors (Table 7). The first extensions are often localized to lymph-node regions adjacent to those that were involved clinically at the beginning of treatment.

Of 94 patients with local disease first seen during 1944—1965 (Table 8), 29 showed no extension. The first extensions were exclusively nodal in about half the patients, and usually localized to regions adjacent to those initially involved; in 20% of patients the first extension involved extranodal sites. When different modes of spread after the initial treatment were analyzed with regard to the different histological types (Table 9), no significant differences could be detected between the histological types, but the numbers were small.

Table 7. Reports on location of first extension after initial treatment in localized Hodgkin's disease

	Number of patients	First extension	
		in a group adjacent to the initial site	at distant sites
CROSBIE [2]	42	15 (17)	19
PETERS [21]		with few exceptions	
SCHEER [27]	68	21	
NEWALL [20]	36	20	16
JELLIFFE [8]	18	12	6
ROSENBERG and KAPLAN [26]	90	22	4
HAN and STUTZMAN [6]	106	54	26
BANFI *et al.* [1]	79	57	22

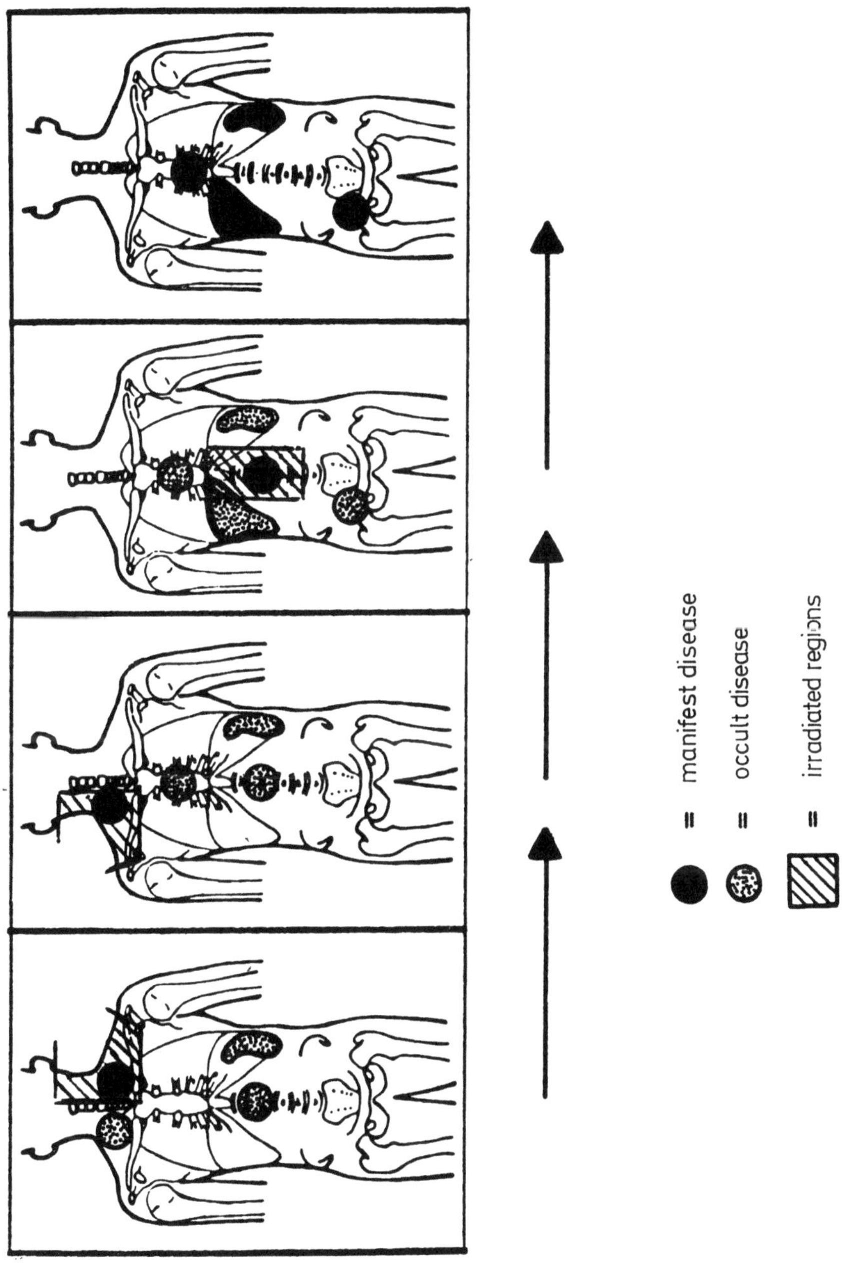

Fig. 3. Example of clinical progression of Hodgkin's disease treated with radiation therapy restricted to overtly involved regions

Table 8. Location of first extension after initial treatment in 94 patients with localized Hodgkin's disease. Lund 1944—1965

	Number of patients	%
No extensions noted	29	31
First extension in		
lymph node groups on the same side of the the diaphragm	34	36
lymph node groups on the other side of the diaphragm	8	9
lymph node groups on both sides of the diaphragm	4	4
tissues outside the lymph node groups	12	13
tissues outside the lymph node groups + in lymph node groups	7	7

Table 9. Location of first extension distributed among different histologic types in 94 patients with localized Hodgkin's disease. Lund 1944—1965

Histological type	No extensions noted	First extension only in lymph-node groups	outside lymph-node groups
Lymphocyte predominance	8 (40%)	9 (45%)	3 (15%)
Nodular sclerosis	9 (30%)	17 (57%)	4 (13%)
Mixed cellularity	12 (30%)	18 (45%)	10 (25%)
Lymphocyte depletion	0	2 (50%)	2 (50%)

Post-Mortem Findings

The post-mortem findings in Hodgkin's disease are greatly influenced by the therapy given. Table 10 shows the results of post-mortem examination in 31 patients first treated in the period 1944—1960. There was frequent involvement of the spleen, liver, lymph nodes in the mediastinum and retroperitoneum, and of the skeleton. Lymphomas in the superficial regions were much rarer, but this may have been an effect of therapy.

In conclusion, Hodgkin's disease is primarily a disease of the lymphatic system. It may be unilocular at the beginning and then spread at first locally in the lymphatic system. Spread via the blood stream seems to be more frequent with advancing disease, but may occur early. Direct overgrowth to extranodal sites may also occur in the course of the disease.

Table 10. Location of Hodgkin's disease at post-mortem examination in 31 patients. Lund 1944—1960

Spleen	28
Liver	23
Lymph nodes in mediastinum	23
Lymph nodes in retroperitoneum	20
Skeleton	17
Lymph nodes in axilla	10
Lymph nodes in mesentery	10
Lymph nodes in neck	7
Lymph nodes in groin	6
Kidney, lung, pleura, etc., per site	<5

References

1. BANFI, A., BONADONNA, G., CARNEVALI, G., OLDINI, C., SALVINI, E.: Preferential sites of involvement and spread in malignant lymphomas. Europ. J. Cancer 4, 319 (1968).
2. CROSBIE, J.: A clinical study of Hodgkin's disease. In: Progress in radiation therapy (BUSCHKE, F., Ed.). New York-London: Grune & Stratton 1962.
3. DORFMAN, R. F.: Relationship of histology to site in Hodgkin's disease. Cancer Res. 31, 1786 (1971).
4. ENGESET, A., BRENNHOVD, I. O., CHRISTENSEN, I., HAGEN, S., HOEG, K., HØST, H., LIVERUD, K., NESHEIM, A.: Sternberg-Reed cells in thoracic duct lymph of patients with Hodgkin's disease. Blood 31, 99 (1968).
5. FARRER-BROWN, G., BENNETT, M. H., HARRISON, C. V., MILLET, Y., JELLIFFE, A. M.: The pathological findings following laparotomy in Hodgkin's disease. Brit. J. Cancer 25, 449 (1971).
6. HAN, T., STUTZMAN, L.: Mode of spread in patients with localized malignant lymphomas. Arch. intern. Med. 120, 1 (1967).
7. HASS, A. C., BRUNK, S. F., GULESSERIAN, H. P., GIVLER, R. L.: The value of exploratory laparotomy in malignant lymphoma. Radiology 101, 157 (1971).
8. JELLIFFE, A. M.: The present place of radiotherapy in the cure of Hodgkin's disease. Clin. Radiol. 16, 274 (1965).
9. JELLIFFE, A. M., MILLET, Y. L., MARSTON, J. A. P., BENNETT, M. H., FARRER-BROWN, G., KENDALL, B., KEELING, D. H.: Laparotomy and splenectomy as routine investigations in the staging of Hodgkin's disease before treatment. Clin. Radiol. 21, 439 (1971).
10. KADIN, M. E., GLATSTEIN, E., DORFMAN, R. F.: Clinicopathologic studies of 117 untreated patients subjected to laparotomy for the staging of Hodgkin's disease. Cancer (Philad.) 27, 1277 (1971).
11. KAPLAN, H. S.: On the natural history, treatment, and prognosis of Hodgkin's disease. The Harvey Lectures, series 64, p. 215. New York-London: Academic Press 1970.
12. KAPLAN, H. S.: Contiguity and progression in Hodgkin's disease. Cancer Res. 31, 1811 (1971).
13. LANDBERG, T., LARSSON, L.-E.: Studium des klinischen Verlaufs bei Sternbergscher Erkrankung. Radiol. Aust. 18, 197 (1968).
14. LANDBERG, T., LARSSON, L.-E.: Hodgkin's disease. Retrospective clinico-pathologic study in 149 patients. Acta radiol. Ther. Phys. Biol. 8, 390 (1969).
15. LANDBERG, T.: Clinical course of Hodgkin's disease treated with radiotherapy. Acta radiol. Ther. Phys. Biol. 8, 487 (1969).
16. LANDBERG, T.: Hodgkin's disease. An analysis of a clinical material with respect to staging, histologic typing, clinical course and radiosensitivity. Lund: Studentlitteratur 1970.
17. LUKES, R. J., BUTLER, J. J., HICKS, E. B.: Natural history of Hodgkin's disease as related to its pathologic picture. Cancer (Philad.) 19, 317 (1966).

18. MUSSHOFF, K., RENEMANN, H., BOUTIS, L., AFKHAM, J.: Die extranoduläre Lymphogranulomatose. Fortschr. Röntgenstr. 109, 776 (1968).
19. MUSSHOFF, K.: Prognostic and therapeutic implications of staging in extranodal Hodgkin's disease. Cancer Res. 31, 1814 (1971).
20. NEWALL, J.: The management of Hodgkin's disease. Clin. Radiol. 16, 40 (1965).
21. PETERS, M. V.: A study of survivals in Hodgkin's disease treated radiologically. Amer. J. Roentgenol. 63, 299 (1950).
22. PETERS, M. V.: The need for a new classification in Hodgkin's disease. Cancer Res. 31, 1713 (1971).
23. PROSNITZ, L. R., NULAND, S. B., KLIGERMAN, M. M.: Role of laparotomy and splenectomy in the management of Hodgkin's disease. Cancer (Philad.) 29, 44 (1972).
24. RAPPAPORT, H., STRUM, S. B.: Vascular invasion in Hodgkin's disease. Cancer (Philad.) 25, 1304 (1970).
25. RAPPAPORT, H., STRUM, B., HUTCHISON, G., ALLEN, L. A.: Clinical and biological significance of vascular invasion in Hodgkin's disease. Cancer Res. 31, 1794 (1971).
26. ROSENBERG, S. A., KAPLAN, H. S.: Evidence for an orderly progression in the spread of Hodgkin's disease. Cancer Res. 26, 1225 (1966).
27. SCHEER, A. C.: The course of stage I malignant lymphomas following local treatment. Amer. J. Roentgenol. 90, 939 (1963).
28. SCHWARZ, G.: The role of lymphography. Hodgkin's disease. J. Amer. med. Ass. 190, 912 (1964).
29. SLAUGHTER, D. P., ECONOMOU, S. G., SOUTHWICK, H. W.: Surgical management of Hodgkin's disease. Ann. Surg. 148, 705 (1958).
30. SMITHERS, D. W.: Spread of Hodgkin's disease. Lancet 1970 I, 1262.
31. WESTLING, P.: Studies of the prognosis in Hodgkin's disease. Acta radiol. (Stockh.) Suppl. No. 245 (1965).

Reticulosarcoma and Lymphosarcoma, Pattern of Relapse and Spread

B. VAN DER WERF-MESSING

Summary

In a retrospective study of 142 cases of loco-regional lympho-reticulosarcoma, data have been collected concerning survival, local recurrence, regional extension and distant spread. Based on these data a trial was started in the O.E.R.T.C., comparing "loco-regional irradiation" with "loco-regional + lumbar irradiation".

The European Cooperative Group on Radiotherapy and Chemotherapy decided in 1970 to start a cooperative study on patients with reticulosarcoma and lymphosarcoma. A retrospective study was therefore undertaken of all patients with lymphosarcoma and reticulosarcoma treated at the Rotterdam Radiotherapy Institute between 1953 and 1963.

The patients were retrospectively staged according to the Rye Classification. No lymphography had been performed. All histological slides were reviewed. All patients had been treated by irradiation of the affected area; no prophylactic treatment was applied to the regional lymph nodes.

The actuarial survival according to stage is presented in Fig. 1. These data are in agreement with those reported by ENNUYER *et al.* [3], SCHEER [8] and DANCOT [1].

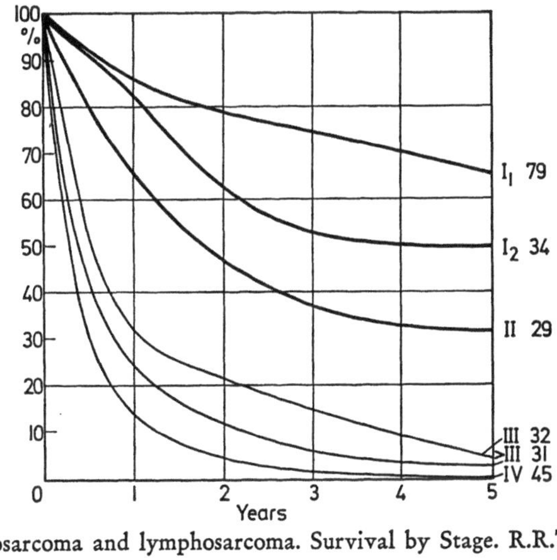

Fig. 1. Reticulosarcoma and lymphosarcoma. Survival by Stage. R.R.T.I. 1953—1963

Apart from intercurrent death, patients died of local recurrence, regional extension and distant metastases.

In order to improve initial prognosis, a local recurrence has to be prevented. For this purpose, a dose-response curve was constructed on the basis of our radiotherapy data (Fig. 2). From this curve it is evident that the curative dose range varies from 2000 rad distributed over five irradiation sessions to 4000 rad in 20—30 sessions.

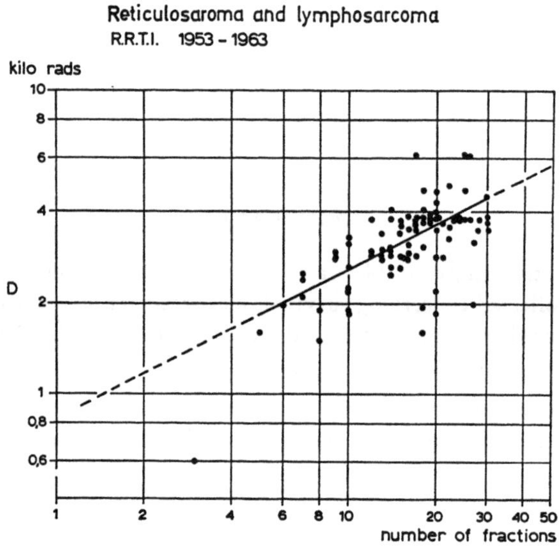

Fig. 2. Reticulosarcoma and lymphosarcoma. Relation between dose (in rad) and number of fractions for local cure. R.R.T.I. 1953—1963

To determine a useful prophylactic irradiation protocol, the pattern of spread for each primary location was assessed according to stage. Based on the results of this analysis, the potential survival rate offered by prophylactic regional irradiation could be assessed (Table 1). As a mediastinal skip could be demonstrated [9], the mediastinum was not included in the prophylactic irradiation region.

In a high percentage of cases, the first relapse after treatment of a supradiaphragmatic primary occurred in the lumbar-hepatosplenic region; therefore, potential survival rate was also calculated for prophylactic irradiation of this region (Table 2).

The potential survival rate after this type of prophylactic irradiation is similar to the potential survival after regional prophylactic irradiation.

By combining the advantages of both prophylactic irradiation procedures, potential survival after 5 years is about 80% in Stage I_1 (10% improvement), about 80% in Stage I_2 (30% improvement) and in Stage II about 75% (0% improvement; Table 3).

With modern supervoltage machines, it is not difficult to deliver a tumor-lethal dose of 4000 rad to all lymphatic regions above the diaphragm and an additional dose of 3500 rad to the subdiaphragmatic lumbar region. The European Radiotherapy Group, therefore, decided to start a randomized trial. Patients with a lymphosarcoma or a reticulosarcoma Stage I or II located above the diaphragm, are allocated at random to two treatment groups:

Table 1. Reticulosarcoma and lymphosarcoma R.R.T.I 1953—1963 possible benefit of restricted prophylactic regional irradiation (1st site above diaphragm)

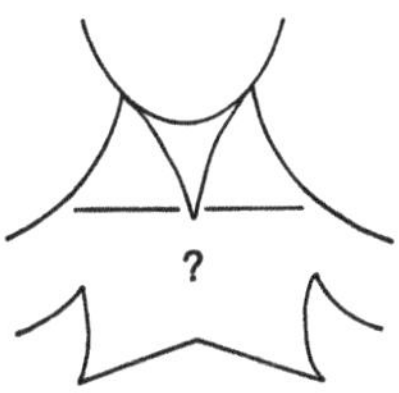

Stage	N	Actual 5-years survival	Predicted 5-years survival
I_1	64	70%	74% (+0) [a]
I_2	33	50%	60% (+6%) [a]
II	29	35%	58% (+3%) [a]

[a] Additional benefit of mediastinal spedition.

Table 2. Reticulosarcoma and lymphosarcoma R.R.T.I. 1953—1963 possible benefit of prophylactic combined restricted regional and liver-spleen-epigastric irradiation (1st site above diaphragm)

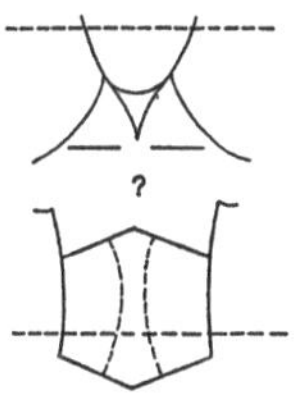

Stage	N	Actual 5-years survival	Predicted 5-years survival
I_1	64	70%	83%
I_2	33	50%	81%
II	29	35%	75%

Table 3. Reticulosarcoma and lymphosarcoma R.R.T.I. 1953—1963 possible benefit of prophylactic irradiation of liver-spleen-epigastric region (1st site above diaphragm)

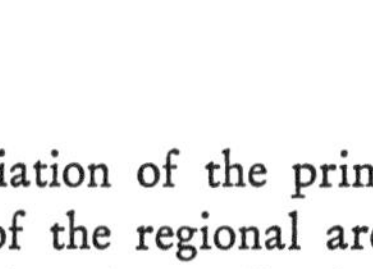

Stage	N	Actual 5-years survival	Predicted 5-years survival
I_1	64	70%	74%
I_2	33	50%	69%
II	29	35%	51%

A. Irradiation of the primary focus with a dose of 4000 rad in 4 weeks, and irradiation of the regional areas above the diaphragm with a dose of 3500 rad in 4 weeks. Unless the mediastinum is involved, the mediastinal area is not irradiated.

B. As A but, in addition, a prophylactic dose of 3500 rad in 4 weeks is delivered to the lumbar region.

Until now, 40 cases have been included in this trial. Within 5 to 10 years it will be possible to assess whether the actual survival rate corresponds to the predicted potential survival rate.

References

1. Dancot, H.: Étude du prognostic des lymphosarcomes et des réticulosarcomes. J. belge Radiol. 49, 264 (1966).
2. Dancot, H.: Personal communication.
3. Ennuyer, A., Helary, J., Bataini: Résultats de la radiothérapie des lymphoréticulosarcomes des voies aérodigestives supérieures. Bull. Ass. franç. Cancer 50, 413 (1963).
4. Ingold, J. A., Reed, G. B., Kaplan, H. S., Bagshaw, M. A.: Radiation hepatitis. Amer. J. Roentgenol. 93, 1268 (1966).
5. Kaplan, H. S., Rosenberg, S. A.: Extended-field radical radiotherapy in advanced Hodgkin's disease: short-term results of 2 randomized clinical trials. Cancer Res. 26, 1286 (1966).
6. Kaplan, H. S.: Personal communication.
7. Peters, V.: The contribution of radiation therapy in the control of early lymphomas. Amer. J. Roentgenol. 90, 956 (1963).
8. Scheer, A. C.: The course of stage I malignant lymphomas following local treatment. Amer. J. Roentgenol. 90, 939 (1963).
9. Tin Han, Stutzman, L.: Mode of spread in patients with localized malignant lymphoma. Arch. intern. Med. 120, 1 (1967).
10. Werf-Messing, B. van der: Reticulum cell sarcoma and lymphosarcoma. A retrospective study of potential survival in loco-regional disease. Europ. J. Cancer 4, 549 (1968).

Staging in Malignant Lymphoma

Hodgkin's Disease and Non-Hodgkin Lymphomas

K. Musshoff

Summary

The currently recognized staging classification of malignant lymphoma, which was formulated in Ann Arbor in 1971, is a result of the revision and extension of the 1965 Rye Classification.

It can be distinguished from the latter, *first* by a division of staging determination into two parts, the "Clinical" and the "Pathological", *secondly* by the inclusion of findings which make it possible to apply staging classification not only to Hodgkin's disease, as was the case with the Rye Classification, but also to all malignant lymphoma, and *thirdly* by the incorporation of new findings gained in the meantime.

ad 1: While the previous clinical staging classification was based on the results of predominantly clinical investigation methods (clinical, radiological, laboratory and primary histological), pathological staging additionally emphasized surgical investigation methods, especially laparotomy combined with splenectomy in the evaluation.

ad 2: The fact that the origin of the disease in extranodal organs, as is frequently the case with non-Hodgkin's as opposed to Hodgkin's lymphomas, has nearly the same prognosis as a primary lymph node finding permits the ranking equally of both forms of primary nodal and primary extranodal involvement.

ad 3: The following points, established after 1965, were included in the staging classification:

a) There are two forms of secondary organ involvement: locally limited organ involvement, which is caused by invasion of the disease from neighbouring involved lymph nodes and which has the same prognosis as lymph node involvement of the same extent, and disseminated organ involvement, arising from hematogenous dispersal and with an unfavourable prognosis.

b) As the spleen is a preferred starting-point for hematogenous dispersal, it plays a particular role regarding the spread of the disease.

c) In contrast to weight loss, itching has no prognostic significance.

The indication for and the extent of any local tumor therapy depends upon an adequate staging of the disease. This applies as much to malignant lymphomas as to other malignant tumors.

The modern practice is to apply local irradiation to malignant lymphomas, although by means of the mantle and reversed-Y method the whole system of lymph nodes and lymph channels is included. That is its simultaneous strength and weakness. It is its strength because it can be used in doses which can destroy foci in restricted regions of the body, and its weakness because of the risk of treating only part of the diseased tissue. The more exactly the primary diagnosis defines the severity and extent of the disease, the greater the chance that local therapy can make an impact on the disease and cure it. Thus, present efforts to improve the staging of malignant lymphomas are particularly concerned with more exact methods of diagnosis.

The efforts to produce a viable clinical classification of malignant lymphomas, in particular Hodgkin's disease, have been promoted by [4, 5, 8, 10, 11, 12, 16, 17, 18, 20, 21, 22, 25] and by Symposia in Paris [26], Rye, New York, 1965 [27] and Ann Arbor, 1971 [28].

In discussing the present state of staging, I shall mention the historical development only as far as is necessary for the understanding of the present situation. In 1965 a clinical staging classification was suggested at the Symposia for the control of Hodgkin's disease in Paris (organized by Tubiana), and in Rye, New York (sponsored by the National Cancer Institute and the American Cancer Society). The Rye Staging Classification has received world-wide recognition.

Table 1. Rye staging classification [24]. All stages will be subclassified as "A" or "B" to indicate the absence or presence, respectively, of systemic symptoms. The following recorded symptoms, otherwise unexplained, are significant: (a) fever; (b) night sweats; (c) pruritus

Stage	
I [a]	Disease limited to one anatomical region or to two contiguous anatomical regions on the same side of the diaphragm.
II	Disease in more than two anatomical regions or in two non-contiguous regions on the same side of the diaphragm.
III	Disease on both sides of the diaphragm, but not extending beyond the involvement of lymph nodes and spleen with or without Waldeyer's ring.
IV	Involvement of the bone marrow, lung parenchyma, pleura, liver, bone, skin, kidneys, gastrointestinal tract, or any tissue or organ in addition to lymph nodes, spleen, or Waldeyer's ring.

[a] Some centers will prefer to continue to distinguish patients with disease limited to one anatomical region. For those centers wishing to make this distinction, the following subdivision of stage I is recommended: Stage I_1, disease limited to one anatomic region; stage I_2, disease limited to two contiguous anatomical regions on the same side of the diaphragm.

The Rye Staging Classification (Table 1) sub-divides the disease into 4 stages, 3 of which are stages with different degrees of lymph-node involvement. The local Stage I affects one lymph-node group; Stage II affects two or more lymph-node regions on one side of diaphragm and Stage III affects some or all of the lymph-node regions above or below the diaphragm. The spleen counts as a lymph-node region. In Stage III, the disease is, by definition, limited to these topographically connected organ systems and can therefore not be considered a generalized form of the disease. Only the Rye Stage IV, which includes any extra-nodal or tissue involvement, would be unanimously recognized and defined as generalized Hodgkin's disease.

The view that any extra-nodal or extra-lymphatic organ and tissue involvement is to be considered as dissemination entailing distant metastases is associated with the Ann Arbor Symposium of 1971 [28].

The basis for this view were the findings by [19, 20], [25] as well as our own [12, 14, 16, 19], which agreed that in a number of cases with organ involvement the disease has to be considered as locally limited and not generalized. This localized organ involvement we called organ involvement per continuitatem (Stage IV p. c.) because it develops by spread from affected neighbouring lymph nodes, in contrast to disseminated organ involvement, which was called Stage IV per disseminationem (IV p. d.) [12, 16, 17]. Localized organ involvement has a statistically better prognosis under present therapeutic conditions than disseminated organ involvement. This is demonstrated in Fig. 1 which shows part of the Freiburg patients series. Of those

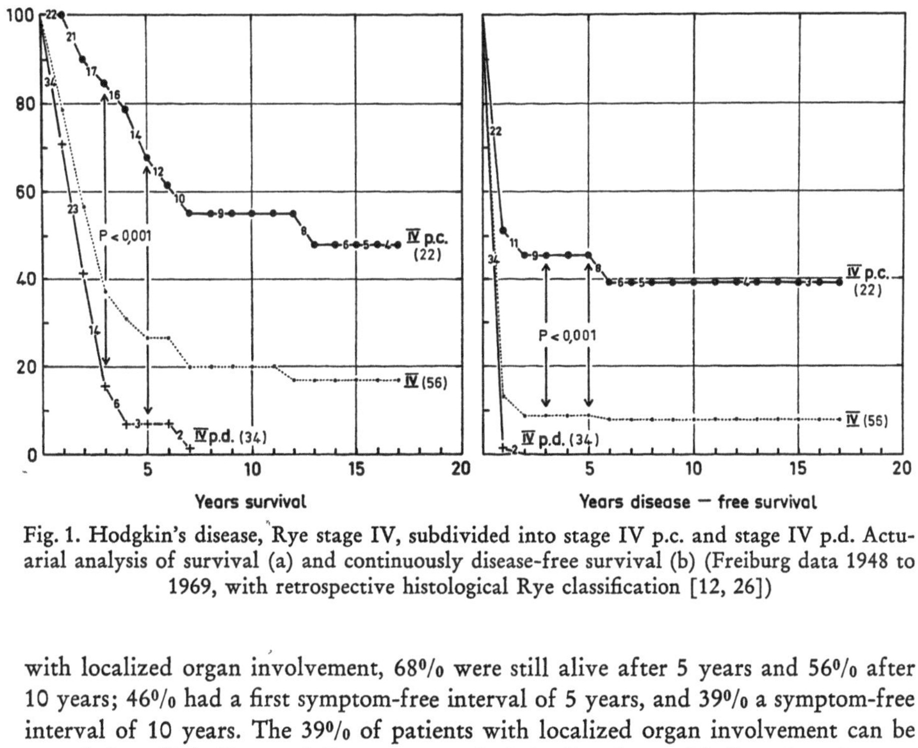

Fig. 1. Hodgkin's disease, Rye stage IV, subdivided into stage IV p.c. and stage IV p.d. Actuarial analysis of survival (a) and continuously disease-free survival (b) (Freiburg data 1948 to 1969, with retrospective histological Rye classification [12, 26])

with localized organ involvement, 68% were still alive after 5 years and 56% after 10 years; 46% had a first symptom-free interval of 5 years, and 39% a symptom-free interval of 10 years. The 39% of patients with localized organ involvement can be regarded as clinically cured. In contrast, only 7% of patients with disseminated organ involvement reached the 5-year-survival limit, and no patient survived for 10 years. A completely symptom-free survival period was achieved in very few cases.

If we compare Stage II and III patients with the same degree of lymph-node involvement, one group having an additional localized organ involvement and the other not, we find that the survival and remission rates are actually better in the group with additional organ involvement, though this difference may not be statistically significant. Thus locally limited organ involvement does not have an unfavorable effect on the prognosis, provided it can be treated in the same way as the affected lymph nodes (Fig. 2).

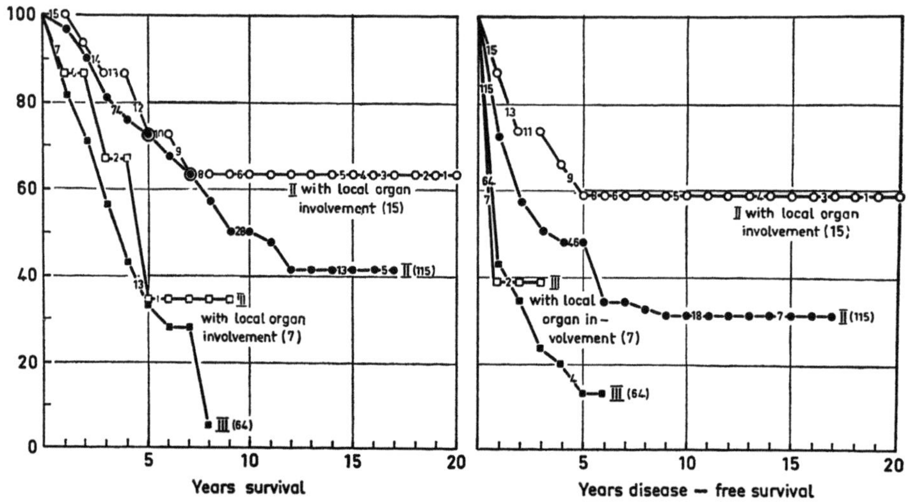

Fig. 2. Hodgkin's disease, stages II and III, with and without localized involvement of extranodal non-lymphatic organ or site. Actuarial analysis of survival and continuous disease-free survival. (Freiburg data 1948 to 1969, with retrospective histological Rye classification [12, 26])

The prognosis for localized organ and lymph-node involvement of the same degree is the same, and identical therapy is indicated. This could, therefore, be the basis for staging these two modes of spread in the same way, i. e. to classify the localized organ involvement together with the local regional lymph node Stages II and III. Table 2 gives our suggestions for a classification which would not apply only to Hodgkin's disease. The reason for this will be discussed later.

At the Ann Arbor Symposium [28] a revised form of the Rye Staging Classification was proposed (Table 3), in which the involvement of the spleen, in contrast to the recommendations of Paris and Rye, is itself considered to be an important event, since it had meanwhile been accepted that the spleen has a special role in the spread of

Table 2. Staging classification, applicable to all malignant lymphomas (K. Musshoff *et al.*, 1971; 18). In Hodgkin's disease each stage will be divided into A without signs and symptoms of active disease, and B with such signs and symptoms

Stage	Involvement
I	Disease limited to (1) one lymphatic region, nodal or extranodal (Waldeyer's ring, spleen) or (2) one non-lymphatic region.
II	(1) Disease in two or more lymphatic regions on the same side of the diaphragm (2) including localized non-lymphatic organ involvement which is either primary or in conjunction with lymph node involvement (p.c.).
III	(1) Disease in lymphatic regions on both sides of the diaphragm (2) including localized non-lymphatic organ involvement which is either primary or in conjunction with lymph node involvement (p.c.).
IV	Disseminated non-lymphatic organ involvement (p.d.) with or without lymphatic involvement.

Table 3. Ann Arbor staging classification (CARBONE *et al.*, 1971; 1). Each stage will be subdivided into categories A and B: B for those with defined general symptoms and A for those without. The B classification will be given those patients with (a) unexplained weight loss of more than 10% of the body weight in the 6 months prior to admission; (b) unexplained fever with temperatures above 38°; and (c) night sweats

Stage	Involvement
I	Involvement of a single lymph-node region (I) or of a single extralymphatic organ or site (I_E).
II	Involvement of two or more lymph-node regions on the same side of the diaphragm (II) or localized involvement of extralymphatic organ or site and of one or more lymph-node regions on the same side of the diaphragm (II_E). An optional recommendation is that the numbers of node regions involved be indicated by a subscript e. g., II_3.
III	Involvement of lymph-node regions on both sides of the diaphragm (III), which may also be accompanied by localized involvement of extralymphatic organ or site (III_E) or by involvement of the spleen (III_S), or both (III_{SE}).
IV	Diffuse or disseminated involvement of one or more extralymphatic organs or tissues with or without associated lymph-node enlargement. The reason for classifying the patients as stage IV should be identified further by defining the site by symbols.

disease. As in the Rye Classification, Hodgkin's disease patients are divided into Groups A and B, to indicate the absence or presence of one of the three symptoms: a loss of weight greater than 10% of the body weight within the previous 6 months; a rise of temperature to more than 38° C, and night sweat. As against the Rye Classification, pruritus was replaced by weight loss as a Group B symptom because pruritus was shown to be not prognostically significant [3, 15, 28], whereas weight loss is [29].

The Ann Arbor Classification applies both to Hodgkin's disease and to other lymphomas, as suggested in 1969 on the basis of the following findings and considerations. In both lymphosarcoma and reticulum-cell sarcoma the disease can in a percentage of cases originate in an extranodal tissue or organ. This probably never happens in Hodgkin's disease. Primary organ involvement in reticulum-cell sarcoma and lymphosarcoma has a similar prognosis to the involvement of the lymph nodes alone, if the degree of involvement is the same. This applies in the same way to secondary organ involvement in Hodgkin's disease.

The Freiburg series of patients with reticulum-cell sarcoma and lymphoreticular sarcoma during the years 1948—1968 (Table 4) shows that the 5-, 10-, and 15-year survival rates of the local regional Stages I and II are the same or somewhat better in the group with primary organ involvement than in the group with primary lymph-node involvement.

The percentage of survivors with symptom-free periods of more than 10 years in the local regional Stages I and II in the group with primary lymph-node involvement (48%) is similar to that in the group with primary organ involvement (45%) (Table 5).

Assignment of the different malignant lymphomas to one prognostic classification depends on a) localized development in lymph nodes or organs and b) the observation that the locally limited involvement of organs (whether primary, as in reticulum-

Table 4. Reticulum-cell sarcoma and lymphoreticular sarcoma, stages I through IV (n=224). Comparative survival figures for primary lymph-node versus primary organ involvement. (Freiburg 1948—1968); [18]

Stage	Primary site of disease in lymph nodes				in organs			
	Survival rates % in							
		years				years		
	n	5	10	15	n	5	10	15
I	(39)	76	66	59	(13)	61	61	61
II	(42)	28	28	19	(22)	58	58	49
I+II	(81)	50	42	38	(35)	59	59	51
III	(34)	11	11	11	(7)	0	0	0
IV disseminated (p.d.)	(51)	0	0	0	(10)	0	0	0
IV localized (p.c.)	(6)	56	56					
Total	(172)	28	28	23	(52)	36	36	31

Table 5. Reticulum-cell sarcoma and lymphoreticular sarcoma, stages I through IV (n=224). Percentage of patients surviving 10 or more years in complete clinical remission following an initial radiotherapy treatment for disease originating in lymph nodes or disease originating in organs. (Freiburg 1948—1968) [18]

Stage	10 years disease-free survival rates %	
	Primary site of disease in lymph nodes	Primary site of disease in organs
I	67	44
II	27	45
I+II	48	45
III	4	0
IV (p.d.)	0	0
IV (p.c.)	50	
Total	30	31

Table 6. Ann Arbor classification pathological staging symbols [1]

N+ or N−	For other lymph node positive for disease or negative by biopsy
H+ or H−	For liver positive or negative by liver biopsy
S+ or S−	For spleen positive or negative following splenectomy
L+ or L−	For lung positive or negative by biopsy
M+ or M−	For marrow positive or negative by biopsy or smear
P+ or P−	For positive or negative pleural involvement by biopsy or cytological examination
O+ or O−	For positive or negative bone involvement by biopsy
D+ or D−	For positive or negative skin involvement by biopsy

cell sarcoma, or secondary, as in Hodgkin's lymphoma) has the same or even better prognosis than lymph-node involvement of the same clinical degree.

The Ann Arbor Conference made diagnostic procedures an intrinsic part of staging classification. In addition to the diagnostic procedures used for clinical staging (primary histology, laparoscopy, bone-marrow biopsy, X-ray and laboratory investigations), the staging method was extended to include more radical diagnostic procedures, in particular, laparotomy with splenectomy (Table 6). To give an example: a clinical Stage II A patient with involvement of three lymph-node regions underwent laparotomy with splenectomy. Findings were positive in the spleen and abdominal lymph nodes, and negative in the liver and bone marrow. This is written:

$$\text{CS II A}_3\ \text{PS III}_{S+N+H-M-}\,.$$

Since various surgical explorations of the abdomen have shown, that the peripheral portions of the mesentary, which is not encompassed by the usual radiotherapy technique used in Hodgkin's disease, is more frequently involved in non-Hodgkin lymphomas, as JOHNSON has shown in this volume p. II, it is necessary and advisable to designate these mesenterial lymph nodes in pathological staging by, for instance, the abbreviation "$N_{mes.}$ positive or negative".

The Ann Arbor Classification was discussed at the Hodgkin Symposium organized by KAPLAN in Stanford [9] after a trial period of one year. Its continued use was generally recommended.

A critical assessment of the Ann Arbor Classification with its extensive and radical diagnostic procedures requires consideration of the following points.

1. Hodgkin's disease is a potentially curable condition in a high percentage of cases. To realize this possibility of cure, the extent of the disease must be assessed by every possible diagnostic means. On the basis of our present knowledge, this entails the procedures recommended at Ann Arbor. The spleen cannot reliably be assessed by any method other than splenectomy. Multiple small foci which are asymptomatic and occult can remain silent for years before they progress and extend. The importance of recognizing involvement of the spleen is that according to the Stanford group [2], involvement of the liver (which has a bad prognosis) occurs always, or in a very high percentage of cases via the spleen. Our series also indicates that an untreated spleen can be the source of generalized organ metastases [12, 13]. These clinical observations are supported by the pathohistological findings of RAPPAPORT and STRUM [23], which show that, as the spleen has a higher number of specific vascular invasions than other lymphatic tissues, hematogenous spread may originate from the spleen.

The Stanford series of 272 patients subjected to primary laparotomy shows that at the time of diagnosis the spleen is involved in a third of all cases. All clinical stages and all histological types can occur, in equivalent numbers. In contrast, the involvement of the liver and bone marrow, which carries a poor prognosis, is a relatively rare finding at the time of diagnosis (KAPLAN: 3—4%; DORFMANN: 8%), but its incidence increases with the duration of the disease. Laparotomy with splenectomy has therefore two objects:

a) As a diagnostic procedure it gives the most extensive results and is therefore the safest basis for the optimal use of therapeutic measures.

b) We can expect early splenectomy to be a good prophylactic measure in a relatively high percentage of patients to prevent dissemination of the disease, the risk of which may be present in a third of all cases. This proportion is too high to be disregarded in the therapeutic management of a tumor patient. By comparison, the operative risk, which Dr. Staib has discussed in this volume, p. II, is small.

Johnson [6, 7] has shown in a series of cases that a similar therapeutic improvement to that following splenectomy could also be achieved by radiotherapy of the spleen and the para-aortic lymph nodes in all cases or, if appropriate, by total nodal irradiation.

2. The Ann Arbor Staging Classification has the theoretical and technical advantage that it is applicable to all malignant lymphomas; in this it differs from the Rye Classification. Thus the wide experience gained in diagnosis and treatment of Hodgkin's disease over the last decade can be applied to the other malignant lymphomas and the model used for their further investigation.

This does not, of course, mean that we can transfer our findings in Hodgkin's disease to the other malignant lymphomas without any modification. On the contrary, the differences between these groups must be stated. In this respect, the staging methods will be particularly valuable.

References

1. Carbone, P. P., Kaplan, H. S., Musshoff, K., Smithers, D. W., Tubiana, M.: Report of the committee on Hodgkin's disease staging procedures. Cancer Res. **31**, 1860 (1971).
2. Dorfman, R. F.: Relationship of histology to site in Hodgkin's disease. Cancer Res. **31**, 1786 (1971).
3. Ennuyer, A., Bataini, P., Franiatte, I.: Résultats lointains obtenus par radiothérapie dans la maladie de Hodgkin. Nouv. Rev. franç. Hémat. **6**, 76 (1966).
4. Jelliffe, A. M., Thomson, A. D.: Prognosis in Hodgkin's disease. Brit. J. Cancer **9**, 21 (1955).
5. Jelliffe, A. M.: The place of radiotherapy in the cure of Hodgkin's disease. Clin. Radiol. **16**, 274 (1965).
6. Johnson, R. E.: Irradiation of the spleen in the management of Hodgkin's disease. In press.
7. Johnson, R. E., Glover, M. K., Marshall, S. K.: Results of radiation therapy and implications for the clinical staging of Hodgkin's disease. Conference on Staging in Hodgkin's disease; Ann Arbor, April 1971. Cancer Res. **31**, 1834 (1971).
8. Kaplan, H. S.: Radical radiotherapy of regionally localized Hodgkin's disease. Radiology **78**, 553 (1962).
9. Kaplan, H. S.: International Symposium on Hodgkin's disease. Stanford, California, March 20—24, 1972. National Cancer Institute Monograph 36 (1973).
10. Lukes, R. J., Craver, L. F., Hall, Th. C., Rappaport, H., Ruben, Ph.: Report of the Nomenclature Committee. Cancer Res. **26**, 1311 (1966) .
11. Musshoff, K.: Therapy and prognosis of two different forms of organ involvement in cases of malignant lymphoma (Hodgkin's disease, reticulum-cell sarcoma) as well as a report about stage division in those disease. XII. International Congress of Radiology. Topyo, Oct. 6—11, 1969, Abstracts p. 77. Klin. Wschr. **48**, 673 (1970).
12. Musshoff, K.: Prognostic and therapeutic implications of staging in extranodal Hodgkin's disease. Conference on staging in Hodgkin's disease. Ann Arbor, April 26—28, 1971. Cancer Res. **31**, 1814 (1971).
13. Musshoff, K.: Grundlagen der Strahlentherapie des Morbus Hodgkin, Indikation und Ergebnisse. Deutscher Krebskongreß Hannover 1971. Z. Krebsforsch. **78**, 162 (1972).
14. Musshoff, K., Boutis, L.: Therapy Results in Hodgkin's disease; Freiburg i. Br. 1948—1966. Cancer (Philad.) **21**, 1100 (1968).

15. MUSSHOFF, K., BOUTIS, L., LASZLO, A. M., LASZLA, I.: Prognostische Krankheitssymptome und -zeichen bei Morbus Hodgkin und ihre Bedeutung für die Therapie der Erkrankung. Strahlentherapie **131**, 482 (1966).
16. MUSSHOFF, K., RENEMANN, H., BOUTIS, L., AFKHAM, J.: Die extranoduläre Lymphogranulomatose-Diagnose, Therapie und Prognose bei zwei unterschiedlichen Formen des Organbefalls. Ein Beitrag zur Stadieneinteilung des Morbus Hodgkin. Fortschr. Röntgenstr. **109**, 776 (1968).
17. MUSSHOFF, K., RENEMANN, H., BOUTIS, L., AFGHAM, J.: The differentiation of two different types of stage IV of Hodgkin's disease. II. International Congress of Lymphology Miami, March 15—20, 1968, Abstracts No. 171. In: Progress in Lymphology II, p. 272. Stuttgart: Thieme 1970.
18. MUSSHOFF, K., SCHMIDT-VOLLMER, H., MERTEN, D.: Reticulum cell sarcoma, an oncologic model for a system of classification the malignant lymphomas. Europ. J. Cancer **7**, 451 (1971).
19. PETERS, M. V.: A clinical classification of the malignant lymphomas related to the course of the disease. II. International Congress of Lymphology Miami, March 15—20, 1968.
20. PETER, M. V.: The need for a new clinical classification in Hodgkin's disease: Keynote address. Cancer Res. **31**, 1713 (1971).
21. PETERS, M. V., MIDDLEMISS, K. C. H.: A study of Hodgkin's disease treated by irradiation. Amer. J. Roentgenol. **79**, 114 (1958).
22. PETERS, M. V.: A study of survivals in Hodgkin's disease treated radiologically. Amer. J. Roentgenol. **63**, 299 (1950).
23. RAPPAPORT, H., STRUM, ST. B.: Vascular invasion in Hodgkin's disease: Its incidence and relationship to the spread of the disease. Cancer (Philad.) **25**, 1304 (1970).
24. ROSENBERG, S. A.: Report of the Committee on Staging of Hodgkin's disease. Cancer Res. **26**, 1310 (1966).
25. ROSENBERG, S. A., KAPLAN, H. S.: Hodgkin's disease and other malignant lymphomas. Calif. Med. **113**, 23 (1970).
26. Symposium: La radiothérapie de la maladie de Hodgkin, Paris, 1965. Radiol. Électrol. **47**, Suppl. Nos. 1—2 (1966).
27. Symposium: Obstacles to the control of Hodgkin's disease; Rye, New York, September 13—15, 1965. Cancer Res. **26**, 1043 (1966).
28. Symposium: Staging in Hodgkin's disease; University of Michigan, Ann Arbor, Michigan, April 26—28 1971. Cancer Res. **31**, 1707 (1971).
29. TUBIANA, M., ATTIE, E., FLAMANT, R., GERARD-MARCHANT, R., HAYAT, M.: Prognostic factors in 454 cases of Hodgkin's disease. Cancer Res. **31**, 1801 (1971).

Therapy of Malignant Lymphoma

Radiotherapy of Hodgkin's Disease and Malignant Lymphomas

R. E. Johnson

Summary

The radiotherapeutic management of Hodgkin's disease is approaching optimization with appreciation of the need to extend treatment to include major portions of the axial lymphatic chain. Unequivocal evidence now exists that "prophylactic" irradiation of occultly diseased sites can not only reduce the incidence of relapse but also materially improve survival. Further major advances in the therapy of Hodgkin's disease will depend upon the integration of chemotherapy and radiotherapy in those presentations having a significant risk of clinically undetectable extranodal spread.

Relatively little progress has occurred with radiotherapy of the malignant lymphomas of the non-Hodgkin's types. This reflects lack of definition of the natural history of the lymphomas and the failure to adopt radiotherapy techniques which are relevant. The majority of patients with non-Hodgkin's lymphomas have systemic involvement at the time of diagnosis and the high dose, shaped-field techniques utilized for Hodgkin's disease are ill-advised. More systemic approaches such as whole-body irradiation are required and preliminary experience has yielded encouraging results.

Development of a rational therapeutic program for the malignant lymphomas is contingent upon accurately defining the natural history for each disease in its variable clinical presentation and having methods for locating each patient within the overall spectrum of the disease. These two requirements are mutually interdependent. The clinician can delineate the natural history of any malignancy when and only when techniques exist for evaluating the anatomic extent of involvement with reasonable precision, i. e. "staging" the patient. Similarly, correct interpretation of many diagnostic tests demands and understanding of the disease itself, including both the indirect and direct effects of the neoplasm on the host.

The biologic behavior of Hodgkin's disease is now sufficiently well defined to facilitate treatment decisions. Although the exact extent of lymphatic spread in any patient cannot be reliably determined with current "staging" approaches, involvement often remains confined to the lymphatic system long enough to enable "prophylactic" radiotherapeutic measures to be effectively employed. The guidelines for evaluation and management of the lymphoreticulosarcomas are more obscure. The histopathologic classification remains in a stage of flux, "staging" procedures are less reliable than with Hodgkin's disease, the anatomic patterns of spread are often unpredictable, and there is extremely wide variation in biological behavior. As a consequence, there is substantial doubt as to whether the radiotherapeutic approaches used for Hodgkin's disease have any major relevance for the majority of patients with lymphomas of other histologic types.

Hodgkin's Disease

Two concepts form the basis of modern radiotherapy in Hodgkin's disease, namely the concept of "tumoricidal dose" and the concept "prophylactic irridiation". Both of these concepts were in essence espoused by GILBERT [1] nearly three decades ago and have simply become progressively refined in the interim.

Tumoricidal radiotherapy in Hodgkin's disease pertains to the administration of that radiation dose which prevents subsequent local recurrence with high probability. Numerous reports [2—4] have documented the tumoricidal effect of doses exceeding 3500 rad. However, the time-dose data has been misinterpreted to suggest that such doses must be delivered within an elapsed time of three to four weeks for therapeutic effectiveness. Relationship of dose and time are not very rigid for Hodgkin's disease [5, 6], and equally efficient tumor control can be achieved with greater protraction, including split-course irradiation. The latter serves to attenuate the severity of normal tissue reactions and virtually eliminates delayed complications in normal tissue.

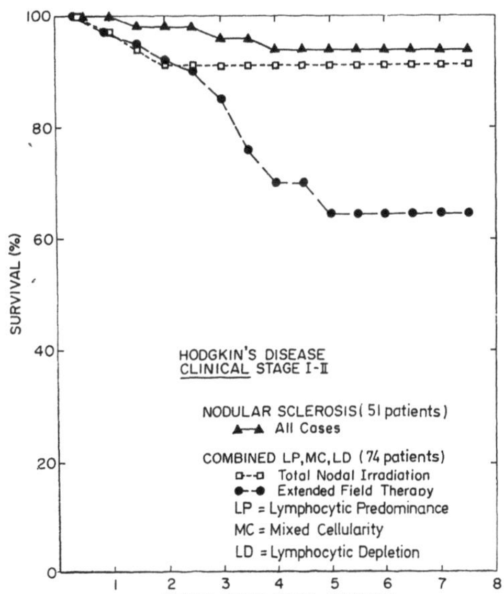

Fig. 1. Actuarial survival curves for stage I—II A and B patients assigned to extended(adjacent)-field versus total nodal irradiation by random selection. The minimum and mean observation periods are three and more than five years respectively

Prophylactic irradiation is essential in the radiotherapy of Hodgkin's disease because clinical evaluation of the extent of disease is not sufficiently reliable to guide planning of treatment. Radiation fields limited to obviously involved sites permit a high relapse rate by extension of disease [1, 7]. These relapses in non-irradiated sites are often not detectable clinically until wider dissemination has taken place, and the opportunity for cure with secondary treatment is thereby lost [7—9]. Thus, prophylactic irradiation of clinically uninvolved sites serves not only to reduce the incidence of relapse but, more importantly, recently has been shown for the first time to reduce the mortality rate. In a prospective, random, controlled study at the National Cancer Institute, extensive prophylactic irradiation yielded the highest survival rates thus far reported for patients with local regional involvement (Fig. 1).

Comprehensive lymph-node irradiation does not afford protection against one mechanism of relapse, namely extranodal extension. In some cases, the presence of occult foci of Hodgkin's disease in extranodal sites is not clinically detectable by current methods prior to treatment, and this cause for failure of treatment can only be remedied with a systemic approach. The combined use of chemotherapy and radiotherapy is presently under investigation in many centers [10—12], in our opinion it should be restricted to cases considered to have a significant risk of extranodal relapse [13]. Such a combined attack would appear to offer the potential for improving the results achievable with radiotherapy alone, and results of our own three years experience with sequential MOPP chemotherapy and radiotherapy are beginning to suggest an advantage (Fig. 2).

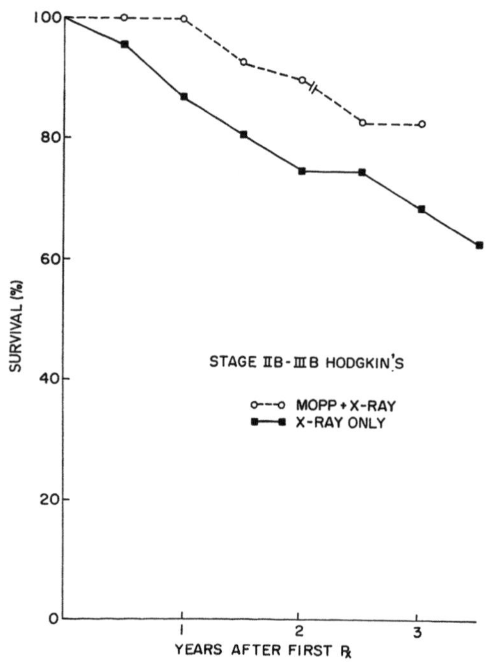

Fig. 2. Actuarial survival curves for matched stage II B—III B groups treated by extensive radiotherapy alone or in combination with adjuvant four-drug (MOPP) chemotherapy. The chemotherapy consisted of six cycles administered prior to initiation of radiotherapy

Lymphoreticulosarcoma

The non-Hodgkin lymphomas have a range of natural histories which differ greatly from Hodgkin's disease. The exception are those lymphoreticulosarcomas of extranodal origin which follow a similar pattern of behavior to Hodgkin's disease, frequently spreading to regional lymph nodes in a predictable fashion during the early clinical phase. However, the majority of patients initially present with lymph-node manifestations and have a marked propensity for disseminated involvement at the time of diagnosis. In retrospect, it is obvious that lack of clinical determination of the extent of disease at diagnosis has been responsible for the absence of progress in the radiotherapeutic management.

A relatively small fraction of patients have localized extranodal presentations of lymphoreticulosarcoma, and conventional radiotherapy techniques effect appreciable control in these cases [14—16]. As already mentioned, the majority of newly diagnosed patients have more extensive, if not systemic disease, and this observation has stimulated the investigation of total-body irradiation at the National Cancer Institute. Preliminary experience indicated excellent remissions in lymphosarcoma patients presenting with generalized lymph-node involvement [17—19], and it has been observed that neither response rates nor survival has been materially affected by histologic involvement of extranodal sites such as the bone marrow or liver. The

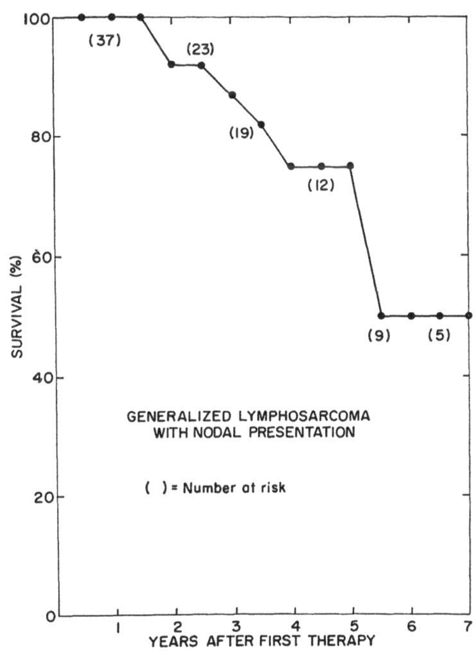

Fig. 3. Actuarial survival curves for lymphosarcoma patients initially presenting with clinically generalized involvement and managed primarily with ultrawide-field radiotherapy (usually whole-body irradiation). Approximately one-half of the cases with nodal presentation had documented microscopic invasion of the bone marrow or liver, or both. The latter has not influenced response to treatment or survival to a significant extent

prognosis is strikingly less favorable when the major clinical manifestation is visceral dissemination or a leukemic phase of the disease. Our data for survival of lymphosarcoma patients presenting with clinically generalized involvement at diagnosis are given in Fig. 3. Wide-field radiotherapy techniques, particularly whole-body irradiation, clearly deserve increased consideration in the management of generalized lymphoproliferative disorders. Any corresponding improvement in chemotherapy demands that the role of "systemic radiotherapy" be re-evaluated by means of comparative clinical trials.

Discussion

The impressive success in the radiotherapeutic management of Hodgkin's disease during the past decade reflects an enhanced understanding of the natural history of disease and the consequent adoption of relevant treatment techniques. Other advances, such as megavoltage radiotherapy, have also contributed to improved survival rates, but are of secondary importance. In contrast, there has been a relative lack of progress in the management of the non-Hodgkin lymphomas. This is attributable to the ill-defined natural history of many lymphoreticulosarcomas, combined with inadequate methods for clinically establishing the true extent of involvement. One factor has become increasingly apparent, however, namely the marked propensity for systemic involvement when patients present with lymph-node manifestations of lymphoreticulosarcoma. This demands the adoption of more systemic radiotherapeutic techniques or the utilization of chemotherapy as an adjunct to conventional radiotherapy rather than the irrelevant treatment methods utilized for Hodgkin's disease.

References

1. Gilbert, R.: Radiotherapy in Hodgkin's disease. Amer. J. Roentgenol. **41**, 198 (1939).
2. Jelliffe, A. M., Thomson, A. D.: The prognosis in Hodgkin's diseaese. Brit. J. Cancer **9**, 21 (1955).
3. Scott, R. M., Brizel, H. E.: Time-dose relationships in Hodgkin's disease. Radiology **82**, 1043 (1964).
4. Kaplan, H. S.: Evidence for a tumoricidal dose level in the radiotherapy of Hodgkin's disease. Cancer Res. **26**, 1221 (1966).
5. Landberg, T., Forslo, H.: Radiosensitivity of mediastinal lymphomas in Hodgkin's disease treated with split-course radiotherapy. Acta Radiol. (Stockh.) **9**, 177 (1970).
6. Johnson, R. E.: Total nodal irradiation of Hodgkin's disease: Technical and clinical aspects. In: Textbook of Radiotherapy (Fletcher, G., Ed.). Philadelphia: Lea & Feibiger.
7. Johnson, R. E., Glover, M. G., Marshall, S. K.: Results of radiation therapy and implications for the clinical staging of Hodgkin's disease. Cancer Res. **31**, 1834 (1971).
8. Kaplan, H. S.: Prognostic significance of the relapse-free interval after radiotherapy in Hodgkin's disease. Cancer (Philad.) **22**, 1131 (1968).
9. Seydel, H. G., Wizenberg, M. J., Bloedorn, F. G.: Results of radiotherapeutic treatment of relapsing Hodgkin's disease. Cancer (Philad.) **23**, 1033 (1969).
10. Moore, M. R., Bull, J. M., Jones, S. E., Rosenberg, S. A., Kaplan, H. S.: Combined radiotherapy and chemotherapy in the treatment of Hodgkin's disease. Ann. intern. Med. **77**, 1 (1972).
11. De Vita, V. T., Johnson, R. E.: Unpublished data.

12. Leukemia Cooperative Group B: Unpublished data.
13. Johnson, R. E., Thomas, L. B., Chretien, P.: Correlation between clinico-histologic staging and extranodal relapse in Hodgkin's disease. Cancer (Philad.) **25**, 1071 (1970).
14. Van der Werf-Messing, B.; Reticulum cell sarcoma and lymphosarcoma. A retrospective study of potential survival in Loco-regional disease. Europ. J. Cancer **4**, 549 (1968).
15. Wang, C. C., Fleischli, D. J.: Primary reticulum cell sarcoma of bone. Cancer (Philad.) **22**, 994 (1968).
16. Banfi, A., Bonadonna, G., Ricci, S. B., Milani, F., Molinari, R., Monfardini, S., Zucali, R.: Malignant lymphomas of Waldeyer's ring: Natural history and survival after radiotherapy. Brit. med. J. **1972 III**, 140.
17. Johnson, R. E.: Evaluation of fractionated total body irradiation in patients with leukemia and disseminated lymphomas. Radiology **86**, 1085 (1966).
18. Johnson, R. E., O'Conor, G. T., Levin, D.: Primary management of advanced lymphosarcoma with radiotherapy. Cancer (Philad.) **25**, 787 (1970).
19. Johnson, R. E.: Remission induction and remission duration with primary radiotherapy in advanced lymphosarcoma. Cancer (Philad.) **29**, 1473 (1972).

Chemotherapy and Radiotherapy in the Management of the Malignant Lymphomas

A. M. JELLIFFE and Y. L. MILLETT

Summary

This paper is restricted to discussion of malignant lymphomas originating primarily in the lymph nodes. During the last decade there has been a dramatic change in the management of patients with lymphomas, due to improvements in radiotherapy, in chemotherapy, in investigations to determine the extent of the disease, and above all to our acceptance that lymphomas are not always fatal.

It is now accepted that many patients with Hodgkin's disease are curable by radiotherapy. We believe that many patients with lymphosarcoma and reticulosarcoma can also be cured. The efficiency of modern radiotherapy and cancer chemotherapy makes it sometimes difficult to select the best method of treatment for a particular patient.

Histological Classification

It is important to define the groups of malignant lymphomas referred to in this paper. The classification used is that specified by the Pathology Panel of the British National Lymphoma Investigation.

Hodgkin's Disease

We recognize four types of Hodgkin's disease: lymphocyte predominant, nodular slerotic, mixed cellularity, and lymphocyte depleted. The essential common feature is presence of the Sternberg-Reed cell, which is an absolute requirement for diagnosis of Hodgkin's disease.

Lymphosarcoma

We recognize four types of lymphosarcoma. The first is follicular lymphoma. The characteristic features of this tumor were described by [2, 4].

The second is diffuse lymphosarcoma in which the nodal architecture is diffusely replaced by mature lymphoid cells. There may be some residual follicular pattern, but when most of the node shows diffuse involvement, it is classified as diffuse lymphosarcoma.

The third is lymphoblastic lymphosarcoma. Here, there is diffuse replacement by more primitive lymphoid cells.

The fourth, nodular sclerotic lymphosarcoma, was recently described [1]. In this type there are prominent fibrous bands dividing part or all of the lymph node into irregular nodules. The fibrous bands vary in thickness from ten to several hundred, are doubly refractile, and contain many reticulin fibres. The background cellular pattern may be that of lymphoblastic lymphosarcoma, diffuse lymphosarcoma, or follicular lymphoma (Fig. 1).

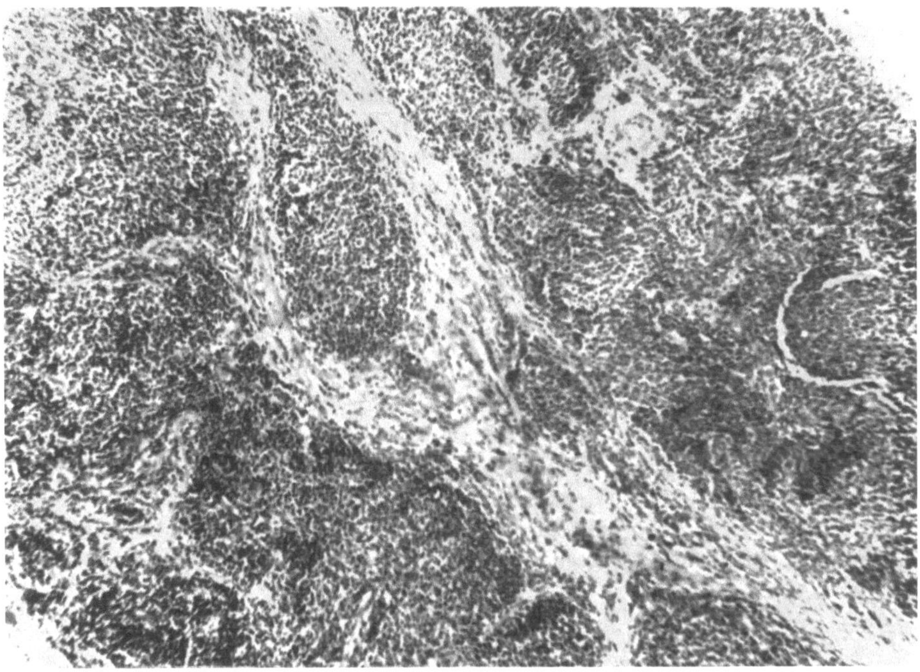

Fig. 1. Nodular sclerotic lymphosarcoma. Well-marked fibrous bands and diffuse pattern with both mature and immature lymphoid cells. (Clin. Radiol. 20, 340 (1969). Reproduced with permission of the Editor and Authors [1])

Reticulum-Cell Sarcoma

The lymph node shows replacement with sheets of cells larger than lymphoid cells, with large vesicular nuclei and pale cytoplasm. The term reticulum-cell sarcoma has been retained by our Pathology Panel because it is well recognized and because there is as yet no proof that the cell of origin is the histiocyte.

Choice of Treatment

Radiotherapy is more effective when a lymphoma is localized. Cytotoxic drugs are indicated more often in the presence of widespread disease, particularly when there is extranodal invasion of other organs. The indications for either treatment method may sometimes depened upon the histological type of lymphoma. But whatever the histological appearance, it is of the greatest importance that he extent of the disease be determined as accurately as possible.

Hodgkin's Disease

Over the last 2$^{1}/_{2}$ years in the United Kingdom, the Cooperative Clinical Cancer Therapy Group [1], involving 17 centres throughout the country, has been investigating the treatment of this condition. The data presented here are based on the work of this group, and we are grateful to our colleagues for their permission to publish this information.

Mandatory investigations include clinical examination, chest X-ray and abdominal lymphogram, hematological and biochemical investigations. Half of the collaborating clinicians favor diagnostic laparotomy. These routine investigations frequently demonstrate advanced disease in patients who would otherwise have been thought to have localized lymph-node involvement. In our experience, the histological type of Hodgkin's disease does not affect the choice of treatment.

Stages I and II

When disease is localized to one half of the body, radiotherapy is the method of choice. We believe that the extent of prophylactic irradiation indicated in patients who have been investigated radically, is as yet unknown. Of the 301 patients accepted for our investigation, 50% were classified as stage I or II. One half received irradiation to the affected region only, and the other half prophylactic irradiation to adjacent areas. So far there has been no difference in rate of recurrence or survival between the two groups.

Stage III

In this stage, with lymph-node involvement both above and below the diaphragm and without extranodal invasion, we are comparing the effects of total-node irradiation, as advocated by KAPLAN, with intensive combintaion chemotherapy, as originally suggested by CARBONE and DE VITA. Trends are appearing: 46 patients without systemic manifestations have been treated, and appear to respond equally well to total-node irradiation *or* combination chemotherapy. A difference may become apparent, but at present, both methods appear to be equally effective.

Systemic manifestations were present in 26 patients. We have the impression that cytotoxic drugs may be preferable to total-node irradiation in this group.

Stage IV

When the disease involves extranodal tissues, combination chemotherapy is the treatment of choice. We are at present comparing one group of patients treated by

[1] Prospective Trials organized by this Group started in February 1970. In the 2$^{1}/_{2}$ years since then 301 patients with Hogkin's disease have been accepted.

the MOPP regime with a second group of patients who are receiving the same combination of drugs, but without prednisone. We had expected to find that prednisone was protecting the bone marrow and preventing some of the unpleasant immediate side-effects that are encountered in this type of combination chemotherapy, but we have so far discovered no difference between the two groups of patients. However, long-term follow-up may demonstrate whether prednisone is advantageous or disadvantageous. Seventy percent of all stage IV patients are in remission.

Lymphosarcoma and Reticulum-Cell Sarcoma

In this group, the histological pattern is of greater importance than in Hodgkin's disease in determining the initial method of treatment.

Radiotherapy

In a series of 325 patients treated principally only by local radiotherapy, and reviewed in 1969 [3], long-term survivors were found in all four histological subgroups (Fig. 2). The survival rate was best in patients with nodular sclerotic lymphosarcoma and follicular lymphoma, even when the disease was generalized. The survival rate was lower in the diffuse lymphocytic lymphosarcoma group and very poor in the lymphoblastic group. Permanent cure does appears to be possible in some cases of lymphosarcoma. Twenty-one patients who had survived 5 years without clinical recurrence were analyzed. Survival for up to 20 years was seen in this group. Three 5-year survivors with localized lymphoblastic lymphosarcoma are included in this group. In cases of this highly malignant tumor, generalized disease is likely to occur within 1 to 2 years after initial treatment if the patient is not cured. Survival for

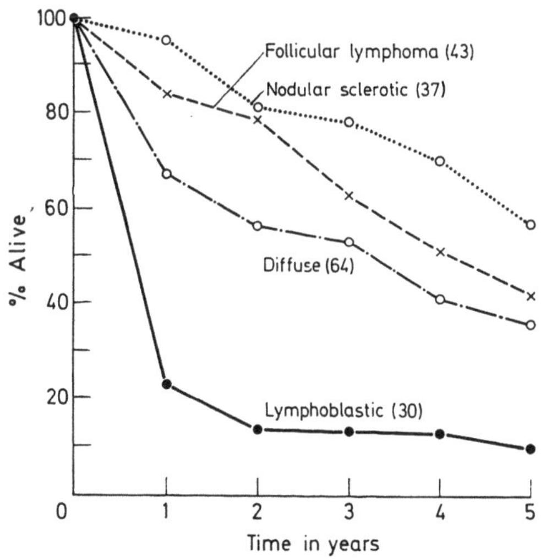

Fig. 2. Five-year-survival rates of 174 patients with lymphosarcoma. With nodular sclerotic lymphosarcoma, 56% survive for 5 years. (Brit. J. Cancer 23, 686 (1969). Reproduced with the permission of the Editor and Authors [3])

only 2 years probably means permanent cure. This suggests that localized disease should be treated with radiotherapy, regardless of the histological group. The value of prophylactic irradiation is as yet undetermined. It is possible that cytotoxic drugs should be used after local radiotherapy with the more malignant lymphomas. The British group is considering these problems at the present time.

The one exception to this general principle is in those patients who present in the first two decades of life (Table 1). In patients under the age of 20, lymphosarcoma is particularly vigorous. Of these 19 patients, only 1 with diffuse lymphosarcoma had survived. Four others with follicular lymphoma or nodular sclerotic lymphosarcoma were alive and well after 11, 12, 17 and 19 years. The other patients with diffuse lymphosarcoma or lymphoblastic lymphosarcoma survived for only short periods. This suggests that all young patients with localized lymphoblastic or lymphocytic sarcoma should be considered for energetic chemotherapy, either alone or after local radiotherapy.

In lymphosarcoma and reticulum-cell sarcoma it is extremely important to investigate the nasopharynx, the bone marrow and the liver. Bone-marrow invasion is frequent in lymphosarcoma. Liver involvement is easier to detect by a closed liver biopsy because of the diffuse nature of the infiltration.

When the disease is generalized, involving lymph nodes both above and below the diaphragm, this can be treated effectively with total-node irradiation or cytotoxic

Table 1. Analysis of 19 patients with lymphosarcoma who presented before the age of 20. Apart from 1 patient with localized diffuse lymphosarcoma, only 4 patients have survived for a long time and all have low grade lymphosarcoma. (Brit. J. Cancer **23**, 686 (1969). Reproduced with the permission of the Editor and Authors.) From [3]

Histological group	Patients	Age	Sex	Extent of disease at presentation	Survival in years
Lymphoblastic lymphosarcoma	SD	11	M	Generalized	7/12—AW
	JF	5	M		7/12—D
	MF	17	M		3/12—D
	BM	19	M		3/12—D
	DM	16	M		2/12—D
	MM	16	F		9/12—AR
	MK	12	M		10/12—D
	JG	17	M		18 days—D
	GM	9	M	Localized	4/12—AW
	EC	14	M		6/12—D
Diffuse lymphosarcoma	EH	19	M	Generalized	4 days—D
	JJ	12	F		15/12—D
	MS	8	M		3/12—D
	RO	16	M		10/12—D
	MS	19	M	Localized	8 years—AW
Follicular lymphoma	GF	19	M	Generalized	20 years—AW
	RD	11	M	Localized	5 4/12—AW
Nodular sclerotic lymphosarcoma	GF	9	M	Localized	19 years—AW
	MA	8	F		17 years—AW

AW: alive and well AR: alive with recurrence D: dead

drugs. At present total-node irradiation should be considered only when treating follicular lymphoma, nodular sclerotic lymphosarcoma, and perhaps diffuse lymphocytic lymphosarcoma. In lymphoblastic lymphosarcoma and reticulum-cell sarcoma it is likely that the disease has already progressed too far to allow both halves of the body to be irradiated with a reasonable chance of success. It may prove preferable to treat the patient with cytotoxic drugs, or with whole-body irradiation, as recommended by JOHNSON in the previous paper.

Chemotherapy — Low-Grade Lymphosarcoma

With generalized lymphosarcoma of low activity there are two possible approaches using cytotoxic drugs. In the past, patients have been treated satisfactorily with small doses of alkylating agents such as chlorambucil for long periods of time. This approach is based upon the belief that the disease is always fatal, but that long survival is usual and cannot be improved by energetic treatment. We believe that such pessimism is wrong. Over the last 2 years we have treated a small number of patients with generalized low-grade lymphosarcoma with repeated courses of combination therapy using cyclophosphamide, vincristine, prednisone and sometimes procarbazine (Table 2). Of the 4 patients with follicular lymphoma treated in this way, all are in complete remission. Two patients with diffuse lymphosarcoma have been treated with combination chemotherapy and both are in complete remission (Table 3).

Repeated courses of combination therapy may be necessary, and patients treated in this way may do no better than with chlorambucil maintenance therapy. It is necessary to carry out a controlled investigation to compare the two methods.

It is possible that single-agent maintenance therapy may prove to be a valuable method of treatment in *low-grade* lymphosarcoma. But careful clinical assessment of individual patients is essential. The histological report may suggest a low-grade lymphosarcoma while rapid progression of the disease and infiltration of extranodal

Table 2. Combination therapy used with Hodgkin's disease, similar to the original MOPP regime. Prednisone was used with each individual course of treatment

Day 0	Vincristine	1.4 mg/m²
and		
Day 7	HN 2	6 mg/m²
Day 0—10	Natulan	100 mg/m²
Day 0—14	Prednisone	25 mg/m²

Table 3. Combination therapy used with lymphosarcoma and reticulum cell sarcoma, similar to original MOPP regime. Prednisone was used with each individual course of treatment

Day 0	Vincristine	1.4 mg/m²
and		
Day 7	Cyclophosphamide	600 mg/m²
Day 0—7	Natulan	100 mg/m²
Day 0—7	Prednisone	25 mg/m²

structures indicates a more malignant process. In such cases, better control is probably obtainable with combination therapy. We have recently treated 2 patients with generalized follicular lymphoma with chlorambucil maintenance therapy. One is very fit, though still with active disease, but the other responded poorly and died. This second patient had bone invasion when first seen.

Chemotherapy: Lymphoblastic Lymphosarcoma: Reticulum-Cell Sarcoma

Many of the more anaplastic tumors of lymph nodes grow so rapidly that the use of single cytotoxic drugs in low dosage is ineffective. Combination chemotherapy is more likely to induce remission, and we have used this technique in 15 patients. Among the 5 patients with generalized lymphoblastic lymphosarcoma, the disease has been controlled for 11 and 17 months in 2 cases. Of 10 patients with generalized reticulum-cell sarcoma, 2 have been controlled for 5 and 11 months by one course of combination chemotherapy, and 1 is being controlled (after 18 months) by repeated courses (Table 4). These results may represent an improvement, but they are not good, and we hope that other drug combinations will prove more effective.

At present, when standard combination therapy fails, we try continuous infusions with methotrexate or with a mixture of adriamycin, cytosine arabinoside and vin-

Table 4. Relative value of combination chemotherapy in a small number of patients with non-Hodgkin's lymphoma. Of 6 patients with follicular lymphoma and diffuse lymphosarcoma, all have achieved complete remission. With lymphoblastic lymphosarcoma, 2 out of 5 patients are in remission. With reticulo sarcoma 2 remissions have been obtained and 1 patient of a total of 10 patients treated with combination therapy has been kept in remission with maintenance combination therapy

Treatment	Cases	Cases controlled
Follicular lymphoma		
Combination chemotherapy	4	4 (8, 13, 14, 15 [d])
Chlorambucil	2	0 (1 [c], 1 [b])
Radiotherapy	1	0 (1 [b])
Diffuse lymphosarcoma		
Combination chemotherapy	2	2 (14, 15 [d])
Radiotherapy	1	1 (15 [d])
Lymphoblastic lymphosarcoma		
Combination chemotherapy	5	2 (11, 17 [d]) (1 [c], 2 [b])
Reticulum-cell sarcoma		
Combination chemotherapy	10	3 (5, 11, 18 [d]) (5 [c], 2 [b])
Radiotherapy	2	0 (2 [c])

[a] Alive; no disease
[b] Alive with lymphoma
[c] Dead
[d] Months

cristine. Control of the more malignant forms of these diseases remains a very difficult problem, and we see little hope of curing many patients with the cytotoxic drugs available at present.

The Future

We need to be able to select for each patient the method of treatment which offers the greatest chance or cure with the least risk. This aim will be achieved only by the use of prospective controlled clinical trials, in which there is very close cooperation between radiotherapists and physicians.

Acknowledgements

We are very grateful to our colleagues in Birmingham, Cambridge, Cardiff, Cheltenham, Coventry, Harefield, Leeds, Liverpool, London, Northwood, Plymouth, Southampton, Southend and Truro for permission to refer to the research programme in which we are collaborating, and to the members of our Pathology Panel, Professor C. V. Harrison, Dr. M. H. Bennett and Dr. G. Farrer-Brown for their constant help.

We are indebted to Mr. M. Turney, Mr. P. Drury and the Department of Medical Illustration for the preparation of illustrations, and to Mrs. Audrey Taylor for secretarial assistance.

This work has been supported financially by the Aitchison Charitable Trust, the Batchworth Trust, The Cancer Research Campaign, the J. S. Fraser Trust Fund, Eli Lilly & Co. Ltd., the New Court Charitable Trust, the Peggy Russell Memorial Fund and many other generous individuals and families.

References

1. Bennett, M. H., Millett, Y. L.: Clin. Radiol. 20, 339 (1969).
2. Harrison, C. V.: In: Recent Advances in Pathology, No. 8, p. 232. (Harrison, C. V., Ed.) London: Churchill 1966.
3. Millett, Y. L., Bennett, M. H., Jelliffe, A. M., Farrer-Brown, G.: Brit. J. Cancer **23**, 683 (1969).
4. Rappaport, H.: In: The lymphoreticular tumors in Africa, p. 174. (Roulet, F. C., Ed.) Basel: Karger 1963.

Clinical Trials of the European Organization for Research on Treatment of Cancer (E. O. R. T. C.)

Survey presented by BRIGIT VAN DER WERF-MESSING,
President of the organization (on behalf of all cooperative centres)

Chairmen of E.O.R.T.C.: M. TUBIANA (1964—1967), K. BREUR (1967—1969), B. VAN DER WERF-MESSING (1969—1971). General Secretary: A. LAUGIER. Statistician: M. HAYAT.

Cooperative Centres in France: C. A. C. Bordeaux (C. LAGARDE), C. A. C. Caen (S. ABBATUCCI, Lyon (J. PAPILLON, L. REVOL), Paris: Hôtel-Dieu (J. BOUSSER), C. A. C. Rouen (H. PIGUET), Villejuif (G. MATHÉ, M. TUBIANA, J. L. AMIEL); in Belgium: Brussels Institut Jules Bordet (J. HENRY), Liège (R. LEMAIRE), Louvain (A. WAMBERSIE); in The Netherlands: Amsterdam (K. BREUER, M. BURGERS), Leyden (P. THOMAS), Nimmegen (C. HAANEN), Rotterdam (B. VAN DER WERF-MESSING, W. F. STENFERT KROESE).

Members of the histology review committee: R. GÉRARD-MARCHANT, J. VAN UNNIK; lymphography review committee: R. W. KROPHOLLER, J. D. PICARD, P. MARKOVITS, J. L. CHASSARD.

Summary

A brief outline is given of clinical trials, run by European Cancer Centres: morbus Hodgkin stage I and II, nodular supradiaphragmatic reticulumcellsarcoma stage I and II, Ewingsarcoma and osteosarcoma.

In 1964 the Cancer Centers of France, Belgium and Holland decided to start a cooperative study on patients with Hodgkin's disease stages I and $II_{A,B}$. The purpose was to assess whether additional chemotherapy after a full course of irradiation could improve prognosis.

All patients were investigated according to a fixed scheme, including lymphography. In all cases the histological preparations were reviewed by an international board of pathologists. Lymphographies were similarly reassessed by an international group of lymphography experts. In no instance was a diagnostic laparotomy performed.

Patients were randomly allotted to one of the following two treatment schedules:

A. A complete course of irradiation, mantle technique or inverted-Y technique, delivering 4000 rad in 4 weeks to the affected region and 3500 rad in the same period as prophylactic treatment.

B. The second group received a similar radiotherapy treatment followed by vinblastine intravenously once weekly for 2 years (10 mg in patients with a leukocyte count more than 5000; 5 mg with leukocyte 3000—5000; no vinblastine with leukocyte less than 3000).

In 1971, 296 cases had been admitted and the preliminary results were evaluated (Fig. 1). It appeared that additional vinblastine therapy improved both the actuarial survival rate and the actuarial relapse-free survival rate. Detailed analysis showed that histology, sex, mediastinal involvement, systemic symptoms and age had an im-

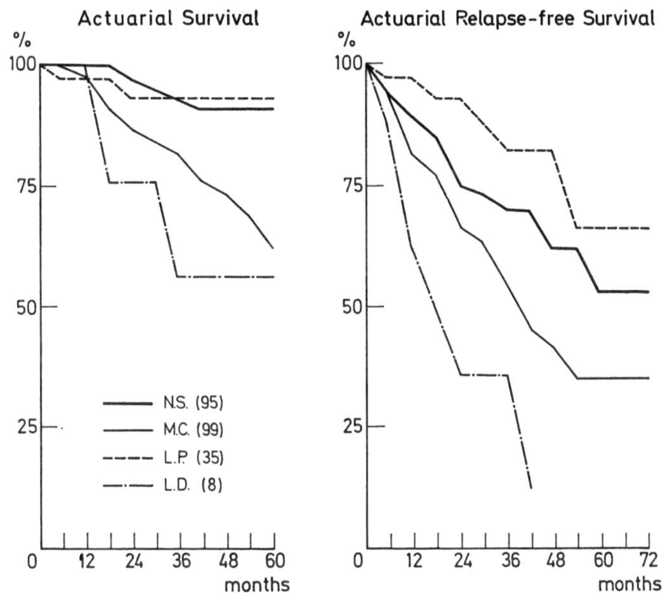

Fig. 1. Effect of radiotherapy (RX) with and without vinblastine (VBL) in 269 HD patients (stages I and II)

portant bearing on prognosis (Table 1). Histologic type appeared to be the most significant factor, and the prognostic influence of other factors could be explained by their relation to histology (Fig. 2). Additional vinblastine improved prognosis in all analyzed sub-groups but was most influential in the histological sub-group mixed cellularity (Fig. 3).

A new European trial has been designed, based on these data. The value of splenectomy will be assessed by randomly allotting patients to laparotomy with splenectomy followed by radiotherapy, or to radiotherapy only. As the previous trial demonstrated that the majority of recurrences appeared in the lumbar region after mantle-technique irradiation (Table 2), all patients in the new trial will receive irradiation to the lumbar nodes (and to the spleen in cases in whom no laparotomy has been performed) in addition to the mantle treatment. As additional chemotherapy was most effective in the histological sub-group mixed cellularity, all patients with disease of this histological type will receive additional chemotherapy again in a randomized trial: either vinblastine once weekly, or vinblastine plus Natulan.

Table 1. Effect on survival of sex, age, systemic symptoms, mediastinal involvement, and histologic type of HD in 269 patients (stages I and II). Actuarial survival and actuarial relapse-free survival of HD patients in relation to various tumor and host factors

	Total number	3-Year % Survival	3-Year % Relapse-free survival	5-Year % Survival	5-Year % Relapse-free survival
Male	183	85	55	80	40
Female	113	90	70	75	55
≧ 30 years	133	90	55	70	35
< 30 years	163	80	65	80	55
Systemic symptoms "B"	39	70	45	55	45
No systemic symptoms "A"	257	90	65	80	50
Stage I+II$_{A,B}$ above diaphragm					
Mediastinum involved	102	95	60	80	55
Mediastinum not involved	180	80	60	70	40
Stage I+II$_{A,B}$ below diaphragm	14	85	50	80	30
Histology [a]					
Lymhocytic Predominance	35	94	83	93	65
Nodular Sclerosis	95	94	68	91	53
Mixed Cellularity	99	82	53	63	38
Lymphocytic Depletion	8	75	37	57	13
					(after 42 months)

[a] At the time of this evaluation all histological slides had not been reviewed.

Table 2. Hodgkin's disease: Site of relapse after mantle irradiation with and without vinblastine (269 patients)

	X-ray only		X-ray +vinblastine
Local recurrence (in irradiated area or marginal recurrence)	6		5
Transdiaphragmatic extension	23	←——→	7
Visceral extension or dissemination	13		17
All relapses	42	←——→	29

←——→ : Statistical significance

In 1966 the cooperative centres (also) decided to conduct a trial for patients with Ewing's sarcoma. After a full course of irradiation (6000 rad in 6 weeks to the whole affected long bone or 4000 rad in 4 weeks to the flat bone), the effect of additional chemotherapy (Endoxan) on prognosis was determined in a randomized trial. The preliminary results show poorer prognosis in the chemotherapy group after 6 months. This effect disappears after 1 year (Fig. 4).

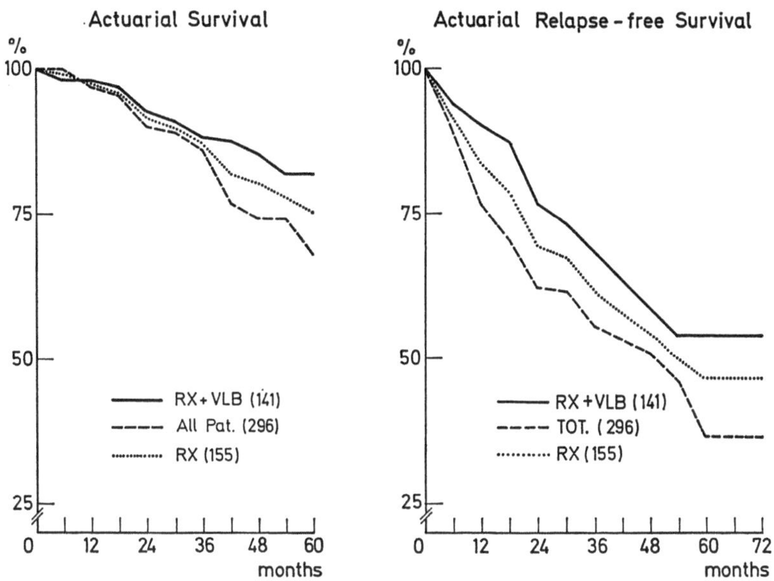

Fig. 2. Influence of histologic type of HD on survival

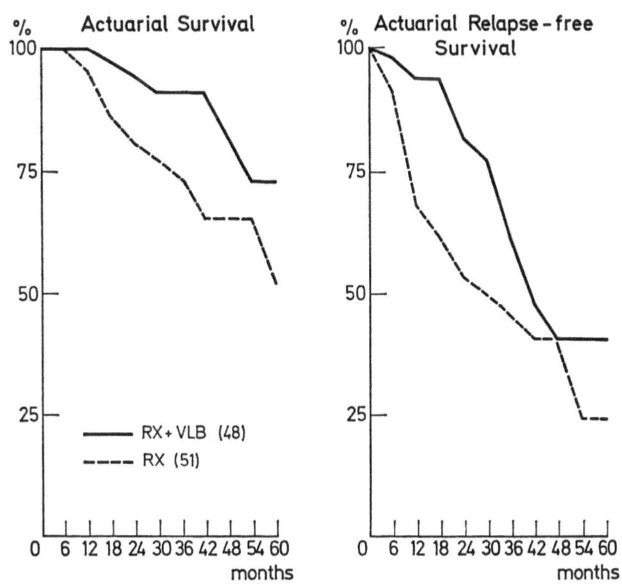

Fig. 3. Effect of radiotherapy with and without vinblastine in cases of mixed cellularity type

In 1970 a trial was started for patients with reticulum-cell sarcoma and lymphosarcoma stages I or II with a glandular lesion above the diaphragm. The purpose was to assess whether additional irradiation to the lumbar nodes could improve prognosis after radiotherapy to the lymphatic region above the diaphragm (mantle-technique excluding the mediastinum, 4000 rad in 4 weeks to the affected area, 3500 rad to adjacent regions). Until now, 40 patients have been admitted. The number is still too small to assess preliminary results.

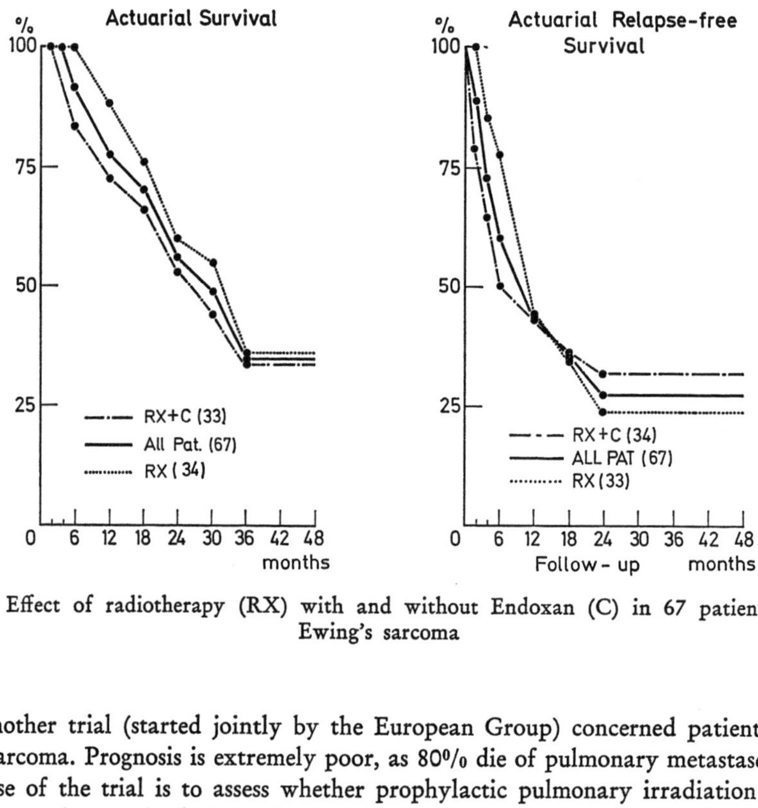

Fig. 4. Effect of radiotherapy (RX) with and without Endoxan (C) in 67 patients with Ewing's sarcoma

Another trial (started jointly by the European Group) concerned patients with osteosarcoma. Prognosis is extremely poor, as 80% die of pulmonary metastases. The purpose of the trial is to assess whether prophylactic pulmonary irradiation might eradicate microscopic foci in the lungs, thereby preventing the development of pulmonary metastases. Twenty-seven patients have been admitted. Here again, the number is still too small to enable evaluation of the preliminary results.

The latest trial is devoted to Hodgkin's disease stage III_B. The treatment modalities are either chemotherapy alone (MOPP) or in combination with radiotherapy. Until now only a few cases have been admitted.

The European Centers hope jointly to provide answers to the various problems within 5 to 10 years. In addition to the scientific and hence therapeutic benefits of these trials, cooperation has promoted mutual respect and understanding amongst specialists at the various European centers. Thus, cooperation is a sound basis for continued joint efforts to improve the treatment of cancer patients.

Therapeutic Results in Malignant Lymphoma

The Curability of Hodgkin's Disease

J. Papillon

Summary

The curability of Hodgkin's disease is based not only on long-term survivors, but also on the notion that patients properly treated may have the same expectation of life as that of the normal population. The most reliable criterion of curability is the recurrence-free survival over 10 years following the first treatment. Using data drawn from a series of 282 patients primarily treated between 1939 and 1962, and followed for more than 10 years, the cure rate is 15%. This rate is essentially related to patients treated before the era of supervoltage radiation therapy and of lymphangiography. Cure rate is 44% in stage I and II A, 17% in stage II B. Stress is placed on the most favorable clinical presentations and on the management of these forms. Télécobalt-therapy, lymphangiography and chemotherapy are improving the long-term results and the curability of Hodgkin's disease.

The possibility of cure in Hodgkin's disease has now been recognized, as was predicted by Gilbert [1]. Even then Gilbert thought that early and intensive radiation therapy might sometimes give very long, even definitive remissions. Many physicians knew of long-time survivors, yet refused to believe that Hodgkin's disease could be permanently cured. In medicine, established beliefs are often hard to change.

In 1966 Peters [3, 4] remarked that survival for a very long period — 15 to 20 years — without detectable signs of Hodgkin's disease argued strongly in favor of the curability of the disease. Easson and Russell [2] were the first to demonstrate that, in a group of patients who survived for 10—15 years, expectation of life could be shown to be similar to that of the normal population of the same sex and age. He was the first to offer proof of the cure of patients treated for Hodgkin's disease.

Curability is gratifying for the physician, but for the patient it spells the hope of a completely normal life with no restrictions at all.

On the basis of data from the literature and an analysis of our own statistics based on 282 patients initially treated between 1939 and 1962 and followed up for more than 10 years, we would like to discuss:

1. criteria of curability
2. rate of cure
3. clinical factors in prognosis
4. management of Hodgkin's disease, when the prognosis was good.

1. Criteria of Curability

What is the Basis for Assessing whether a Patient has a Chance of Being Cured?

Peters was the first author to point out the necessity of an assessment after 10 years. In all the studies, some patients who lived more than 10 years after the first treatment died from the disease between the 10th and the 20th year. Almost all these patients had one or more recurrences before the 10th year.

Heilmeyer, Musshoff [5, 6] demonstrated that among the criteria for cure, the best and most convenient one is survival without recurrence for 10 years following first treatment. If a patient is alive and in complete remission after more than 10 years, the likelihood of recurrence is negligible and the patient can be said to be cured. In a very few cases, a recurrence is observed after periods of remission of 10 to 15 years. The definition of "first treatment" must be such as to include any second treatment necessary soon after the first, because lesions in the area marginal or adjacent to the primary location can be considered as a continuation of the first treatment rather than a true recurrence. Peters had already suggested this concept. Our group of cured patients contained three who had such early relapses.

Kaplan [7, 9] considered 10 years too long and thought it possible to use an earlier indicator of ultimate prognosis, since patients with Hodgkin's disease who remain relapse-free for 5 years after radiotherapy have at least a 95 percent chance of permanent cure. [8] also stressed an interval of 5 years as a useful indicator.

In 1970 we examined our statistics for the percentage of relapse-free patients after 10 and 5 years, respectively. We concluded that a patient who remains relapse-free for more than 5 years has a more than 80 percent chance of being permanently cured.

2. Rate of Cure

Peters estimated the overall cure rate in her patients as 20 percent, and in [6] it is 20.9 percent.

In Lyons, 68 of the 282 patients (23%) followed for more than 10 years, are still alive. Of these, 44 (15%) have been in complete remission since the first treatment. These 44 patients, disease-free for 10 to 33 years, may be considered as probably cured.

The percentages, based on the notion of long-term relapse-free survival, are related to patients treated long before the introduction of lymphangiography and before (or at the beginning of) the advent of supervoltage radiation. These facts must be kept in mind since the figures quoted here cannot be compared with those published in 1972 by Kaplan relating to patients treated with modern procedures for whom actuarial analysis reveals an overall 10-year survival rate of 58 percent.

3. Clinical Factors in Prognosis

The analysis of these 44 cases reveals which features of Hodgkin's disease are associated with the best prognosis.

The prognosis is significantly better in females than in males, i. e. the cure rate is 22% and 10%, respectively, in our series. MUSSHOFF has shown that the differences within stages are not significant; the better prognosis for females is essentially due to the percentage of unfavorable stages (II B, III and IV) being smaller than in males.

Obviously, staging is of prognostic value. The cure rate is 44% in stages I and II A, 17% in stage II B and only 1% in stages III and IV.

All systemic symptoms are not of the same significance, e. g. pruritus is not as bad a sign as fever or loss of weight.

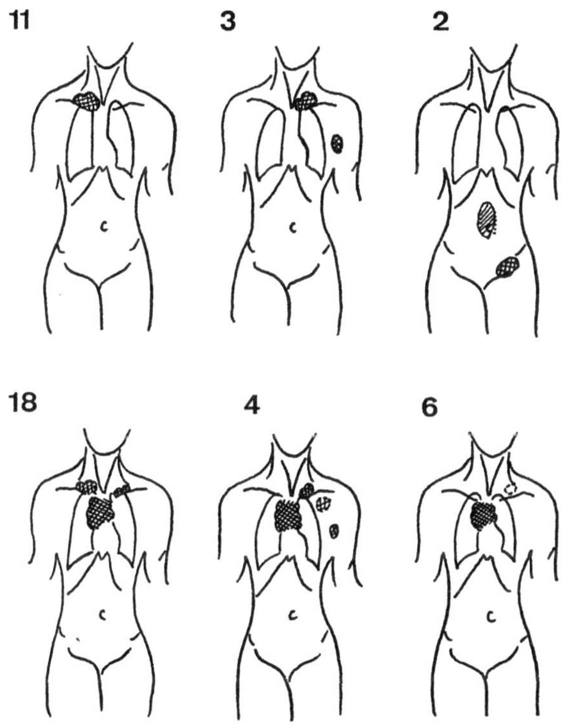

Fig. 1. Primary clinical presentation in 44 recurrence-free 10 year survivors among 282 patients with Hodgkin's disease seen at Lyons (1939—1962) and followed for more than 10 years

The locations of the nodes found to be involved at the first examination in our group of 44 cured patients are indicative of the more favorable presentations. Fig. 1 shows the primary clinical presentations of these patients:

early supraclavicular location was present 36 times out of 44;
the upper neck was not usually involved clinically;
all involvements of the axilla (6 cases) occurred in patients who had also invasion of the supraclavicular area;
the axilla alone was never invaded. (It is well known that axillary presentations are prognostically unfavorable and often display evidence of dissemination.)

The mediastinum was radiologically invaded in 28 cases (63%).

We found it necessary to compare 2 different locations in the mediastinum: involvement of the upper and anteriour mediastinum (i. e., the paratracheal chains and the internal mammary chains) and involvement of the hilar nodes (i. e., the peribronchial nodes). The prognosis of these locations is completely different: in the hilar presentations, whether or not combined with the upper mediastinum, the average survival is 38 months and the average duration of the first remission is 13 months. In contrast, the figures are respectively 62 months and 38 months in the upper mediastinal presentations.

Among the 44 cured patients, both hila were generally not invaded (except in two cases) while the involvement was located in the upper mediastinum. Hilar involvement is almost always synonymous with spread of the disease into the lung, whereas the involvement of the upper mediastinum is not prognostically bad.

In 6 of the 44 cured patients, the first location was in the mediastinum only. This is proof that Hodgkin's disease is curable even if the first presentation is situated in the thorax.

We would like to draw attention to the involvement of the internal mammary chain at the first examination, which has been seldom reported in Hodgkin's disease. Of 421 patients primarily treated from 1939 to 1966, we observed 25 patients who had Hodgkin's disease which had spread to this particular area. It is interesting to study its prognostic value. In the history of the disease the first symptoms mentioned were:

in 10 cases, a parasternal swelling;
in 6 cases, cervical node and a simultaneous parasternal swelling;
in 7 cases, parasternal swelling appeared a few weeks after that of the cervical nodes;
in 2 cases, initial involvement of the internal mammary chain was found during the thoracotomy for mediastinal lymphoma. The prognosis of the latter presentation is not very favorable. After 5 years 11 out of 25 patients are alive (4 are relapse-free). After 10 years 4 out of 16 are alive (2 are relapse-free).

4. Management of the Favorable Presentations

Taking all these factors into consideration, it is possible to try to predict the course and the outcome in the individual case and to define the most favorable presentations.

The therapist should realize that a patient with localized Hodgkin's disease has a good chance of being cured if the treatment is adequate. It has been proved that vigorous local therapy can eradicate the disease and yield long-term survivors without recurrence. The main consideration is the form of therapy of patients should receive.

The value of irradiation in localized Hodgkin's disease has been clearly established. There is now universal agreement that the dosage to the sites of involvement should be intense, and minimal levels of 3500 rads in four weeks are generally advocated. In Lyons, we have long been convinced of the advantage of prophylactic irradiation of uninvolved adjacent node-bearing areas at a dosage of 3000 rads over 4 weeks, but we have never practised "total nodal irradiation". For the stages I and II above the diaphragm (normal lymphangiography) we do not irradiate the abdominal chain with cobalt.

For the past 6 years we have been using radioactive lymphangiography systematically in the first investigations of the new patients. Phosphorus-32 was used at a dose of 4 mCi during the first period from 1966 until June 1969 and at a dose of 8 mCi since July 1969. We are fully aware that this endolymphatic beta-therapy is not homogenous and is unable to sterilize large foci of Hodgkin's tissue in a lymph node. Although some para-aortic and iliac nodes are not impregnated, we think that this method may be of some value of prophylactic irradiation of normal or subnormal abdominal lymph nodes.

We consider, the purpose of radioactive lymphangiography to be twofold:

1. to avoid the systematic irradiation of the abdominal chains in case of normal lymphangiography;

2. to avoid irradiation of the ovaries in young women when lymphangiography shows an involvement of the upper para-aortic nodes. In these cases, irradiation is limited to the lumbar area and we rely on endolymphatic beta-therapy to irradiate the iliac chains prophylactically.

Between 1966 and February 1971, 123 ^{32}P lymphangiographies were carried out. The results fell into two groups: 1. negative or equivocal; 2. positive.

When the lymphogram was negative or equivocal, external cobalt irradiation below the diaphragm was not always performed. In this group of 53 patients followed from 18 months to 6 years we observed only 6 recurrences in the abdominal area. These 6 patients have had lymphangiographies with only 4 mCi of ^{32}P. So far, no other patients have developed abdominal recurrences.

Seventy lymphangiographies were positive and the patients received an irradiation to the abdominal chains at a dosage of 3500 rads. With 13 women the irradiation was limited to the para-aortic area; the iliac chains, which were apparently normal, were not irradiated. No recurrence in the pelvic area was observed clinically.

It is too early to assess the place of radioactive lymphangiography in the management of Hodgkin's disease. Although the delay of follow-up is too short for some cases, we think that the percentage of abdominal recurrences is especially low and that this is a provisional proof of the prophylactic efficacy of the radioactive lymphangiography on the abdominal chains.

There are a number of, as yet, unanswered questions.

What is the role of splenectomy in the curative treatment of localized Hodgkin's disease? Should laparotomy be routine in early cases? On the other hand, is caution advisable in selection of patients for laparotomy, as is our present practice? Is chemotherapy of value in radical treatment, especially of the mixed cellularity cases?

In conclusion, the literature and the present study offer proof that it was possible to cure some patients with Hodgkin's disease before the era of lymphangiography and the supervoltage radiation therapy. We now have more sophisticated methods of investigation and powerful tools of treatment. Kaplan, and many other authors [8] have demonstrated that the 3- and 5-year relapse-free survival rate has progressively improved, and it is likely that the rate of remission for more than 10 years will also increase.

Among the several possibilities for planning treatment, the major problem will be: what is the optimal procedure for each individual patient? In other words, which treatment will give him the best chance of cure with the minimum risk of recurrence or complications?

I do not believe that a systematic approach to the treatment of Hodgkin's disease is possible. Between an intensive and extensive method, with very high risk of complications, and a too timid approach, a compromise adapted to each individual patient must be found. This choice is difficult. It can only be made with the close collaboration of physicians, hematologists and radiotherapists.

References

1. Gilbert, R.: Radiotherapy in Hodgkin's disease (malignant granulomatosis). Amer. J. Roentgenol. **41**, 198 (1939).
2. Easson, E. C., Russell, M. H.: The cure of Hodgkin's disease. Brit. med. J. **1963 I**, 5347 1704, 1077.
3. Peters, M. V.: Long-term results of radical radiotherapy of Hodgkin's disease. Cancer Res. **26**, 1253 (1966).
4. Peters, M. V., Middlemiss, K. H.: A study of Hodgkin's disease treated by irradiation. Amer. J. Roentgenol. 79—114 (1958).
5. Heilmeyer, L.: Neues über Diagnostik und Therapie der Lymphogranulomatose. Münch. med. Wschr. **108**, 349 (1966).
6. Musshoff, K., Boutis, L.: Therapy results in Hodgkin's disease. Freiburg i. Br. 1948—1966. Cancer (Philad.) **21**, 1100 (1968).
7. Kaplan, H.: Prognostic significance of the relapse-free interval after radiotherapy in Hodgkin's disease. Cancer (Philad.) **22**, 1131 (1968).
8. Lauwers, L., Dancot, H.: Relation entre le degré d'activité de la maladie d'Hodgkin au cours des cinq premières années et le devenir des malades survivants à 5 ans. Nouv. Rev. franç. Hémat. **6**, 98 (1966).
9. Kaplan, H.: Hodgkin's disease. Cambridge, Mass: Harvard University Press 1972.

The Curability of Lympho- and Reticulosarcomas

H. DANCOT and W. FEREMANS

Summary

1. A study of the fate of patients treated for lympho- or reticulosarcomas and living without recurrence at the end of the 5th year after treatment. At the end of the 10the year since the treatment only 3% had experienced a recurrence (3 on 89), and at the end of the 20th year, only 6% (3 on 47). A comparison of the frequency of late recurrences of patients treated for cancer of the uterine cervix and apparently cured 5 years after treatment is made.

2. A comparison of the evolution of lympho- and reticulosarcomas recurring at any time after treatment (from 6 months to 17 years) is made in order to determine whether there is any difference in this evolution after the first recurrence: no distinct difference does appear.

It is now generally agreed that lympho- and reticulosarcomas are not infrequently curable. We first discuss the fate of 89 patients (58 with lymphosarcoma, 31 with reticulosarcoma) who were alive without recurrence at the end of the 5th year after treatment. The time elapsed since treatment is now 10 to 33 years. The primary locations were: lymph nodes, tonsils, nasopharynx, stomach, intestine, skin, orbit, etc. Secondly, we discuss lympho- and reticulosarcoma recurrences at any time after treatment to see whether there is any difference in the prognosis with early or late first recurrence.

Patients Apparently Cured at 5 Years

The results at 10, 15, 20 and 25 years for patients apparently cured 5 years after their treatment are given in Table 1. We stress that, of the 89 cases, 71 (80%) were alive and free of disease at the end of the 10th year, 15 (17%) had died of intercurrent disease between the 5th and the 10th years, and only 3 (3%) had experienced a recurrence during this period.

In Table 2 the patients are subdivided in two groups according to their age at the time of treatment (averages respectively 32 years 6 months; 64 years). Obviously, deaths due to intercurrent disease are much more frequent in the second group.

The frequency of recurrences during each subsequent 5-year period is summarized in Table 3 for 105 patients, including the 89 in Table 2. For comparison with Table 1, we now show the fate after 5 years of 300 epitheliomas of the uterine cervix, all without recurrence at the end of the 5th year and all with an interval of 25 years or

Table 1. Lympho- and reticulosarcomas. Results at 10, 15, 20 and 25 years for patients apperently cured 5 years after treatment

Years after treatment	Number of cases	Cured	Deaths due to intercurrent diseases	Recurrences
10	89	71—80%	15—17%	3— 3%
15	73	47—64%	22—30%	4— 6%
20	47	22—47%	22—47%	3— 6%
25	29	10—35%	16—55%	3—10%

Table 2. Lympho- and reticulosarcomas. Patients of Table 1 subdivided in two groups according to age at time of treatment

A. Patients 50 years old or less (Average: 32 Y. 6 M.)				
Years after treatment	Number of cases	Cured	Deaths due to intercurrent diseases	Recurrences
10	33	31—94%	1— 3%	1— 3%
15	24	22—92%	1— 4%	1— 4%
20	16	14—88%	1— 6%	1— 6%
25	12	7—58%	4—34%	1— 8%
B. Patients older than 50 years (Average: 64 years)				
10	56	40—71%	14—25%	2— 3%
15	49	25—51%	21—43%	3— 6%
20	31	8—26%	21—68%	2— 6%
25	17	3—18%	12—70%	2—12%

Table 3. Lympho- and reticulosarcomas. Frequency of recurrences for each 5-year period

Periods	No. of patients alive and without recurrence at beginning	at end	Recurrences during period each 5-yr [a]
5 to 10 years	105	71	3—4% (approx.)
10 to 15 years	71	47	3—5% (approx.)
15 to 20 years	47	22	1—3% (approx.)
20 to 25 years	22	10	0
after 25 years (up to 33 years)	10	6	0

[a] 4 R. Sarcomas, 3 L. Sarcomas.

more (Table 4). For comparison with Table 2, we have arranged the same patients in Table 5 according to age at time of treatment (averages 42 years and 63 years 5 months). It may be seen that the same differences appear between the results of the two groups as for lympho- and reticulosarcoma.

Table 4. Cancer of the uterine cervix. Results at 10, 15, 20 and 25 years for patients apparently cured 5 years after treatment

Years after treat-ment	Number of cases	Cured	Deaths due to intercurrent diseases	Recurrences
10	300	230—77%	35—11,5%	35—11,5%
15	300	177—59%	77—26 %	46—15 %
20	300	147—49%	107—39 %	46—15 %
25	300	111—37%	143—48 %	46—15 %

Table 5. Cancer of the uterine cervix. (Same patients as in Table 4.) Patients subdivided in two groups according age at time of treatment

A. Patients 50 years old or less (Average: 42 Years)				
Years after treat-ment	Number of cases	Cured	Deaths due to intercurrent diseases	Recurrences
10	142	124—87%	7— 5%	11— 8%
15	142	110—78%	15—10%	17—12%
20	142	102—72%	23—16%	17—12%
25	142	84—59%	41—29%	17—12%
B. Patients older than 50 years (Average: 63 Y. 5 M.)				
10	158	106—67%	28—18%	24—15%
15	158	67—42%	62—39%	29—19%
20	158	45—28%	84—53%	29—19%
25	158	27—17%	102—64%	29—19%

Recurrences after Treatment

We now discuss lympho- and reticulosarcomas recurring at *any* time after treatment in order to determine whether there is any difference in the case histories when first recurrence appears early or late (from 6 months to 17 years). When we examine survival time after this first recurrence (Fig. 1 and Table 6), we can see that there is no distinct difference.

In Table 7, we have shown the histories after the first recurrence for the patients who had more than 3 years of survival after this recurrence. Here too, the prognosis is the same whether the first recurrence appeared early or late.

Table 6. Lympho- and reticulosarcomas. Conclusion: The difference between B and C (19%, 27%) is not sufficient to confirm that there are two quite different forms of the same affection when the first recurrence appears early or late

Time elapsed between the treatment and the 1st recurrence	Survival after the 1st recurrence a) Less than 3 Years	b) Longer than 3 Years
A. 6 months to 1 year (30 cases)	28	2 (7%)
B. 1 to 3 years (32 cases)	26	6 (19%)
C. 3 years or more (17 yr.) (11 cases)		3 (27%)

Table 7

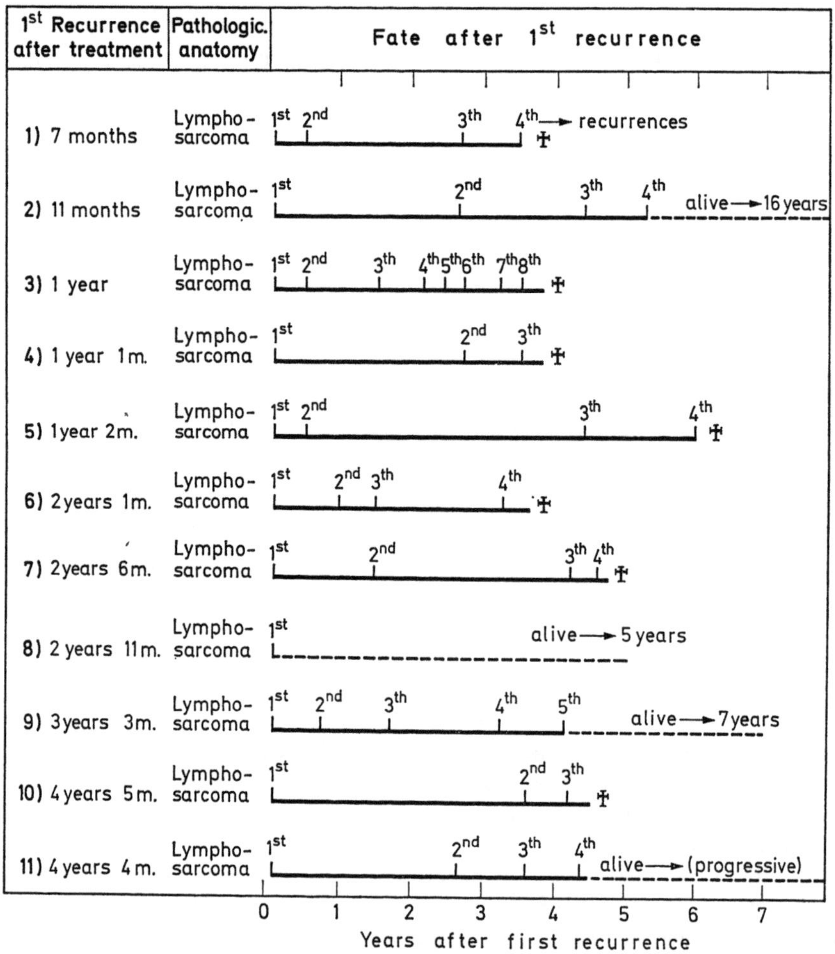

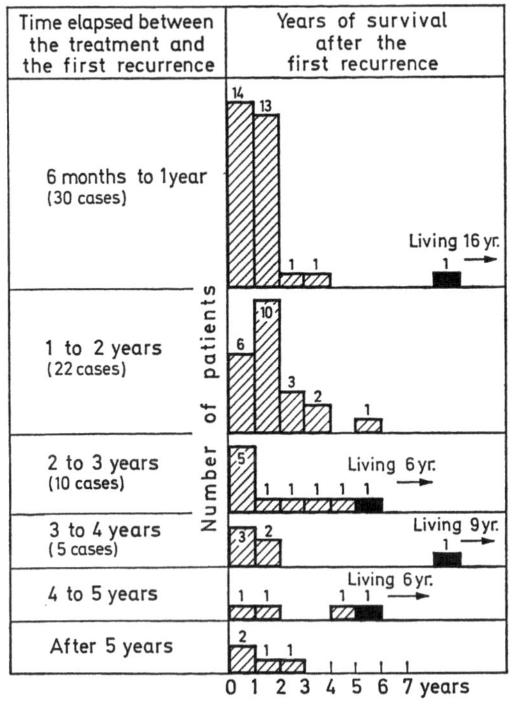

Fig. 1. Lympho- and reticulosarcomas. Survival after the first recurrence

Conclusions

The prognosis for lympho- and reticulosarcoma cases surviving at the end of the 5th year without recurrence during the 5 years is the same as for epithelial tumor cases under the same conditions:

a) The frequency of recurrence after 5 years is not high.

b) As with epithelial tumors, a late recurrence does not mean that subsequent progress will be slower than with earlier recurrence.

There are, therefore, no clinical reasons for thinking that lympho- and reticulosarcomas are not curable.

Results of Therapy in Hodgkin's Disease: Freiburg i. Br. 1964—1971

K. Musshoff, C. Hartmann, B. Niklaus, and R. Rössner

Summary

A series of comparative investigative studies has shown that radiotherapy between the years 1964—1971 developed from local radiation to radiation of extended fields and finally to total nodal radiation including the spleen or spleen extirpation. Thus the total results of this treatment period are the results of a continual development of the treatment methods prevalent at that time.

The 5-year survival rates of this period amount to 70% in the total collective, to 100% in stage I of the Ann Arbor Clinical Staging Classification, 81% in stage II, 63% in stage III, 79% in stages I—III A and to 60% in stages I—III B.
The prognosis is dependent on:

1. the therapy
2. the clinical stage of the Ann Arbor Classification including the B-Symptomatic
3. the histological Rye Classification and
4. the age of the patient collective.

The better prognosis of the collective with first full remission following the first radiation treatment in contrast to the collective with partial remission, and of the latter in contrast to the collective without remission, applies not only to the length of the first remission but also to the prognosis of the first recidive: recidives following full remission have a better prognosis after the second radiation treatment than do manifest recidives following partial remission.

If a full remission is again obtained by means of a renewed radiation treatment of the first recidive, then this full remission has a favorable prognosis comparable to the first full remission.

Introduction

In 1964 the technique of irradiating affected lymph-node groups in H. D. patients separately was replaced by a system of irradiation of contiguous fields. This allowed not only single groups but also large parts or the whole of the lymph-node system to be irradiated if necessary [9]. This method has been described by Jelliffe [3] and Kaplan [4] and has now, under the names of supradiaphragmatic mantle irradiation and infradiaphragmatic inverted-Y irradiation, become the standard method for radiotherapy of malignant lymphomas. A focal dose of 4000 rad is generally given within 4—5 weeks.

From 1964 until 1969, however, this method of treatment was not applied in the same way to all cases because the method was still under clinical trial and some of the specific disease mechanisms were unknown.

1. To assess the clinical value of prophylactic irradiation of adjacent, but as yet unaffected regions in stages I and II, we used either radiotherapy limited to the affected region or extensive radiotherapy of all lymph-node regions on the same side of the diaphragm.

2. In stage III, total nodal irradiation was carried out in 80% of the cases. In the other 20%, extensive but not total nodal irradiation was used; this did not include lymph-node regions without clinical symptoms. In two thirds of all cases in stage III (30 of 46), the spleen showed no clinical signs and was not irradiated.

After 6 years, an analysis of the results of this method was carried out [7, 8]. The findings were:

a) In stage I, and particularly in stage II, the results of local irradiation treatment are not as good as those of extensive irradiation which includes clinically unaffected regions. The diaphragm should not be taken as a limit for the extension of the radiotherapy fields.

b) In stage III, any form of partial irradiation of the lymphatic system is inferior to total nodal irradiation including the spleen.

3. In spite of these reservations, the new method of treatment produced significantly better results than the conventional orthovolt radiotherapy used before 1964. The 5-year survival rate rose from 42% in 1948—1964 to 66% in 1964—1969. Symptom-free 5-year survival after the first course of treatment increased significantly from 19% to 36% (Fig. 1).

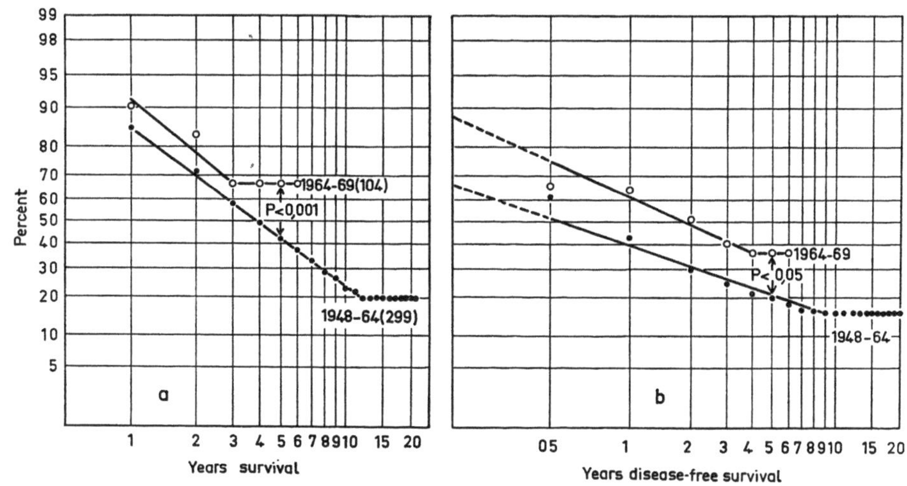

Fig. 1 a and b. Hodgkin's disease: a Actuarial survival, b disease-free survival in the periods 1964 to 1969 and 1948 to 1964. (403 previously untreated cases, all stages). (Reprinted from Musshoff, 1973)

Methods and Patients

After our 1969 analysis of results of irradiation, we agreed on the following treatment procedure, which we have employed as far as possible during the last 2 years:

1. in the localized regional stages I and II (with the exception of some selected cases in stage I) irradiation of all supradiaphragmatic regions and the para-aortic lymph nodes of the abdomen and the spleen (or splenectomy);
2. in stage III, total nodal irradiation including splenic irradiation (or splenectomy).

After a new staging classification, which includes several substantial changes from the Rye Classification, had been introduced in Ann Arbor [2], we subdivided our patient series from 1964—1971 according to this new classification. Besides the survival rates, we investigated the prognostic significance of the different kinds of remissions and relapses. The series includes 175 previously untreated patients.

Results

1. Concerning the New Ann Arbor Classification

a) The 175 untreated patients in the years 1969—1971 were staged as follows: stage I = 9%, stage II = 42%, stage III = 44% and stage IV = 5% of the patient collective.

b) A substantial deviation from the Rye Classification is the smaller percentage of B-cases. This is due to a change of criteria for the B-symptomatology: the prognostically irrelevant symptom of pruritis has been replaced by the symptom of weight loss of more than 10% of the body weight in the 6 month previous to admission, which has great prognostic significance. The B-group, according to the Ann Arbor Classi-

Table 1. Hodgkin's disease. Distribution of the 175 untreated (new) patients by the clinical stages of the Ann Arbor Classification (Freiburg i. Br., 1964—1971)

Stages	Patients			
	No.	%	No.	%
I A	15	8.5	15	8.5
B	0			
II A	55	31.0		
B	13	7.5	73	41.7
II_E (A+B)	5	2.9		
III A	46	26.5		
B	25	14.5	78	44.6
III_E (A+B)	7	4.0		
IV A	2	1.1	9	5.2
B	7	4.0		
Total	175	100.0	175	100.0

Table 2. Hodgkin's disease. Distribution of 175 patients by symptoms A or B (Freiburg data, 1964—1971)

Classification	Patients	No.	Group distribution			
			A No.	B No.	A %	B %
Rye	1964—1969	104	47	57	45	55
Ann Arbor	1964—1971	175	125	50	71	29

fication, has a higher concentration of cases with bad prognosis than the Rye Classification B-group (Table 2).

2. Concerning the Survival and Remission Rates

There was a further slight increase in the results of the 1964—1971 series compared to the 1964—1969 series:

a) The 5-year survival rate of the whole series was 70% and the 5-year symptom-free remission rate was 40%.

b) The 5-year survival rates are in stage I = 100%, in stage II = 81%, and in stage III = 63%. The 5-year symptom-free remission rates are in stage I = 91%, in stage II = 42% and in stage III = 32%. In this series the marked improvement of results in stage III should be emphasized. In the previous series, the results in stages I

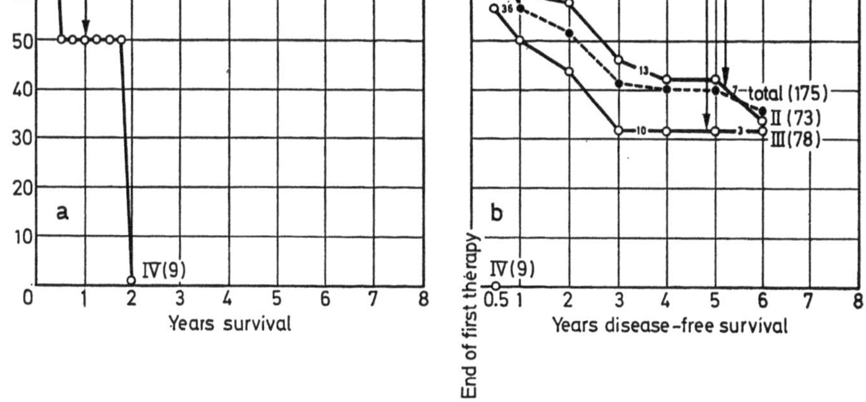

Fig. 2. Hodgkin's disease stages I, II, III, and IV (Ann Arbor Classification). Actuarial survival and disease-free survival in the different stages and in the whole group. (175 previously untreated cases of the period from 1964 to 1971)

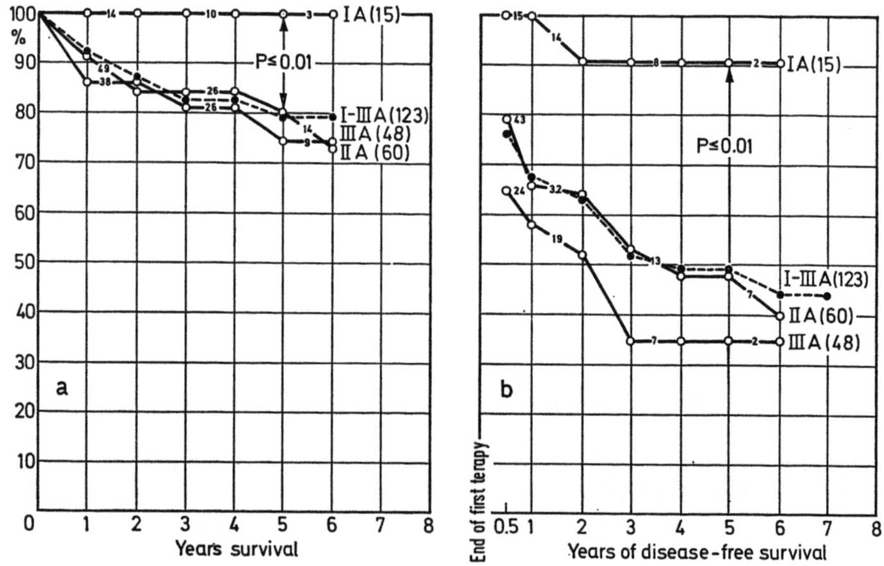

Fig. 3 a and b. Hodgkin's disease stages I A, II A and III A (Ann Arbor Classification). a Actuarial survival, b disease-free survival. (123 previously untreated cases of the period from 1964 to 1971)

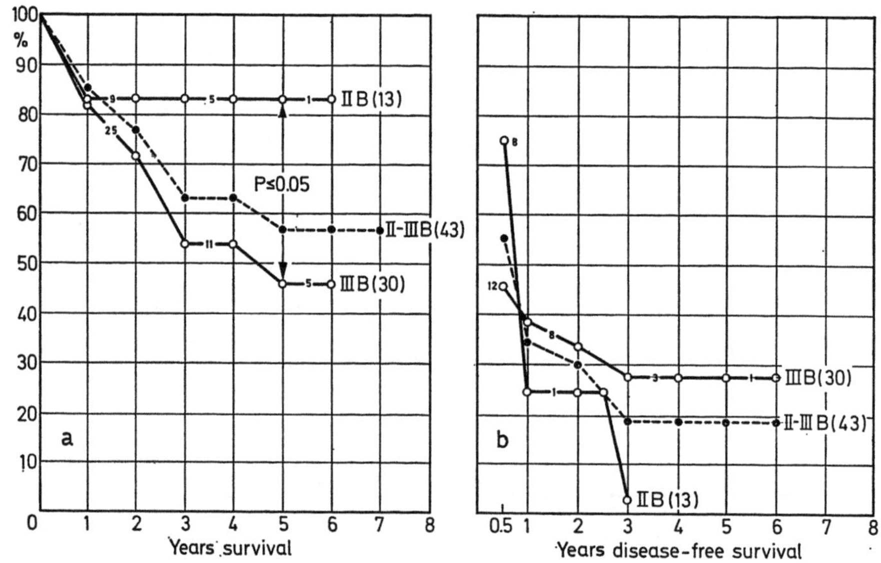

Fig. 4 a and b. Hodgkin's disease stages II B and III B (Ann Arbor Classification). a Actuarial survival, b disease-free survival. (43 previously untreated cases of the period from 1964 to 1971)

and II were similar or even identical, but now the results in stage II and stage III had become similar (Fig. 2).

This unexpected similarity becomes even more apparent when the A and B forms are compared: The 5-year remission rate is 35% in stage III A; 48% in stage II A (Fig. 3).

In stage III B, 30% of patients are still symptom-free within 5 years. In contrast to this, no patient in stage II B has reached a symptom-free remission of 5 years. All

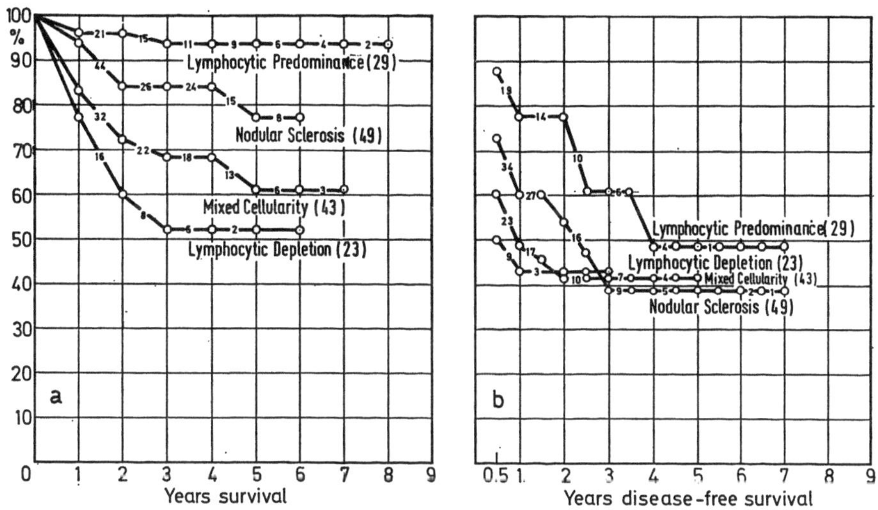

Fig. 5 a and b. Hodgkin's disease, Rye histopathological classification. a Actuarial survival, b disease-free survival related to histology. (144 previously untreated cases of all clinical stages with histopathological typing in the period from 1964 to 1971)

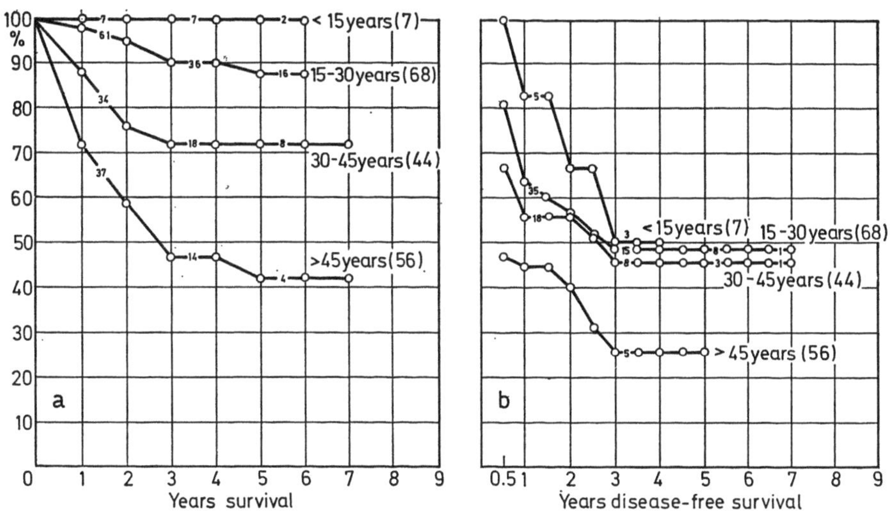

Fig. 6 a and b. Hodgkin's disease: a Actuarial survival, b disease-free survival in the age groups under 15 years, from 15 to 30 years, from 30 to 45 years and over 45 years. (175 previously untreated cases of all stages in the period from 1964 to 1971)

patients relapsed after 3 years at the latest. The large number of relapses in stage II B within first 3 years after radiotherapy contrasts with the high survival rate of 83% after 1—7 years. These apparently contradictory results are due to the specific character of the recurrence, which we shall discuss later, and to the incomplete radiation therapy technique in stage II-patients with the diaphragm as borderline (Fig. 4).

c) The survival rates of the whole collective are determined not only by the therapy and the clinical form A and B, but also by the histological type (Fig. 5) and the age of the patients (Fig. 6).

3. Concerning the Different Types of Remissions

When evaluating the results of tumor therapy we have to distinguish (a) a full remission from (b) a partial remission or (c) absence of a remission.

In this series we define full remission as normalization of all symptoms and signs of the disease. The patient can be regarded as healthy judging by subjective and objective criteria. When there are no manifestations of the disease such as enlarged lymph nodes or organ involvement, but at the same time there are still signs of activity of the disease, we consider this a partial remission. We state the absence of a remission when the disease is found to progress during therapy or immediately after therapy is discontinued.

In this series of 175 patients, full remission occurred in 65%, partial remission in 22% and no remission in 13% of the cases (Table 3). The further history of the disease in the 3 groups with different types of remission differs significantly: The 5-year survival rate in the patient group with full remissions is 96%, in the patients group with partial remissions 33%, and in the patients group without remission 9%. In the full remission group, 59% of patients were still in their first remission after 5 years. In the partial remission group, only 10% were in their first remission after 1 year and 0% after 2 years (Fig. 7).

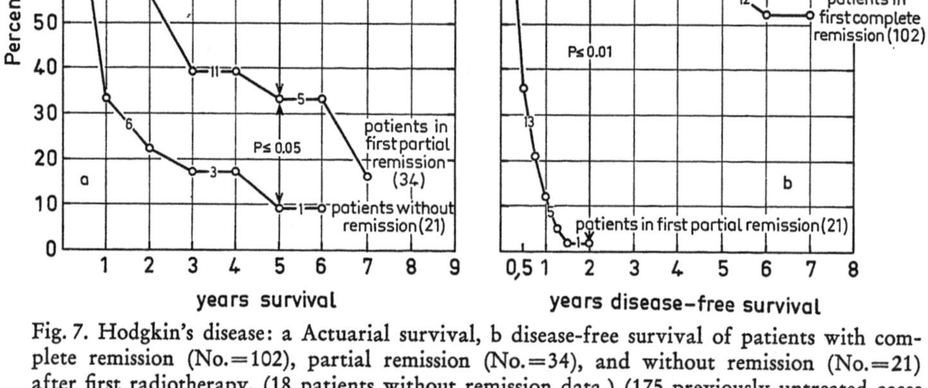

Fig. 7. Hodgkin's disease: a Actuarial survival, b disease-free survival of patients with complete remission (No.=102), partial remission (No.=34), and without remission (No.=21) after first radiotherapy. (18 patients without remission data.) (175 previously untreated cases of all stages in the period from 1964 to 1971)

The chance of achieving a first full remission by radiotherapy not only depends on the method of therapy but also on the clinical stage and histological findings (Tables 4 and 5).

The relationship between onset of a remission after therapy and the survival and remission rates becomes clearer when we look at the various forms of recurrences which occur after full or partial remissions.

Table 3. Hodgkin's disease results of first radiotherapy, all stages

	Patients	
	No./No. [a]	%
Complete remission	102/157	65
Partial remission	34/157	22
No remission	21/157	13
without data	18/175	

[a] No. of patients in remission / No. of patients at risk.

Table 4. Hodgkin's disease: Complete remission after the first radiation treatment in relation to the clinical stages of the Ann Arbor Classification (Freiburg data 1964—1971, 175 patients)

Clinical stage		No. of patients			Complete remission		Death	
		total	without data	with data	No.	%	No.	%
I	A	15		15	15	100	0	0
II	A	60	5	55	43	78	3	5.5
	B	13	2	11	8	73	0	10
III	A	48	8	40	24	60	4	10
	B	30	2	28	12	43	7	25
IV	A B	9	1	8	0	0	5	63
		175	18	157	102	66	19	12

Table 5. Hodgkin's disease: complete remission after first radiation treatment in relation to the Rye Classification histology (Freiburg data 1964—1971; 144/175 patients with histological Rye Classification)

Histological type	Total	Without data	With data	Complete remission	
	No.	No.	No.	No.	%
Lymphocytic predominance	29	7	22	19	86
Nodular sclerosis	49	2	47	34	72
Mixed cellularity	43	3	40	23	58
Lymphocytic depletion	23	3	20	9	45
	144	15	129	85	66

4. Concerning the Different Forms of Recurrences

a) Nomenclature of recurrences. When assessing manifest recurrences, we have to distinguish the following types shown in Table 6.

b) Distribution of recurrences. In the two groups with full, respectively partial remission (1.) the number, (2.) the time of appearance, and (3.) the localization of recurrences are different:

1. In the full remission group, 32/102 patients (31%) had a recurrence during the observation period. In the partial remission group, 34/34 (100%) patients had a recurrence.

2. a) Recurrences after full remissions are found within the first 5 years after treatment: About half occurred in the first year, one third in the second and third year and the remaining rest in the third to fifth year.

b) In the partial remission group, all manifest recurrences occurred within the first 2 years; 33 of 34 of these appeared in the first year (Table 7).

3. a) Recurrences after full remissions were found in 59% of cases in non-irradiated lymph nodes regions and spleen and 17% in non-lymphatic organs. In 24% the recurrences were local or marginal. (The local recurrences rate in our 102 patients with full remission, worked out for the number of patients, not of irradiated regions, is 9,5%.)

Table 6. Hodgkin's disease: the different kinds of recurrences

1. Recurrence in previously treated areas
   a Local recurrence
   b Marginal recurrence
   c Recurrence in prophylactically irradiated areas
2. Recurrence in lymph nodes outside the previously treated area
   a on the same side of the diaphragm
   b on the other side of the diaphragm
3. Recurrence in the spleen
4. Recurrence in non-lymphatic organs
   a by direct extension (per continuitatem [p.c.])
   b by dissemination (per disseminationem [p.d.])

Table 7. Hodgkin's disease: the frequency of relapses subsequent to complete or partial remission and the timetable of relapses (Freiburg data 1964—1971)

Remission	No. of patients in remission	No. of patients with relapses						
		total	period between the end of radiotherapy and the development of relapses (years)					
			< 1	1	2	3	4	5
Complete	102	32 (31.5%)	16	5	9	1	0	1
Partial	34	34 (100%)	29	5				

Table 8. Hodgkin's disease: location of relapses after the first remission (Freiburg data 1964—1971)

Remission		Patients with relapses	Relapses								
				Lymph nodes in irradiated areas		in non-irradiated areas				Spleen	Organs
			total	local	marginal	in prophyl-actically irradiated areas	contiguous: same side of diaphragm	contiguous: opposite side of diaphragm	non-contiguous		
	No.	No.	No.	No.	No.	No.	No.	No.	No.	No.	No.
Complete	102	32	41	5	5	0	6	6	4	8	7
				10/41 = 24%			24/41 = 59%				7/41 = 17%
Partial	34	34	65	13	0	5	9	4	6	6	22
					18/65 = 27%				25/65 = 39%		22/65 = 34%

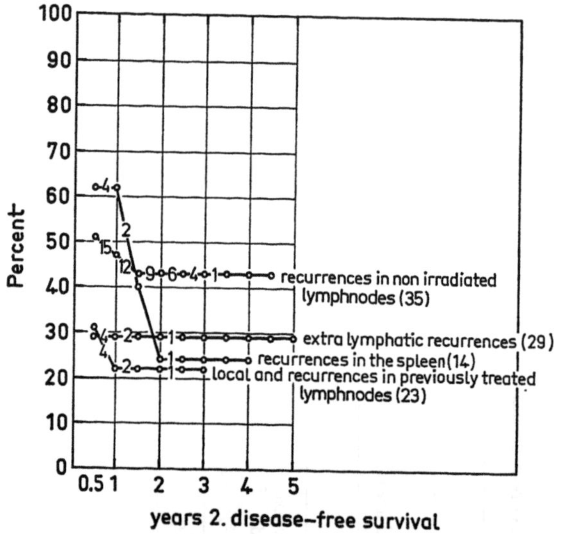

Fig. 8. Hodgkin's disease: Results of radiotherapy in relapses. Second disease-free remission of patients with relapses of different topography after second radiotherapy: Twenty-three patients with recurrences in previously treated areas (5 marginal recurrences not included), 35 patients with recurrences in non-irradiated lymph nodes, 14 recurrences in the spleen, and 29 extralymphatic recurrences. (66 patients of all stages with a total of 101 different relapses after first complete or partial remission)

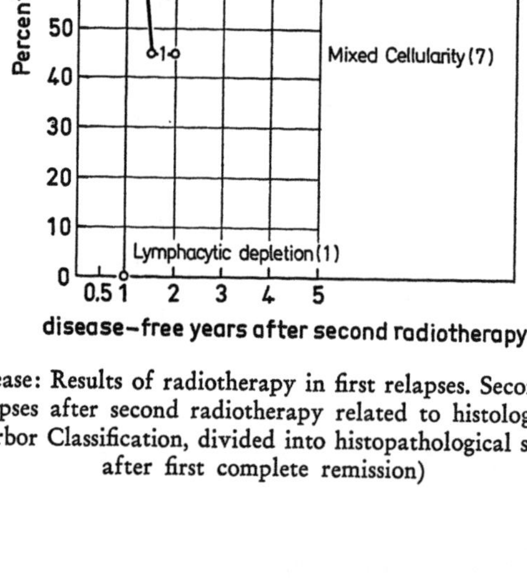

Fig. 9. Hodgkin's disease: Results of radiotherapy in first relapses. Second complete remission of patients with relapses after second radiotherapy related to histology. (24 of 32 patients stage I to III Ann Arbor Classification, divided into histopathological subtypes, with relapses after first complete remission)

After partial remission, manifest recurrences are found in 39% in non-irradiated lymphatic regions; in 34% in non-lymphatic and in 27% in locally irradiated regions.

In the full remission group, recurrences in the lymphatic system, which carry a fair prognosis, as demonstrated later, are more common than extra-lymphatic and local recurrences. In the partial remission group we find the reverse situation. Recurrences in extralymphatic organs and local recurrences, both with a poor prognosis, are more common than recurrences in non-irradiated lymphatic organs (Table 8).

c) Prognostic value of first recurrences. 1. The prognosis of the different types of recurrences after a remission is not the same. Recurrences in lymph nodes which have not so far been irradiated have a better prognosis than local or marginal recurrences and the spread of the disease in spleen and non-lymphatic organs (Fig. 8).

2. The histopathology has a definite influence on the prognosis of the first recurrence. After another course of radiotherapy, recurrences in the lymphocytic predominance group have a better prognosis than those in the nodular sclerosis group, which have still a better prognosis than the mixed cellularity group. (When we evaluate these results we have to consider the relatively small number of patients and the fact that some patients have several recurrences so that the prognosis is determined by many factors in these cases.) (Fig. 9).

5. Concerning the Prognosis of the Second Remission

Finally some remarks about the prognosis of the first recurrence after a second course of radiotherapy (second remission):

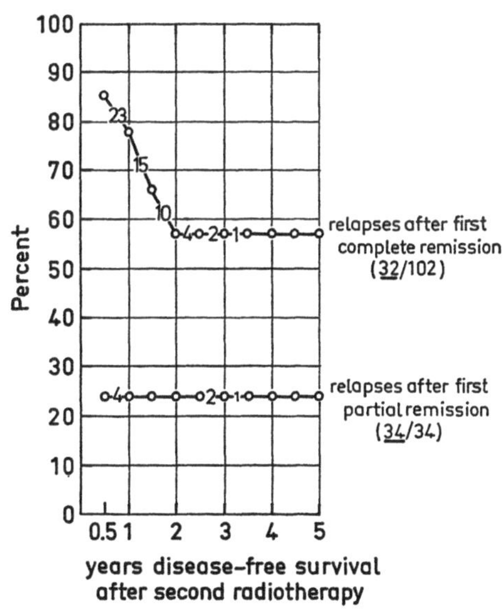

a

Fig. 10. Hodgkin's disease: Results of radiotherapy in first relapses. (a) Second complete remission of patients with relapses after first complete remission (No. 32) and first partial remission (No. 34) after second radiotherapy, (b) second complete remission rate of the first relapses group as a whole. (27/66 patients with second complete remission after first relapse)

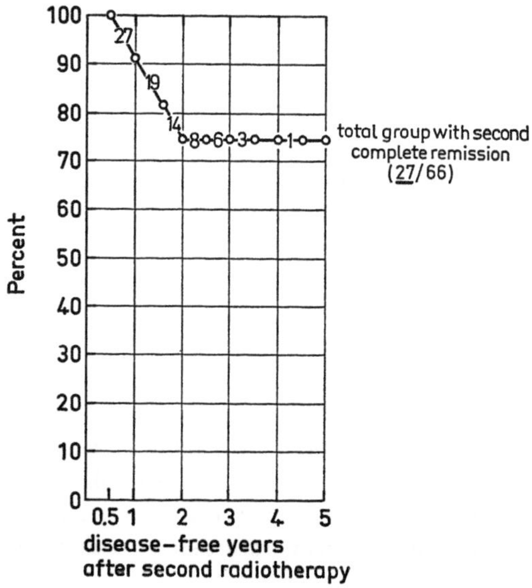

Fig. 10 b

1. 32 out of 102 patients had a recurrence after their first full remission. 86% of these had a second full remission after a second course of treatment. In 57% this second remission lasted for another 5 years.

2. Of the 34 patients with partial remission, all 34 had a manifest recurrence. 24% had a second remission, which was now a full remission, after a second course of treatment. In these 24% the full remission has lasted for an observation period of, so far, 5 years (Fig. 10 a).

These findings indicate that the better prognosis in the full remission group also applies to later recurrences in this group. They also show that in the poor prognosis group with a first partial remission a lasting full remission can be induced in a small percentage of cases. When after a recurrence a full remission can be induced by a second course of radiotherapy, the prognosis for these cases is very good. After 2 years 74% of this group stayed in this second full remission for an further observation period of, so far, 5 years (Fig. 10 b).

Discussion

Our results lead to the following conclusions:

1. The Ann Arbor Classification achieves a better selection of cases with poor prognosis by giving a new definition of stage IV, which limits this stage to cases with genuine metastases, and also by replacing pruritus by weight loss in the group B criteria.

2. A relatively large percentage of cases designated stage II in the Ann Arbor clinical staging are actually stage III cases. In radiotherapy of stage II, this means that irradiation of only one side of the diaphragm is not sufficient.

3. Our results after the first course of radiotherapy suggest that a group of patients with Hodgkin's disease can be divided into 2 subgroups with a different prognosis. Patients who reach a full remission have a relatively good prognosis. Those in whom full remission is not achieved have a poorer prognosis, and results indicate that there is still an active disease process which cannot be localized at the time, but will, as a rule, become manifest within a short while.

4. In the group with better prognosis (a) the progress of the disease is mainly by continuous spread, whereas in the other group (b) non-continuous and metastatic spread is most usual.

Group (a) includes patients in stages I A—III B, by our diagnostic and therapeutic criteria, with lesions of all histological types. This prognostically good group contains fewer patients in the higher clinical stages or with a low incidence of lymphocytes in the histological sections. This corresponds to LUKES' order for the Rye Classification [6]: lymphocytic predominance, nodular sclerosis, mixed cellularity and lymphocytic depletion.

Group (b) has poor-prognosis cases in stages II A — IV B belonging to all histological types, except the nodular type of lymphocytic and histocytic proliferation of the original LUKES and BUTLER Classification [5]. All 4 cases of this type — one in stage I, two in stage II, and one in stage III — are still in their first symptom-free remission, and in 2 of these patients the remission has, so far, lasted more than 7 years.

Two thirds of the patients in our series fall into the better-prognosis group. The actual percentage of prognostically good cases in a group of patients is, in fact, higher than this. An analysis could be utilized as a basis for improving methods of radiotherapy. Our therapeutic aim is to increase the percentage of patients with first full remissions, thereby enlarging the group with good prognosis, because one of the oncological characteristics of malignant tumors is the tendency to non-continuous and metastatic spread, which increases with duration of illness.

Even after further improvement in radiotherapy there will still be a group of patients who cannot be controlled by radiotherapy alone. This group includes, in addition to patients in Ann Arbor stage IV, patients in stages II and III in whom dissemination, though undetectable, had already taken place at the time of diagnosis. This is true not only for the clinical but also for the pathological staging. This group of Hodgkin's disease patients needs early chemotherapy.

References

1. CARBONE, P. P., KAPLAN, H. S., MUSSHOFF, K., SMITHERS, D. W., TUBIANA, M.: Report of the Committee on Hodgkin's disease staging procedures. Cancer Res. **31**, 1860 (1971).
2. HAYAT, M.: A randomized study of irradiation and Vinblastine in stages I and II of Hodgkin's disease. Preliminary results. Radiotherapy-Chemotherapy cooperative Group of E.O.R.T.C. Europ. J. Cancer **8**, 353 (1972).
3. JELLIFFE, A. M.: The place of radiotherapy in the cure of Hodgkin's disease. Clin. Radiol. **16**, 274 (1965).
4. KAPLAN, H. S.: Role of intensive radiotherapy in the management of Hodgkin's disease. Cancer (Philad.) **19**, 356 (1966).
5. LUKES, R. J., BUTLER, J. J.: The pathology and nomenclature of Hodgkin's disease. Cancer Res. **26**, 1063 (1966).

6. LUKES, R. J., CRAVER, L. F., HALL, TH. C., RAPPAPORT, H., RUBEN, P.: Report of the nomenclature committee. Cancer Res. **26**, 1311 (1966).
7. MUSSHOFF, K.: Grundlagen der Strahlentherapie des Morbus Hodgkin, Indikation und Ergebnisse. Deutscher Krebskongreß Hannover 1971. Z. Krebsforsch. **78**, 162 (1972).
8. MUSSHOFF, K.: Survival and relapse data in Hodgkin's disease: Freiburg im Breisgau, 1948—69. International symposium on Hodgkin's disease, Stanford, California, 20.—24. 3. 72. National Cancer Institute, Monograph **36**, 531—539 (1973).
9. STRICKSTROCK, K. H., MUSSHOFF, K., BOUTIS, L : Methode der zusätzlichen prophylaktischen Bestrahlung bei der Lymphogranulomatose. Strahlentherapie **133**, 337 (1967).

Radiotherapy of Reticulum-Cell Sarcoma:

Results and Dose-Time Relationships

W. Erbe, H. D. Franke, and V. Wiebe

Summary

44 out of 165 (= 26.7%) patients with reticulum-cell sarcoma survived 5 years after radiotherapy. The 5-year survival rate was 26.7%. Prognosis was better for patients with localized and regional disease and for manifestations in Waldeyer's lymphatic ring. The time-dose curve for reticulum-cell sarcoma has a steeper slope than the corresponding curves for Hodgkin's disease of other workers.

The biological behaviour of reticulum-cell sarcoma (RCS) is different from that of other malignant lymphomas and poses radiotherapeutic problems which require special consideration. Radiation doses as required by various authors are shown in Table 1. In the past 10 years, general agreement has been reached on a minimum tumor dose of 4000 rads delivered over 3—4 weeks. It is doubtful whether results would be improved by doses in excess of 5000 rads.

Table 1. Radiotherapeutic doses for treatment of RCS as suggested in the world literature

Goes [6]	1953	2500 rad
Bauer [2]	1953	3000 to 4000 rad
Hohn, Neveling and Vieten [9]	1957	4500 to 5000 rad
Gyenes [7]	1967	> 3000 rad
Arndt [1]	1963	4000 rad / 21 d for localized stages
Peters [14]	1963	5000 rad / 4 weeks
Bergsteinova *et al.* [3]	1967	After regression of the tumor the authors give 50% more of the applied dose previously
Fuller [5]	1967	5000 to 6000 rad / 5—6 weeks
Hoppe and Mau [10]	1968	4000 to 5000 rad
Halama and Sziegoleit [8]	1969	4000 to 5000 rad
Tikka and Malmio [18]	1969	4000 to 5000 rad / 4—5 weeks
Newall *et al.* [11]	1970	4500 to 5500 rad / 20—35 days (bone)
		5000 to 6000 rad /25—35 days (head and neck)

In reviewing our cases, we tried to assess the response to irradiation retrospectively. Our review is based on 165 histologically proved cases irradiated between 1947 and 1966 in our department. Distribution of age and sex is similar to that in other series (Fig. 1). There is a 1.5:1 preponderance of males. The anatomical distribution of primary manifestations is characterized by mainly head and neck lesions (Table 2).

Table 2. Site of primary manifestation in our (165 RCS) patients

Tonsils	45
Pharynx (epipharynx)	12
Base of tongue	2
Paranasal sinuses	23
Palate	1
Subramandibular and lacrimal glands	1
Lymph nodes of the neck	33
Skin	20
Inguinal glands	6
Axillary glands	4
Mediastinum	4
Stomach	4
Ileocecal region	2
Bones	2
Retroperitoneal lymph nodes	1
Testes	1
Cerebellum	1
Primary generalization	3
	n=165

Half of the patients died within the first year after irradiation. By the direct method, a 5-year survival rate of 26.7% was calculated for the whole series; 39% of patients with localized and regional disease and 12.5% with generalized disease survived for 3 years. No patient with generalized disease survived for 5 years. No correlation between length of history and survival time was apparent.

Dose-time relationship of local tumor recurrences within irradiated areas were compared with cases which had had no recurrence for one year. No additional treatment had been given in the cases compared, and tumors had regressed completely. Minimum tumor doses are shown in the dose-time graph (Fig. 2). All doses shown were recalculated mathematically and graphically. Differences in therapeutic modalities (ortho- or megavoltage radiation and a mixture of both, different portals or single dose etc.) were not taken into account. Fifteen of the 22 local recurrences occurred within one year of irradiation. Local recurrence was seen in all 8 cases received a tumor dose of less than 2500 rads in 2—3 weeks, while there was only one local recurrence in 10 cases given a dose of over 4000 rads in 4 weeks. [7] regarded 3000 rads in 3 weeks as the critical limit for recurrence. On the basis of our own results, we must set a higher limit.

Dose-time values in 17 of our cases not showing any recurrence were used to calculate a regression line. This is shown in Fig. 3 with corresponding regression lines

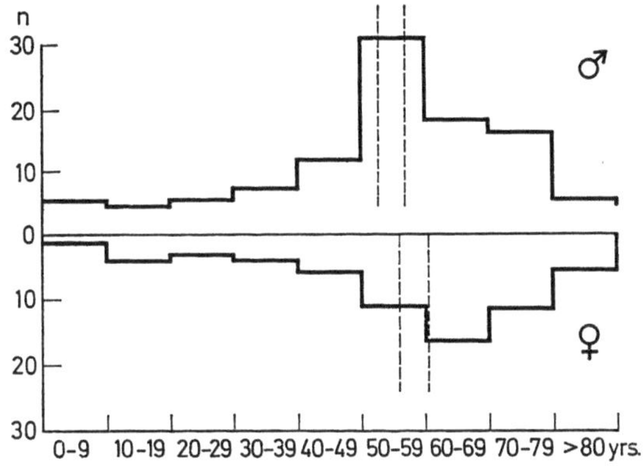

Fig. 1. RCS: Age distribution for males and females

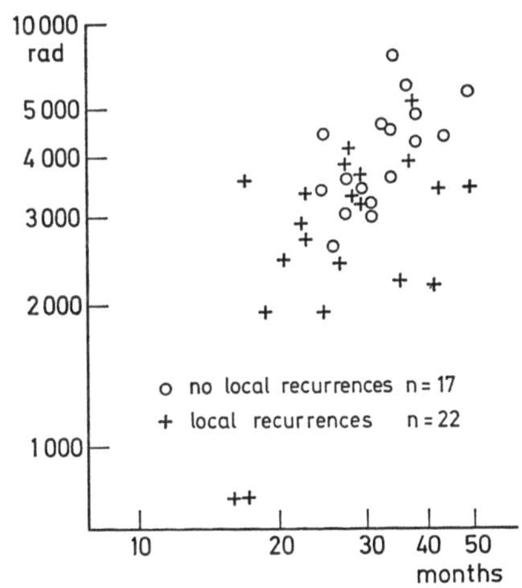

Fig. 2. Dose-time relationship for local recurrences and cases free of recurrences

for cure of carcinoma of the skin, and those of PATERSON [13] and SCOTT *et al.* [16] for "cure" of Hodgkin's disease for comparison. The curve is characterized by a steeper slope (0.72 as opposed to 0.22) demonstrating the better recovery potential of RCS.

Clinical response to irradiation was examined in 138 primary manifestations. There was only partial tumor regression in 9 cases and none at all in 8 cases, 12% resistance to doses of 2500 to 4000 rads administered over 3—4 weeks. Thus it is not possible to maintain that RCS is in general highly radiosensitive, as already mentioned by [13, 15]; our results definitely confirm their observations. There was local recurrence in 36 of our cases. In this group, there were lymph-node manifestations from a high percentage (61%) of the total; however, these usually regressed quickly when irradiated. This illustrates the discrepancy between response to irradiation and

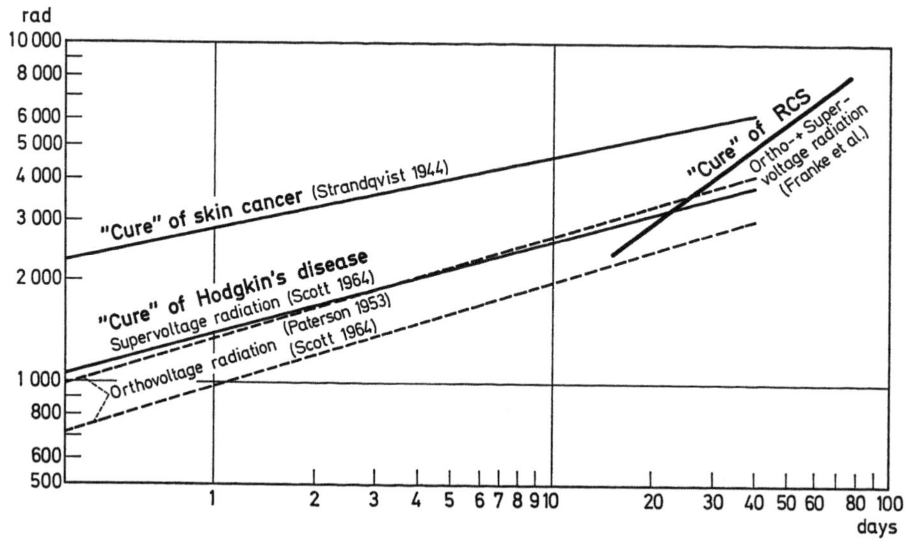

Fig. 3. Slope of time-dose-curve for RCS in comparison with the curves of STRANDQVIST, PATERSON and SCOTT

curability. SAND HANSEN [15], grouping her cases according to irradiation response, found that survival was better in groups that responded more slowly.

Waldeyer's lymphatic ring was the site of the disease in 83% of permanently controlled cases (i. e., without local recurrence). This localization may have a favorable prognosis.

References

1. ARNDT, J.: Radiobiol. Radiother. (Berlin) **4**, 289 (1963).
2. BAUER, R.: Strahlentherapie **91**, 65 (1953).
3. BERGSTEINOVA, V., LINTNER, L., TOPOL, O., ZABOJOVÁ, E.: Radiobiol. Radiother. (Berlin) **8**, 301 (1967).
4. FRANKE, H. D., *et al.:* In press.
5. FULLER, L. M.: Amer. J. Roentgenol. **99**, 340 (1967).
6. GOES, M.: Strahlentherapie **89**, 554 (1953).
7. GYENES, G.: Radiobiol. Radiother. (Berlin) **8**, 401 (1967).
8. HALAMA, J., SZIEGOLEIT, M.: Strahlentherapie **69**, 160 (1969).
9. HOHN, M., NEBELING, R., VIETEN, H.: Strahlentherapie **103**, 428 (1957).
10. HOPPE, D., MAU, S.: Dtsch. Gesundh.-Wes. **31**, 1446 (1968).
11. NEWALL, J., FRIEDMAN, M.: Radiology **94**, 643 (1970).
12. NEWALL, J., FRIEDMAN, M., DE NARVAEZ, F.: Radiology **91**, 708 (1968).
13. PATERSON, R.: Reticulo-Endothelial System. The Treatment of Malignant Disease by Radium and X-Ray. p. 414. London: Edward Arnold 1953.
14. PETERS, V.: Amer. J. Roentgenol. **90**, 956 (1963).
15. SAND HANSEN, H.: Acta radiol. (Stockh.) **8**, 439 (1969).
16. SCOTT, R. M., BRIZEL, H. E.: Radiology **82**, 1043 (1964).
17. STRANDQVIST, M.: Studien über die kumulative Wirkung der Röntgenstrahlen bei Fraktionierung. Stockholm 1944.
18. TIKKA, U., MALMIO, K.: Acta radiol. (Stockh.) **8**, 469 (1969).

Radical Radiotherapy of Hodgkin's Disease. Lund 1944—1956 and 1967—1971

T. Landberg

Summary

In 48 patients with Hodgkin's disease from the years 1944—1956, only a limited abdominal charting of the disease was performed. The patients received radiation therapy to only obviously involved regions. All the 48 patients had clinically localized disease. Thirteen (= 27%) of them are alive 15 years or more after the initial treatment.

In 42 patients from the years 1967—1971, the charting of abdominal disease included in most patients lymphography and scintigraphy of the liver and spleen, but in none staging laparotomy. The 42 patients were considered to have only supradiaphragmatic Hodgkin's disease. Obviously involved lymph node regions as well as the adjacent ones were irradiated. Twenty-nine of the patients have stayed symptom-free after the initial treatment and have been followed for a median of 27 months. Ten patients have shown extensions, which have been seen at a median of 20 months after the beginning of mantle treatment. Three patients have died without demonstrable extensions.

Two different groups of patients with Hodgkin's disease are reviewed.

Group 1

The first group consists of 98 patients with Hodgkin's disease admitted to the Radiotherapy Department in Lund from 1944 to 1956. All patients thus have a possible follow-up of at least 15 years as of January 1972. The patients were described in previous reports [1, 2, 3]. At the beginning of treatment 48 of the 98 patients had clinically localized disease and 50 had advanced disease. The charting of abdominal disease included X-ray examination in only a few cases. The treatment in localized disease was involved-field radiation therapy. Reasonably adequate absorbed doses were given. Patients with advanced disease usually received chemotherapy, and in some cases, additional radiotherapy was given with smaller absorbed doses.

Of the 48 patients with clinically localized disease, 23 were still alive 5 years after the beginning of treatment, and 13 were still alive 15 years after the first treatment. Age at the beginning of treatment among the 15-year survivors was between 15 and 40 years: 6 were males and 7 females. Nine of the 13 had initial mediastinal involvement. A review of the initial biopsies (by Prof. C. G. AHLSTRÖM, Department of Pathology, Lund) showed histological types to be: 2 lymphocyte predominance, 9 nodular sclerosis and 2 mixed cellularity. Nine of the 13 15-year survivors had not shown any new manifestations of Hodgkin's disease after the initial treatment, and 7 of them are still alive 16—23 (median 20, mean 19) years after the beginning of treatment. Four of the thirteen 15-year survivors have died. Autopsy was performed in all 4 and showed persisting Hodgkin's disease in two, but no signs in the other two. All 50 patients with advanced disease died within 8 years after the beginning of treatment.

The 15-year survivors from the years 1944—1956 were described in detail elsewhere [4].

Group 2

The second group consists of 42 patients first seen at the Radiotherapy Department during the years 1967—1971. The table shows some of the staging procedures used and the different histological types. X-ray of the chest and a skeletal survey were performed in all 42, lymphography in 33 and scintigraphy of the liver and spleen in 40. No patient was given a staging laparotomy. About half of the patients had either the lymphocyte predominance or nodular sclerosing type, and the rest mixed cellularity. All 42 were considered to have only supradiaphragmatic Hodgkin's disease, and mantle treatment was considered to be the proper therapy.

Table. Staging procedures and histologic types of biopsy specimens in 42 patients with supradiaphragmatic Hodgkin's disease treated with the mantle technique

Mantle treatment of supradiaphragmatic Hodgkin's disease Lund 1967—1971		
42 patients; no laparotomies; lymphography in 33 patients; scintigraphy of the liver and spleen in 40 patients.		
Histologic types	Lymphocyte predominance	15 patients
	Nodular sclerosis	7 patients
	Mixed cellularity	20 patients
	Lymphocyte depletion	— patients

Mantle treatment (Fig. 1 [5, 6]) was given with ^{60}Co with two opposed fields. The treatment was given in a split course, with two-thirds of the total absorbed dose in the first series and an interval of about 4 weeks between the two series. The total absorbed dose in the target area usually amounted to 4000 rads in 24 fractions in 60 days. A preliminary report of the side effects and early results appeared in 1971 [7].

Staging laparotomy was included in the charting of Hodgkin's disease at the Department only from 1972. Group 2 thus consists of patients considered (without surgical abdominal sampling) to have only supradiaphragmatic Hodgkin's disease and hence were treated with extended-field radiation therapy.

Fig. 2 gives the follow-up for each of the 42 patients and also the details regarding patients in whom extensions have been seen. No local recurrences have been noted clinically. Of the 42 patients, 29 are alive and symptom-free after the initial treatment. These 29 have been followed for 7—59 (median 27, mean 31) months. In 10 patients extensions have been noted. These 10 have been followed for 19—62 (median 42, mean 42) months. One of the (KV) has died. In one (BL) an extension to one lung was verified cytologically 21 months after beginning of treatment. In the

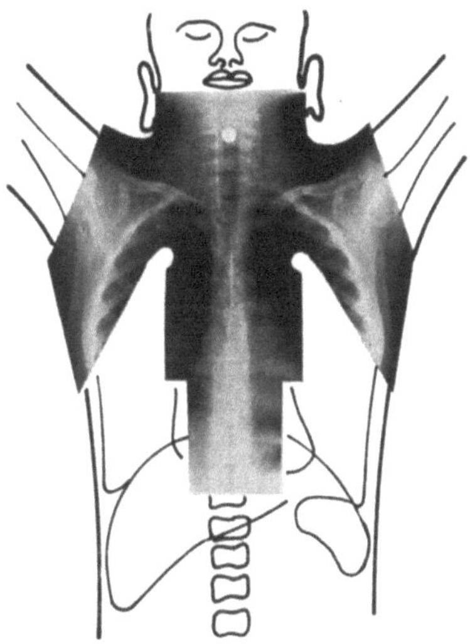

Fig. 1. Example of a ventral mantle field in the radiotherapy of supradiaphragmatic Hodgkin's disease

other 9, the extensions were localized at first to abdominal tissues, and were then diagnosed 4—42 (median 20, mean 22) months after the beginning of mantle treatment. The first abdominal extensions localized to lymph nodes were seen in 4 patients (OI-B, DJ, VR and AR). In 4 patients, involvement of abdominal lymph nodes was seen in addition to other involvements, namely of a vertebral in one (JI), of the spleen in one (JE-B), of the gastric wall in one (RB), and of the spleen and liver in one (HG). In one patient (KV), the initial abdominal extensions were clinically localized to the spleen and the liver. Of the 10 patients with extensions, 2 had the lymphocyte predominance, 4 the nodular sclerosis and 4 the mixed cellularity type. All 9 patients in whom abdominal extensions were seen had a lymphography before the beginning of mantle treatment; in 5 of them (OI-J, JI, RB, HG and KV) the ESR was more than 25 mm/h. Two of the patients with extensions (OI-B and HG) had constitutional symptoms before the beginning of mantle treatment, but in the remaining 40, such symptoms were lacking or not clearcut.

Three patients died 3—10 months after the beginning of mantle treatment. The exact cause of death in these cases is not known, since they died at other hospitals and relevant data were not obtained.

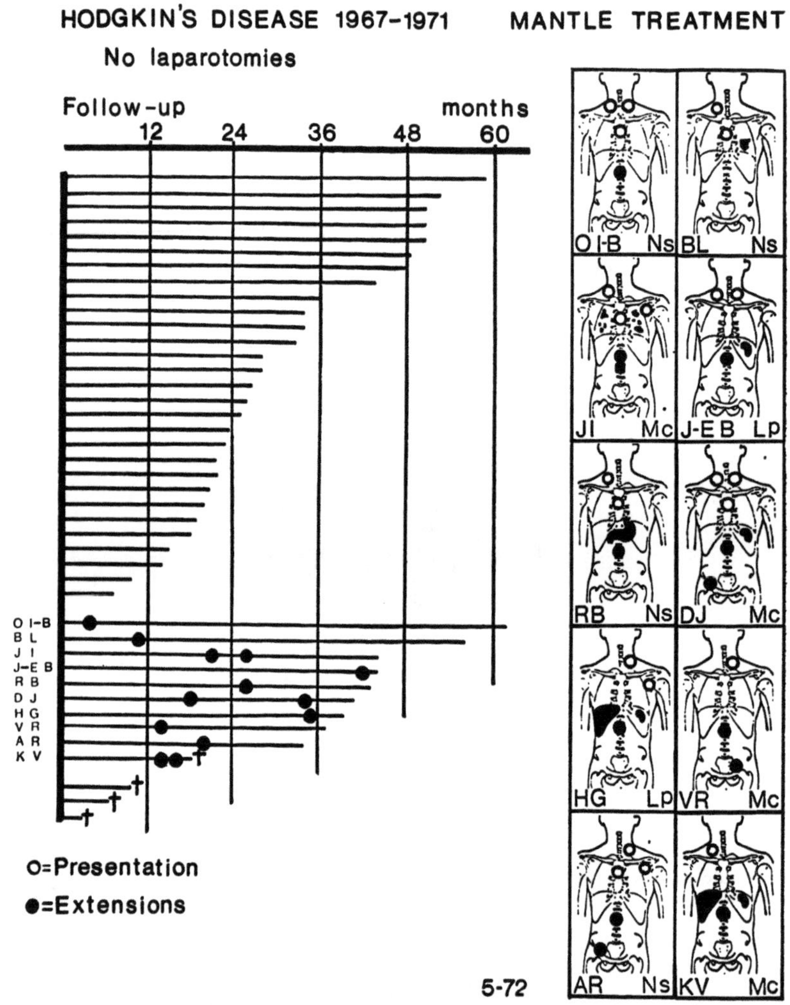

Fig. 2. Follow-up in 42 patients with supradiaphragmatic Hodgkin's disease treated by the mantle technique. The localization of extensions in 10 patients is shown. Lp = Lymphocyte predominance, Ns = Nodular sclerosis, Mc = Mixed cellularity

References

1. Landberg, T., Larsson, L.-E.: Hodgkin's disease. Retrospective clinico-pathologic study in 149 patients. Acta radiol. (Stockh.) **8**, 390 (1969).
2. Landberg, T.: Clinical course of Hodgkin's disease treated with radiotherapy. Acta radiol. (Stockh.) **8**, 487 (1969).
3. Landberg, T., Forslo, H.: Radiosensitivity of mediastinal lymphomas in Hodgkin's disease treated with split-course radiotherapy. Acta radiol. (Stockh.) **9**, 177 (1970).
4. Landberg, T., Ahlström, C. G.: 15-year survivors in Hodgkin's disease. Acta radiol. (Stockh.) **12**, 21 (1973).
5. Svahn-Tapper, G.: Dosimetric studies of mantle fields in cobalt 60 therapy of malignant lymphomas. Acta radiol. (Stockh.) **9**, 190 (1970).
6. Svahn-Tapper, G., Landberg, T.: Mantle treatment of Hodgkin's disease. Technique and dosimetry. Acta radiol. (Stockh.) **10**, 33 (1971).
7. Landberg, T., Svahn-Tapper, G., Wintzell, K.: Mantle treatment of Hodgkin's disease. Preliminary report of side effects and early results. Acta radiol. (Stockh.) **10**, 176 (1971).

Results of Radiotherapy of Malignant Lymphomas

F. HESS, H. K. PEMSEL, and J. W. PLASS

Summary

We observed 105 patients with lymphogranulomatosis, who were divided in two treatment groups:

1958—1964: local irradiation with numerous incidents of recurrence.

1965—1968: large-field radiotherapy with coverage of the adjacent lymph nodes with better prognosis.

We observed a 5-year survival rate of 70% and a 10-year survival rate of 47% in stages I and II, if the mediastinum was free of disease. In case of infiltration of the mediastinal nodes only 58% survived fot more than 5 years, resp. 28% for more than 10 years.

Reticulosarcomas vary greatly in formation of metastasis and speed of spread. Rapid onset portends an early death. The 5-year survival rate is 14,6% in fast-onset groups and 41,2% for those with slow onset. The most appropriate treatment was surgery and radiotherapy with tumor doses which exceed 3000 rad. When chemotherapy is added the results fall rapidly. Finally we discussed 4 patients with lymphosarcoma similar BURKITTS lymphoma.

In hardly any field of oncology has there been such a profound change in theories about nosology in recent years as in that of the malignant lymphomas. This change is closely linked with diagnostic and therapeutic advances.

We report here the significant results of our recent practical clinical experience, with special reference to lymphogranulomatosis, reticulosarcomas and lymphosarcomas. These diseases all have an initial unilocular origin and later a more or less rapid tendency towards generalized disease, somewhat resembling leukemia. In many cases we find relations to the immune response, so that we can advance the hypothesis of a viral etiology. With regard to lymphogranulomatosis, we refer to three meetings [1, 2, 3] at which the histological and clinical staging of lymphogranulomatosis was thoroughly discussed. We follow the recommendations made there and during the present meeting.

From 1958 to 1968 we observed 105 patients who were divided into two treatment groups:

1958—1964: local irradiation of recognized tumor manifestations.

1965—1968: large-field radiotherapy with coverage of adjacent lymph nodes.

The second period was marked by improved diagnostic methods in the form of mediastinoscopy and abdominal lymphography.

There were very early and numerous incidents of recurrence in the first group, with wide differences in time, and predominantly in the vicinity of the primary focus. In the second group, we observed recurrences mainly during the first two years after radiotherapy and distant from the primary focus. The cause of this failure of therapy is the occult spread of the disease across the diaphragm. Today we know that universally applied pre-therapy diagnostic procedures, including exploratory laparotomy, can detect stage III in 20 to 40% of the cases clinically diagnosed as stages I and II. The danger of unrecognized spread beyond the diaphragm is particularly great in case of secondary mediastinal involvement. This observation is confirmed by the success rate: we observed a 5-year survival rate of 70% and a 10-year survival rate of 47% of all patients in stages I and II, provided the mediastinum was free of disease. In case of infiltration of the mediastinal nodes, only 58% survived for more than 5 years, and only 28% for more than 10 years. The combined 5-year survival rate amounted to 64% in 76 cases in stages I and II; the 10-year survival rate was 40%. Of 29 patients in stages III and IV, only one third survived longer than 5 years.

Reticulosarcomas are similarly tumors of the lymphocytes or lymphocyte-derived cells; however, they are obviously pathogenetically different. The average age at onset is distinctly higher than with lymphogranulomatosis. Formation of metastases and speed of spread are also obviously different and vary greatly in this kind of disease. We observed 98 patients from 1947 to 1968 and found a clustering of cases in the years 1948, 1954/1955, 1958, and 1967/1968; we do not know the reason for this. The age distribution (average 54.6 yr) has one peak for men and two for women. The primary localization was found in the tonsils or the cervical lymph nodes in more than 50% of the patients, which suggests that the triggering factor for this disease may act in this region.

A comparison of duration of onset of disease and success of therapy shows that a rapid onset portends an early death which can rarely be prevented by therapy. Of our patients in whom symptoms of disease had been observed for less than six months prior to the final diagnosis, 48.7% died within a year, whereas when diagnosis was delayed for more than six months, only 15.7% had died after the first year. The 5-year survival rate is 14.6% in the fast-onset group and 41.2% for those with slow onset. Age and time of survival are likewise correlated. In the under-40 age group, 32% survived over 5-year limit; in the group above the age of 40, only 19% survived for more than 5 years. This difference clearly exceeds the natural mortality due to aging. These features were independent of the therapy chosen. In order to determine the most appropriate treatment, we have studied the following combination: surgery + radiotherapy + chemotherapy; surgery + radiotherapy; radiotherapy + chemotherapy; and radiotherapy alone. The rates of survival were calculated for each form of treatment.

Of course, each treatment group includes a different distribution of stages, for in general, only localized tumors are operated on, generalized forms are treated primarily with cytostatic drugs, and localized cases which cannot be operated on for technical or prognostic reasons are treated by radiotherapy. Consequently, the indication for each form of treatment depends on the location of the tumor, its size, whether or not it is spreading and the patient's general condition. We therefore determined the distribution of stages among the various combinations of therapeutic measures and the average 5-year survival rates to be expected from these distributions were calculated from the total patient series.

We compared expected with observed survival rates. The difference can then be attributed to the therapy used. We therefore term the factor by which the theoretically expected value has to be multiplied in order to obtain the observed survival rate the "Therapy Factor". A score above 1 means that the treatment was able to increase the average stage-dependent 5-year survival rate. Factors in excess of unity are found in these groups treated exclusively by radiotherapy or by surgery combined with radiotherapy. When chemotherapy is added, the value falls rapidly to one half to one third of the expected survival rate. On the basis of these results we recommend the most complete possible surgical excision of the tumor followed by radiotherapy. The success of the radiotherapy is determined by the tumor dose, which must exceed 3000 rad. Details are given in the table.

Table. Survival rates related to treatment given

Number of patients and treatment		Expected survival	Actual survival	"Therapy factor"
Radiation alone	30	21.4%	23.3%	1.08
Surgery + irradiation	29	28.2%	45.0%	1.60
Surgery + irradiation + chemotherapy	16	22.8%	6.2%	0.27
Irradiation + chemotherapy	17	19.5%	11.7%	0.60

We would now like to discuss some features of lymphosarcomas in our series which may aid assessment of this disease.

At the end of 1971 we observed 4 lymphosarcoma cases which had atypical histology and course and were remarkable for their uniformity and their coincidence in time. Now malignant lymphomas of the Burkitt type have aroused increasing international interest since they were first described in 1958. In typical cases, Epstein-Barr virus or herpes virus could be isolated directly from this tumor and from cell cultures. Antibodies to one or other of these viruses are also found in Burkitt tumor cases. The concentrated occurrence of Burkitt tumors in Central Africa suggested a correlation with endemic malaria. Children above 2 years of age were mainly affected. The characteristic features were an infection and an unusual tumor reaction verging on lymphoblastic leukemia. Burkitt tumors are rarely found in adults.

Our patients were 23, 32, 47, and 60 years of age. Three had huge mediastinal tumors with rapid onset (a few days); one had a tumor in the left axilla which had grown with similar speed. Histologically, all cases were distinctly dedifferentiated lymphosarcomas, some also showing the typical firmament cells of the Burkitt tumor. The immunoglobulin determinations in all cases showed a diminution of the IgG, IgA, and IgM fractions. The immune electropherogram did not show any peculiarities. The Epstein-Barr antibody titers were not characteristically raised. The results of bone marrow biopsy were rather unspecific. In one case we found an increase in the lymphatic plasmacytes like that seen in a virus infection and immunoblasts, which have also been described in Burkitt tumors. The course was uniform. The tumors regressed within 4 days after telecobalt irradiation with single doses of 50 rad (total 200 rad). During the following two weeks lymphoblastic leukemia developed and in spite of combined chemotherapy following the de Vita Method, 3 patients had died within three months. One patient has been in remission for 6 months.

We are convinced that further knowledge can be gained in the clinical treatment of reticulosarcomas and lymphosarcomas that will influence therapy and improve rates of cure. In spite of the promising progress of recent years, it has not yet been possible to achieve the final aim of a comprehensive, causal therapy for lymphogranulomatosis.

References

1. Symposium: Obstacles to the Control of Hodgkin's disease. Rye, New York, September 13—15, 1965. Cancer Res. **26,** 1043 (1966).
2. Symposium: Staging in Hodgkin's disease. Ann Arbor, Michigan, April 26—28, 1971. Cancer Res. **31,** 1707 (1971).
3. 11. Wissenschaftliche Tagung der deutschen Krebsgesellschaft, Deutscher Krebskongreß Hannover, October 1, 1971. Z. Krebsforsch. **78** (1972).

Present Results in the Treatment of Malignant Lymphomas. Results Obtained in a Series of 317 Cases

K. HOHL

Summary

Abstract. A short survey is given of the long-term results which can be obtained with modern radiotherapy in localized malignant lymphomas. Modern aspects of differential radiology are outlined in relation to the prognosis and clinical form of the disease, and guidelines are laid down for the further improvement of the long-term results.

Introduction and Results

A short survey is given of the long-term results which can be obtained with modern radiotherapy in localized malignant lymphomas. The age and sex distribution of the patients in our series is shown in Figs. 1—4. That for lymphogranuloma (Fig. 1) confirms the presence of two frequency peaks as already observed in various European countries. However, the second age peak and the higher mortality rate in males are not so clearly apparent as SCHINZ and REICH [6] asserted on the basis of the mortality statistics for Switzerland. They claimed that the statistically significant second age peak lies between 60 and 70 years and is higher than the first peak, which lies between 25 and 30. This implies that elderly patients should be less commonly assigned to radiotherapy.

The risk of reticulum-cell sarcoma (Fig. 2) is at its greatest in later life (6th to 8th), whereas lymphosarcoma (Fig. 3) occurs at all ages, but most frequently during middle life. We have too few cases of giant-follicle lymphoblastoma (Fig. 4) to allow us to make a statistically significant statement. According to the data of SYMMERS [7], the risk rises to an asymptote between the ages of 20 and 30, followed by a higher peak in the 6th decade.

In our series, males predominate in all types of malignant lymphoma; according to LENNERT [3], males are in a 2:1 majority among cases of Brill-Symmers disease.

Compared with other published data, the frequency index for our series is at the upper limit of the normal range with 2.7 new cases per 100,000 inhabitants per annum for Hodgkin's granuloma and 2.6 new cases per year for the other malignant lymphomas.

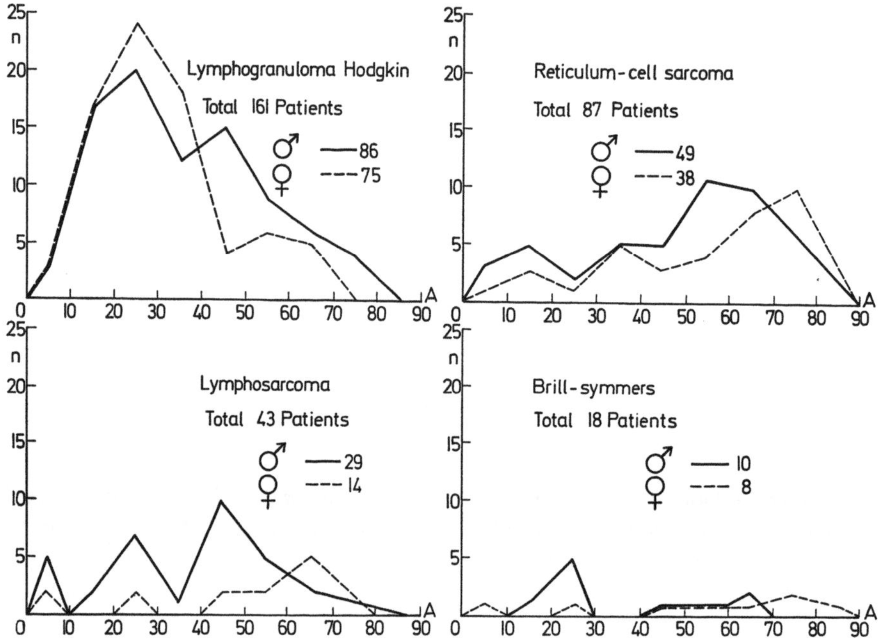

Fig. 1. Lymphogranuloma. Distribution by age and sex. n = No. of patients; A = age in years
Fig. 2. Reticulum-cell sarcoma. Distribution by age and sex
Fig. 3. Lymphosarcoma. Distribution by age and sex
Fig. 4. Brill-Symmers disease. Distribution by age and sex

However, besides our normal catchment area (the cantons of St. Gall, Appenzell, Thurgau), a few patients are sent to the St. Gall treatment center from neighboring districts outside Switzerland (Bavaria and Württemberg in Germany; Vorarlberg in Austria).

In 1951, when we first reported on the results obtained in the treatment of lymphogranuloma on the basis of the Zurich material, we considered (in agreement with [5]) that the extent of spread was of decisive importance for the results of therapy. In general, this opinion is still valid. Since 1965, differential histology as defined by Lukes and Butler [4] has gained in importance with regard to the prognosis of lymphogranuloma. As early as 1947, Jackson and Parker [2] pointed out the important relationship between the histological picture and the long-term prognosis on the basis of the then current classification into the three classes of paragranuloma, granuloma and sarcoma. Today, with the aid of modern histological techniques already widely utilized in Germany, and on the basis of clinical manifestations and mode of spread, clear conclusions can be drawn concerning the form of treatment to be applied and the prospects of cure.

Clearly, histological differentiation by the method of Lukes and Butler [4] is essential for the evaluation and presentation of therapeutic results in a group of patients with malignant lymphoma. Our series was therefore reclassified. The results are shown in Table 1.

Table 1. Histological classification of 161 cases of Hodgkin's disease

	Lymphocytic predominance	Nodular sclerosis	Mixed cellularity	Lymphocytic depletion
Stage I	9.9%	12.7%	8.4%	0%
Stage II	2.8%	11.3%	5.6%	0%
Stage III	1.4%	12.7%	19.7%	1.4%
Stage IV	0%	5.6%	8.5%	0%

Table 2. Malignant lymphoma St. Gall material (1955—1969). Survival table, without age correction

		3 years	5 years	10 years
Lymphogranuloma	161 cases (86 M/75 F)	67%	59%	28%
Reticulum-cell sarcoma	87 cases (49 M/38 F)	38%	26.4%	18.4%
Lymphosarcoma	43 cases (29 M/14 F)	40%	32.6%	19%
Brill-Symmers disease	18 cases (10 M/ 8 F)	78%	61%	50%
Hodgkin's sarcoma	8 cases (7 M/ 1 F)	25%	0%	0%

To estimate the long-term prognosis of malignant lymphoma we refer to Table 2, which shows the survival time of all patients, including those with Hodgkin's sarcoma. Here it can be seen that Brill-Symmers disease and lymphogranuloma run the most favorable course, while lymphosarcoma and reticulum-cell sarcoma are in an intermediate position and Hodgkin's sarcoma has by far the worst prognosis. The percentage survival rates alone allow no conclusions to be drawn as to the therapeutic effects. We therefore applied to our cases of malignant lymphoma the staging criteria of the Rye classification.

Analysis by stages of the St. Gall material shows (Table 3) that the late stages slightly predominate in the lymphogranulomas, in contrast to Brill-Symmers disease, where the early stages account for more than two thirds of cases. The prognosis is particularly poor in reticulum-cell sarcoma and lymphosarcoma, in both of which the

Table 3. Analysis by stages of malignant lymphoma cases in St. Gall (1955—1969). Stage classification after Rye, New York 1965, IX, 13—15

	Total	Stage I	Stage II	Stage III	Stage IV	Early stages	Late stages
Lymphogranuloma	86 M / 75 F =161	30	37	58	36	67=42%	94=58%
Reticulum-cell sarcoma	49 M / 38 F =87	9	10	21	47	19=22%	68=78%
Lymphosarcoma	29 M / 14 F =43	6	4	15	18	10=23%	33=77%
Brill-Symmers disease	10 M / 8 F =18	10	2	2	4	12=66,6%	6=33,3%

late stages account for 78% of cases. This analysis suggests that, in a large proportion of patients, modern systematic large-field layer radiotherapy is not indicated but that a combination of effective cytostatic drugs be given together with palliative irradiation.

Tables 4 and 5 show what even a small radiotherapy center can achieve by modern techniques of curative radiotherapy with simultaneous biochemical support of the tissue recovery processes. The long-term prospects of cure are best in Brill-Symmers disease. Reticulum-cell sarcoma carries the next-best long-term prognosis,

Table 4. Malignant lymphomas St. Gall Material (1955—1969). Patients living and free from symptoms after curative irradiation [a]

	3 years	5 years	10 years	15 years
Lymphogranuloma 94 cases	68%	66%	54%	41%
Reticulum-cell sarcoma 33 cases	88%	83%	75%	40%
Lymphosarcoma 18 cases	58%	56%	53%	30%
Giant follicle lymphoblastoma, 15 cases Brill-Symmers disease	93%	92%	83%	75%

[a] Without age correction.

Table 5. Lymphogranuloma St. Gall Material, 1955—1969, 161 patients (86 M, 75 F)

	Survival table, without age correction 3 years	5 years	10 years	15 years
from Stage I	29 of 30 patients =97%	24 of 27 =89%	16 of 19 =84%	11 of 14 =79%
from Stage II	37 of 37 patients =100%	34 of 35 =97%	18 of 24 =75%	11 of 17 =65%
from Stage III	49 of 58 patients =84%	43 of 58 =74%	6 of 55 =11%	2 of 53 =4%
from Stage IV	4 of 36 patients =11%	1 of 36 =3%	1 of 36 =3%	0 of 36 =0%

Patients alive and free from symptoms following curative irradiation [a], without age correction

	3 years	5 years	10 years	15 years
from Stage I	25 of 30 patients =83%	22 of 27 =81%	14 of 19 =74%	9 of 14 =64%
from Stage II	30 of 37 patients =81%	28 of 35 =80%	17 of 24 =71%	10 of 17 =59%
from Stage III	9 of 27 patients =33%	9 of 27 =33%	4 of 22 =18%	2 of 20 =10

[a] Stage IV was not treated with a curative irradiation.

followed by lymphogranuloma and lymphosarcoma. However, it should be emphasized that stage III cases treated by radiotherapy are included among the lymphogranuloma cases. The detailed results of radiotherapy in the individual stages of lymphogranuloma are shown in Table 5. Here we see that over 74% of stages I and II patients were symptom-free after 5 and 10 years.

Improvement in the cure rate achieved in stage II cases depends on whether we can match the irradiation plan to the clinical course of the disease through a better knowledge of the risk areas. The aim here is to reduce the hazard of late radiation lesions, which it is important not to neglect, particularly after large-area layer irradiation.

Discussion

After a thorough analysis of the material on the basis of our present state of knowledge, we have come to the following conclusions of importance for the treatment of malignant lymphomas.

1. Stage Classification

In all cases, an exact clinical staging classification is essential for planning treatment.

Here it must be borne in mind, particularly for stages I and II, that if the lymphatic system above the diaphragm is affected, a negative lymphogram does not provide absolute confirmation that the system below the diaphragm is affected, since observations of the course of the disease show that, in more than 5 out of 10 patients with negative lymphograms in stages I and II, the disease later affects the lymphatic system below the diaphragm. The exact stage of the disease must be determined, if necessary by exploratory laparotomy and splenectomy .

However, this method does not give absolute certainty, since it will never be possible to carry out an exact biopsy study of all the lymph nodes in the abdomino-retroperitoneal region.

To define the limits of stage IV exactly, we need the assistance of a well-equipped oncological center which can confirm the diagnosis by means of appropriate liver, bone-marrow and organ biopsies.

At present it is still uncertain whether nuclear medicine can make a contribution towards staging classification.

2. Prophylactic Irradiation

Prophylactic irradiation of adjacent lymphatic zones has been much discussed in recent decades. It is still not completely certain whether prophylactic irradiation improves the results of therapy. On the basis of our patient material, we have adopted the following policy: In the "lymphocytic" type (known as paragranuloma in Jackson and Parker's classification) we have so far restricted ourselves to local irradiation of the affected areas with a tumor-destroying dose, and have obtained good results. In cases which could not be controlled therapeutically, a diffuse spread took place; there is thus no exact clinical evidence as to which parts of the body are affected in the event of later recurrence.

By contrast, the "nodular sclerotic" type tends to spread in a typical manner. In stage I, if a upper cervical region is affected, for example, the whole lymphatic system above the diaphragm must be irradiated prophylactically. In stage II, e. g. when the disease affects the cervicomediastinal or axillary area, the whole lymphatic system above and below the diaphragm must be treated with large-field layer or bath irradiation. We have also found that in the nodular sclerotic type (stages I B, II B, III B) the concomitant clinical symptoms (pruritus, fever, sweat, alcoholic pain) produce no statistically significant change in the cure rate.

However, the position is different in the mixed cellularity type. Here the stage, concomitant clinical symptoms and knowledge of the manner of spread are factors that vitally affect the success of treatment. First, it is important to know that in this form the disease hardly involves the mediastinum, at least not until quite a late stage.

Thus, for example, with the mixed cellularity form, when the primary tumor is in the cervical area, prophylactic irradiation will be applied not to the mediastinum but to the abdomino-retroperitoneal space and both axillae. Conversely, after the destruction of a primary tumor in the lymphatic system below the diaphragm, the cervico-supraclavicular and axillary lymph nodes rather than the mediastinum should be irradiated. The future will show whether better long-term results can be achieved with this method.

We have too little clinical experience with lymphocyte-depletion types. However, the relevant literature indicates that these cases are less suitable for local radiotherapy than for treatment with new, modern cytostatic combinations.

In the other malignant lymphomas (reticulum-cell sarcoma, lymphosarcoma, Brill-Symmers disease) we have systematically irradiated the affected lymph nodes and neighboring lymphatic zones with a focus-destroying dose and obtained very satisfactory long-term results.

3. Tumor Doses

Only brief comments need be made on tumor doses. For lymphogranuloma they have been established on the basis of years of experience, although there may be individual and anatomical variations. In the mediastinum and abdominal area we have fixed the dosage at 4000 rads, while the corresponding dose for the neck, axilla, and groin is between 3000 and 4000 rads. The same doses are given for reticulum-cell sarcoma and giant-follicle lymphoblastoma. In our experience, however, lymphosarcoma is considerably more sensitive to radiation, and with due allowance for the time factor, focal doses of 2000 to 3000 rads are sufficient to achieve a lasting destruction of tumor areas.

References

1. Hohl, K., Sarasin, Ph., Bessler, W.: Therapie und Prognose der Lymphogranulomatose. Zürcher Erfahrungen von: 1922—1950. Oncologia 4, 1 (1951).
2. Jackson, H., Jr., Parker, F., Jr.: Hodgkin's disease and allied disorders. New York: Oxford University Press 1947.

3. Lennert, K.: Pathologie der Halslymphknoten. Berlin-Heidelberg: Springer 1964.
4. Lukes, R. J., Butler, J. J.: The pathology and nomenclature of Hodgkin's disease. Cancer Res. **26**, 1063—1081 (1966).
5. Peters, M. V.: A study of survivals in Hodgkin's disease treated radiologically. Amer. J. Roentgenol. 63, 299—311 (1950). Cancer Res. **26**, 1232—1243 (1966).
6. Schinz, H. R., Reich, T. H.: Die Häufigkeit der Todesfälle an Lymphogranulomatose (Morbus Hodgkin) in der Schweiz seit 1931. Dtsch. med. Wschr. **86**, 1054 (1961).
7. Symmers, W. St. C.: Pathology of primary malignant disease of the lymphoreticular system. Cancer (Lond.) **2**, 448—483 (1958 a).

Localization and Prognostic Importance of Post-Radiotherapy Marginal Recurrence of Malignant Lymphomas

H. BÜNEMANN and R. KÖSTER

Summary

None of all marginal relapses seen in this investigation is a proven source of further dissemination. All marginal recurrences developed in the environment of former involved regions; thus it seems recommendable to include a sufficient broad surrounding area of involved peripheral lymphnode-groups into the extended field.

The records of 408 patients with malignant lymphomas (Hodgkin's disease, reticulum-cell sarcoma, lymphosarcoma and Brill-Symmers disease) seen from 1966 to 1971 were retrospectively analyzed. Marginal recurrences after local and "prophylactic extended field" irradiation were noted, especially the localization of these recurrences and their importance for the further development of disease.

The most frequent localization of the marginal recurrence was the upper part of the chain of Lnn. cervicales profundes and the region of the Lnn. axillares pectorales. Progressively less frequent sites were the parahilar region, the retroauricular region, the occipital region and the region below the groin. In some cases marginal recurrences occurred in the preauricular region, in the epipharynx, near the iliac crest and in the paracubital region (the latter was a patient with involvement of the cubital region at the beginning of treatment).

Nearly two thirds of all marginal recurrences appeared at the same time as recurrences in other treated or untreated regions. The solitary marginal recurrences were discovered, without exception, adjacent to regions which were clinically involved at time of starting treatment, and never in the neighbourhood of prophylactically irradiated areas.

The disease-free interval after treatment of solitary marginal recurrence was short (at most 7 months) in all cases not treated with cytostatics; therefore, it is difficult to exclude the possibility of simultaneous, clinically indistinguishable recurrences in other regions when the marginal recurrence was identified. The starting point of dissemination could be proved for none of the marginal recurrences; thus the influence on the further development of the disease is doubtful.

The results show however that it is advisable to include a sufficiently broad margin in the target volume, especially in cases of involvement of a peripheral region in the "extended field".

Author Index

Abbatucci, S. 190
Abbot, A. 29
Abrams, H. L. 97
Afkham, I. 162, 174, 175
Ahlström, C. G. 226, 228
Aisenberg, A. C. 53, 139
Alberto, P. 111
Allen, L. A. 162
Altenbrunn, H.-J. 147
Altmann, D. 75
Amiel, J. L. 88, 190
Amundsen, M. A. 116
Anderson, S. 97
Ando, A. 151
Anger, H. O. 152
Arndt, J. 221, 224
Arvay, N. 74, 75
Aster, R. H. 116
Ause, R. G. 147

Baensch, 75
Bagley, Ch. M. 98
Balint, J. 16
Balkuv, S. 53
Banfi, A. 158, 161, 181
Barcos, M. P. 29
Barge, J. 37
Barker, C. R. 30
Barker, J. R. 151, 152
Bartels, P. 15
Bartok, St. 152
Barth, W. F. 30
Bataini, 162, 174
Bates, D. V. 97
Bauer, R. 221, 224
Bauer, S. 88
Baum, S. 97
Baumal, R. 61
Baumeister, L. 94
Bayindir, S. 152
Beaudoin, D. E. 112
Beck, K. 38, 106, 140
Becker, J. 147
Begemann, H. 111
Belan, A. 75
Benacerraf, B. 54
Bennet, M. H. 43, 134, 139, 161, 189
Benninghoff, D. L. 15, 16, 74
Berard, C. 29, 53, 140
Bergsteinova, V. 221, 224
Berkson, J. 91, 93
Bessler, W. 238
Bismuth, V. 74, 97
Blahut, J. 74
Brase, A. 152
Bloedorn, F. G. 180
Bloom, B. 61
Blümel, I. 112, 113
Böttcher, D. 108, 112, 113
Boiron, M. 93, 140
Bonadonna, G. 161, 181
Boucot, N. G. 97
Bourquin, J. 74
Bousser, J. 190
Boutis, L. 88, 161, 174, 175, 200, 220
Brass, B. 54
Bremer, K. 54
Brennhovd, I. O. 161
Breslow, A. 116
Brettschneider, L. 54
Brizel, H. E. 180, 224
Brostoff, J. 53
Bron, K. M. 97
Brouet, J. 29
Brown, R. S. 53
Bruch, Chr. 54
Brunk, S. F. 132, 161
Brunner, K. 93
Bryan, J. A. 106, 132
Buchner, R. G. 117
Burd, B. L. 152
Bünemann, 240
Bull, J. M. 180
Buono, M. S. 75, 88
Burgers, M. 190
Burkhardt, R. 40, 43, 133, 139
Burn, J. I. 152
Burnet, F. M. 52, 53
Butler, J. J. 29, 88, 93, 140, 161, 219, 239
Byrd, B. L. 152

Camillerie, J. G. 37
Carbone, P. P. 53, 93, 111, 171, 174, 184, 219
Cardis, R. 15
Carlton, J. E. 152
Carnevali, G. 161
Casley-Smith, J. R. 74
Carthcart, R. T. 97
Caylor, H. D. 16
Cervantes, A. 15
Chase, M. W. 43
Chassard, J. L. 97, 190
Chaudri, M. A. 151, 152
Cherry, C. 15
Chretien, P. 128, 181
Christensen, I. 161
Chute, R. 15
Clein, G. P. 30
Close, M. E. 97
Collette, J. M. 74
Collins, R. D. 18, 29, 30
Combes, C. 75
Cooper, J. F. 15
Cordier, G. 15
Corder, M. P. 53
Cottier, H. 93
Cousson, R. T. 117
Craver, L. F. 93, 106, 174, 220
Crosbie, J. 158, 161
Crowther, D. 53, 61
Cuneo, B. 15, 74
Cuneo, M. M. B. 15
Czeizel, E. 15

Dacie, J. V. 117
Dancot, H. 3, 162, 163, 200, 201
Daniel, C. R. 98
Das, B. K. 141
Dargent, M. 97
Davidson, J. W. 15, 74, 88
Dearing, R. 15
Descamps, P. 15, 97
Desprez-Curely, J. P. 74, 97
De Vita, V. T. 53, 93, 106, 139, 140, 180, 184
Diebold, J. 37
Diehl, V. 2, 59, 61
Dietzel, F. 148
Dischler, W. 44, 99, 106
Ditchek, T. R. 74
Dittmann, A. 152
Doddi, O. D. 76
Dolan, P. A. 97
Doll, E. 98
Donaldson, S. S. 44, 139
Dorfmann, R. F. 3, 44, 93, 118, 122, 134, 135, 139, 140, 161, 173, 174
Dormer, A. E. 97
Douglass, C. 53
Dreyer, H. J. 147
Drury, P. 189

Duckert, F. 117
Duhamel, G. 43, 134, 135, 139

Easson, E. C. 195, 200
East, J. 47
Economou, S. G. 162
Edwards, C. L. 148, 152
Ellmann, L. 54
Elmendorf, E. A. 98
Engel, St. 15
Engeset, A. 161
Ennuyer, A. 162, 163, 174
Enright, L. P. 93
Erbe, W. 3, 22

Fabel, H. 95, 97
Fairley, G. H. 53
Farrer-Brown, G. 41, 43, 157, 161, 189
Fass, L. 54
Fehling, H. 152
Feinberg, S. B. 98
Feine, U. 147
Feremans, W. 201
Finstad, J. 29
Fisch, U. 15
Fischer, H. W. 15, 74, 88
Fischer, J. J. 93, 111, 147
Flad, H.-D. 2, 48, 53, 54
Flamant, R. 175
Flandrin, G. 29
Fleischli, D. J. 181
Florey, H. W. 74
Foldi, M. 75
Foley, D.-V. 16
Foley, H. F. 53
Forbes, J. F. 54
Forslo, H. 180, 228
Fraimow, W. S. 97
Frangione, B. 29
Franiatte, I. 174
Franke, H. D. 3, 221, 224
Franssila, K. O. 3, 117, 118
Frey, D. 94
Freireich, E. J. 53
Friedmann, E. A. 16
Friedmann, M. 224
Frischbier, H. J. 74, 76
Frommhold, H. 76
Fuchs, W. A. 15, 74, 88, 89, 93
Fuller, L. M. 118, 122, 221, 224
Futler, J. J. 122

Gage, R. P. 91, 93
Gall, E. A. 29
Gamble, J. F. 122
Gehrmann, G. 117
Geiger, M. T. 115, 117
Georgi, M. 147
Georgii, A. 2, 37, 39
Gérard-Marchant, R. 190
Gergely, R. 74
Gerteis, W. 15, 74, 97
Getzel, L. G. 112
Gilbert, R. 177, 180, 195, 200
Ginestie, J. F. 75
Givler, R. L. 132, 161
Glatstein, E. 39, 43, 93, 105, 106, 132, 140, 161
Glaubitt, G. 147, 152
Glover, M. K. 174, 180
Glueckmann, A. 15
Godard, H. 16
Godwin, H. A. 53
Goes, M. 221, 224
Gold, W. M. 97
Goldberg, M. E. 98
Good, R. A. 29
Gottschalk, A. 152
Gough, J. H. 98, 122
Gough, M. M. 98, 118
Gould, I. 75
Gowan, D. H. 117
Gowans, J. L. 45, 46, 47
Graan, V. 44, 134, 138, 139
Gralnick, H. R. 139
Greaney, E. M. 17
Greaves, M. F. 53
Grebe, S. F. 147, 148, 152
Green, L. 54
Greening, R. R. 76, 97
Greuel, H. 97
Grey, H. M. 29
Gudat, F. 139
Güller, R. 134, 138, 139
Guernsey, J. M. 43, 93, 106, 132
Guiney, E. J. 98
Guinn, G. A. 54
Gulesserian, H. P. 132, 161
Gunz, F. W. 46, 47, 54
Gyenes, G. 221, 224
Gyr, K. 139

Haagensen, C. D. 15, 190
Härtel, M. P. 88, 89, 93
Hafner, E. 76
Hagen, S. 161
Halama, J. 221, 224
Halgrimson, C. G. 29
Hall, T. C. 93, 106, 174, 220
Hallgrimsson, J. 97
Hamann, W. 38, 106, 122
Hamilton, Fairley G. 61
Hammond, W. 54
Hampe, J. 152
Hampton, J. W. 117, 147
Han, T. 158, 161
Hanks, G. E. 106, 132
Harbst, H. 147
Harmsen, D. 117
Harper, P. V. 152
Harrison, C. V. 43, 161, 189
Hartmann, Ch. 122
Hass, A. C. 132, 161
Haubold, V. 141, 147, 152
Zur Hausen, H. 61
Hayat, M. 175, 190, 219
Hayes, R. L. 148, 151
Haynes, H. A. 53
Heger, N. 152
Heilmann, K. 38
Heilmeyer, L. 196, 200
Heimpel, H. 54
Heinzel, F. 74
Helary, J. 162
Hellmann, S. 21, 22, 29
Henle, G. 61
Henle, W. 61
Hennekeuser, H. H. 133, 134, 135, 138
Henrichsen, E. 15
Henry, J. 190
Herb, R. 147
Herbermann, R. B. 54
Hermann, P. G. 15, 16, 74
Hersh, E. M. 53, 54
Herzfeld, V. 147
Hess, F. 3, 229
Hicks, E. B. 29, 88, 161
Higast, T. 152
Hilpert, K. L. 16
Hiraki, T. 152
Hirsch, J. 113, 117
Hisada, K. 151, 152
Hjort, P. F. 117
Hodan, R. P. 108, 111
Hoeg, K. 161
Hör, G. 147, 152
Hoffer, P. B. 152
Hohl, K. 238
Hohn, M. 221, 224
Hollander, L. 152
Hollinshead, W. H. 15
Hoppe, D. 221, 224
Howelt, M. 98
Huber, C. 54
Huget, R. P. 53, 54
Hulu, N. 29
Hundeshagen, H. 152
Hutchison, G. 162

Idanov, D. A. 74
Ikemoto, S. 152
Ingold, J. A. 166
Ingram, G. I. C. 117

Jackson, H. Jr. 234, 237, 238
Jackson, L. 75, 76, 98
Jackson, R. J. A. 15, 98
Jacobsson, S. J. 15, 75
Jahns, E. 147
Jelliffe, A. M. 3, 43, 156, 157, 158, 161, 174, 180, 182, 189, 206, 219
Johansson, S. 88
Johnson, R. E. 3, 93, 128, 132, 140, 173, 174, 176, 180
Johnston, G. S. 152
Jones, S. E. 138, 139, 180
Jossifow, G. M. 15, 75

Kaboth, W. 111
Kadin, M. E. 41, 44, 93, 139, 140, 157
Kaindl, F. K. 75
Kaiser, D. 107
Kalima, T. V. 122
Kaplan, H. S. 3, 43, 90, 93, 106, 107, 111, 118, 122, 132, 134, 139, 140, 157, 158, 161, 162, 166, 173, 174, 175, 180, 184, 196, 200, 206, 219
Karacsonyi, S. 16
Kato, H. 152
Kaufmann, E. 98
Kaufmann, R. M. 116
Kaul, A. 147, 152
Kawat, K. 152
Kay, D. N. 152
Keeling, D. H. 161
Von Keiser, D. 75, 147
Keller, A. R. 118, 122
Kendall, B. 161
Kimmonth, J. B. 75, 98
Kinosita, Y. 152
Kittelson, A. C. 74
Klein, M. 29
Klein, G. 58, 61
Klein, U. 147
Kligermann, M. M. 93, 106, 162
Knight, E. J. 47
Koehler, P. R. 75, 98
Koeppe, P. 147, 152
Koerner, F. 16
Köster, R. 240
Kolc, J. 75
Koller, F. 117
Koppenhagen, K. 147, 152
Kotilainen, H. 117
Kramer, S. 75
Krieger, G. 99
Kröpelin, K. 94, 98
Kropholler, W. 75, 190
Kubik, St. 2, 5, 16, 17, 75, 76
Kunitsch, G. 97

Lacour, J. 88
Lahnhammer, H. 147
Lagarde, C. 190
Lamarque, P. 75
Landberg, T. 3, 118, 122, 153, 161, 180, 225, 228
Langhammer, H. 152
Laning, R. C. 112
Larsson, L. 118, 122, 161, 228
Larson, St. M. 152
Laszla, I. 174
Laszlo, A. M. 174
Laufer, C. 16, 75
Laugier, A. 74, 97, 190
Lauwers, L. 200
Lavender, J. P. 151, 152
Lawrence, H. S. 53, 74
Lawsky, A. R. 117
Lazaro, C. 16
Leadbetter, W. F. 15
Lee, B. J. 93, 98, 140
Lemaire, R. 190
Lennert, K. 26, 29, 30, 140, 233, 239
Leon, A. 147
Leveuf, J. 16
Levin, D. 181
Lewis, P. 97
Liao, K. T. 44, 140
Libre, E. R. 117
Linde, A. H. 139
Linhart, P. 38
Lintner, L. 224
Liverud, K. 161
Lowe, J. 151, 152
Ludwig, J. 16, 75
Lüning, M. 75
Lukes, R. J. 1, 2, 18, 29, 30, 38, 85, 86, 88, 89, 93, 106, 118, 122, 134, 140, 161, 174, 219, 220, 234, 239
Lummus, Z. 29

Mac Leod, M. 38
McAfee, J. G. 147
McBride, J. A. 117
McCready, V. R. 152
McDevitt, H. O. 54
McKee, P. A. 117
McRae, J. 152
Mahorner, H. R. 16
Maier-Borst, W. 147
Malek, P. 75
Malmio, K. 221, 224
Manfredi, O. L. 152
Manlot, G. 75
Mannheimer, E. 75
Mappes, G. 111
Marcille, M. 74
Markovits, P. 190
Marshall, S. K. 174, 180
Marston, J. A. P. 161
Martin, W. J. 54
Masterson, J. G. 16
Mathé, G. 190
Mattingly, R. F. 16
Mau, S. 221, 224
Maurice, P. A. 111
Mayer, K. 44, 139
Meigs, J. V. 16
Mellins, H. Z. 74
Menne, H. D. 54
Merten, 4
Mestdagh, J. 140
Meyers, W. A. 75, 98
Middlemiss, K. H. 200
Mihaesco, E. 29
Milani, F. 181
Milder, M. S. 152
Millett, Y. 43, 161, 183, 189
Mitchell, J. 29
Mitrou, P. S. 23, 29
Möller, G. 54
Molinari, R. 181
Monfardini, S. 181
Moore, F. D. 111
Moore, M. R. 108, 180
Morris, P. J. 54
Moulonguet-Doléris, O. 75
Müftüoglu, A. U. 53
Müller, H. 75
Murata, A. 152
Musshoff, K. 1, 2, 38, 88, 93, 106, 107, 111, 118, 122, 123, 140, 162, 167, 170, 174, 175, 196, 197, 200, 206, 219, 220

Nadel, J. A. 97
Nagel, G. A. 139
Nakamura, I. 152
Nakayama, Y. 152
De Nardo, G. L. 147
Narvaez, F. 224
Nebeling, R. 224
Nelsen, T. S. 118
Nelson, B. M. 152
Nelson, J. H. 15, 16, 74, 98
Nelson, H. P. 16
Nesheim, A. 161
Neveling, 221
Newall, J. 158, 162, 221
Newsome, J. F. 106, 132
Niklaus, B. 122, 206
Nilsson, K. 61
Nicolesco, J. 16
Norris, S. 53
Nossal, G. J. V. 22, 29
Nuland, S. B. 106, 162
Nuss, A. 38, 106, 122

Obrecht, P. 54, 76
O'Conor, G. T. 29, 128, 181
Oehlert, W. 2, 31, 38, 41, 44, 106, 111, 112, 122, 123, 134, 140
Oldini, C. 161
Olson, W. R. 112
Oppenheim, J. J. 53
Order, S. E. 21, 22, 53
Owen, C. A. 116

Pages, A. 75
Palkovich, I. 15
Papamiltiades, T. 15
Papillon, J. 3, 190, 195
Papst, H. W. 147
Paputchis, H. 117
Park, J. K. 29
Parker, F. Jr. 234, 237, 238
Parker, J. W. 29, 30
Parrot, D. M. Y. 45, 47
Parwaresch, M. R. 30
Pataky, Z. 16
Paterson, R. 223, 224
Pattillo, R. A. 16
Pauli-Beisel, Ch. 107, 111, 112, 123
Pemberton, J. 16

Pemsel, H. K. 229
Penick, G. D. 117
Penn, I. 29, 54
Pentl, A. A. 16
Pereira, S. 16
Peters, M. V. 93, 162, 166, 175, 200, 224, 239
Peters, P. E. 77, 88, 155, 158, 195, 196, 221
Pfleger-Schwarz, L. 75
Picard, J. D. 74, 75, 190
Pirofsky, B. 29
Pitney, W. R. 115, 116, 117
Playfair, J. H. L. 53
Pommateau, E. 97
Pool, J. L. 44, 139
Popper, H. 37, 38
Potet, F. 37
Preudhomme, J. L. 29
Propping, D. 88
Prosnitz, L. R. 93, 106, 157, 162
Pujoul, H. 75

Queisser, W. 29
Quinones, J. 152

Rabellino, E. 29
Rafto, J. J. 152
Ramot, B. 29
Rappaport, H. 20, 29, 93, 106, 122, 140, 162, 173, 174, 175, 189, 220
Reddick, R. L. 117
Reed, G. B. 166
Reich, T. H. 233, 239
Reiffenstuhl, G. 16
Renemann, H. 162, 174, 175
Revol, L. 190
Ricci, S. B. 181
Rivera, E. 98
Rizza, G. R. 117
Roberts, H. R. 117
Rodrigues, A. 16
Roedeler, H. D. 147
Römer, M. 148, 152
Rösler, H. 74
Rössner, R. 122, 206
Roitt, J. M. 53
Romanuik, P. A. 75
Roo, I. 75
Rose, R. 54
Rosenberg, S. A. 44, 90, 93, 106, 118, 132, 134, 135, 139, 140, 158, 162, 166, 175, 180
Rossen, R. 54
Roth, J. A. 98
Rouvière, H. 16, 75
Ruben, Ph. 93, 106, 174, 220
Ruettimann, A. 16, 74, 75, 88
Russell, M. H. 195, 200
Rusznyak, J. 75

Salvini, E. 161
Salzman, J.-R. 111
Samim, F. 97
Sanchez, P. D. 152
Sandritter, W. 1, 29
Sand-Hansen, H. 224
Sarasin, Ph. 238
Scott, R. M. 180, 223, 224
Seith, U. 62
Seligmann, M. 29
Senn, H. J. 139
Serell, R. L. 61
Sewell, R. L. 53
Seydel, H. G. 180
Sheybani, M. 147
Shulman, N. R. 117
Silver, R. T. 140
Skelley, D. F. 75
Slanina, 4
Slate, R. W. 112
Slaughter, D. P. 158, 162
Smiley, R. K. 117
Smith, J. L. 30
Smithers, D. W. 93, 111, 162, 174, 219
Söderström, M. 45
Sokoloff, L. 30
Southwick, H. W. 162
Sozuki, S. 152
Spittell, J. A. 116
Sugiyama, M. 152
Sukiennikow, W. 16
Srahn-Tapper, G. 228
Symmers, W. St. C. 233, 239
Szabo, G. 75
Sziegoleit, M. 221, 224
Schaffer, B. 74, 75, 98
Schaffner, F. 37, 38
Scharff, M. D. 61
Scheer, A. C. 158, 162, 163, 166
Scherer, M. 58
Scheurlen, H. 147
Schick, P. 54
Schinz, H. R. 233, 239
Schlotthauer, C. F. 16
Schmiedel, E. 88
Schmidt, C. G. 106, 148
Schmidt-Vollmer, H. 175
Schmitz, H. 2, 55, 58
Schneider, U. 61
Schnellbacher, B. 38, 106, 122
Schoen, H. 152
Van der Schoot, J. B. 147, 152
Schulte-Holthausen, H. 61
Schwartz, R. S. 53, 54
Schwartzendruber, D. C. 152
Schwarz, G. 98, 157, 162
Staib, I. 107, 113, 123, 174
Stalker, A. 38
Starzl, T. E. 54
Stender, H. St. 97
Stein, H. 30
Stenfert-Kroese, W. F. 190
Steckenmesser, R. 152
Sternberg, G. 21, 30
Strandqvist, M. 224
Strazl, T. E. 29
Strickstrock, K. H. 77, 88, 220
Strum, S. B. 162, 173
Stutzmann, L. 134, 135, 158, 161, 166

Taillens, J. P. 16
Talal, N. 30
Tarnuzi, A. 117
Tehranian, N. 152
Terry, L. N. 106, 132
Thaler, H. 38, 106
Theml, 54
Thomas, P. 190
Thomas, L. B. 29, 98, 181
Thomas, M. L. 97
Thompson, J. H. 116, 174
Thomson, A. D. 180
Thornbury, J. R. 74
Thurnher, B. 75
Tikka, U. 221, 224
Tindle, B. H. 29, 30
Tin Han, 166
Tjernberg, B. 75
Topol, O. 224
Torrigiani, G. 53
Tretner, I. H. 152
Triller, I. 89
Tömböl, T. 16
Toendury, G. 17, 75
Torloni, H. 29
Trotter, H. A. 17
Trueblood, H. W. 93
Tubiana, M. 93, 111, 140, 168, 174, 175, 190, 219
Turner, D. A. 152
Turnesco, D. 15
Turney, M. 189
Twomey, J. 53

Uehlinger, E. 140
Uhr, J. W. 54
Ultmann, J. E. 93, 132, 140, 152
Unnik van, J. 190

Varady, K. 16
Vajda, J. 16
Vera, R. 93
Verraust, P. 29
Viamonte, M. 75, 93, 140
Vieten, H. 221, 224
Vincent, P. C. 47, 54
Vizkelety, T. 16
Volpe, J. A. 147
Vykoupil, K. F. 37, 39

Wack, O. 54
Wagenknecht, L. 111
Wagner, H.-N. 147
Wallace, S. 53, 75, 76, 97, 98
Wambersie, A. 190
Wang, C. C. 181
Wann, W. 94
Watkins, D. H. C. 117

Way, S. 15
Webb, D. J. 134, 135, 140
Weber, W. 3
Webster, W. R. 117
Weinberg, J. 17
Weinreich, J. 111
Weiss, A. 75
Weissleder, H. 76, 77, 88
Weitzel, A. 38
Welin, S. 88
Welsh, L. W. 17
Wendland, D. E. 97
Wentz, D. 152
Westerhausen, M. 38, 58
Werf-Messing, B. van der 3, 163, 166, 181, 190
Westling, P. 153, 162
Wettstein, P. 15
Wiebe, V. 221
Wiljasalo, M. 88
Williams, G. R. 117
Willmann, H. 38, 106, 140
Winchell, H. S. 152
Zum Winkel, K. 76, 147
Wintzell, K. 228
Wirth, W. 17, 64, 74, 75, 76
Wizenberg, M. J. 180
Wohl, G. T. 75, 98
Wolf, H. 61, 147
Wolfert, W. 62
Wolodjko, W. P. 17
Würdinger, H. 152
Wunsch, B. 38, 106, 140

Youker, J. 97
Young, R. C. 53

Zabojovà, E. 224
Ziegler, J. 54
Zucali, R. 181

Subject Index

Antigen-induced mitogenic factor of Hodgkin's Disease 49, 50
— — — of lymphocytic leukemia 49, 50
— — — of normal lympho-cytes 49, 50
Antigenic specificities WS and HL-A11 in Hodgkin's Disease 51, 52
— — — and HL-A11 in normals 52

Blood coagulation changes in Factor VIII activity 115, 116
— — — in platelets count after splenectomy 113 ff.
— — — in — after splenectomy 113 ff.
Bone marrow biopsy in malignant lymphoma 133—140
— — — of technique 39
— — in the isolated granulomas 41
— — of mesenchyma and parenchyma 39
— — tumor myelopathy 40, 43
Brill-Symers disease, age and sex distribution 234
— —, clinical stage distribution 235
— —, survival rates 235
Burkitt lymphoma 48, 51
— — and Epstein-Barr virus 51
— — and malaria 51

Chemotherapy, additional-after irradiation 190
— in low-grade lymphosarcoma 187, 188
— in lymphoblastic lymphosarcoma 188, 189
— of malignant lymphoma 182 ff.
— in reticulum cell sarcoma 188—189
Chronic lymphatic leukemia 46, 51
— — —, in cell bearing surface immunoglobulin 51
Chronic lymphatic leukemia, lack of a specific surface receptor 51
Curability, Clinical prognostic factors of — in Hodgkin's disease 196 ff.
—, Criterion of — in Hodgkin's disease 195, 196
— of Hodgkin's disease 195 ff.
— of Lympho- and Reticulosarcomas 201 ff.
— of malignant lymphoma 182
—, management of the favorable presentation for — in Hodgkin's disease 198 ff.
— Rate of — in Hodgkin's disease 196

Endothelium cells role of the lymphocytes within the — 46
Epstein Barr virus (EBV) 55
— — — and Burkitt tumour 55
— — — and Hodgkin's disease 59—61
European organization for Research on Treatment of Cancer (E.O.R.T.C.), Clinical trials of 190
Ewing's sarcoma, effect of additional therapy (Endoxan) on prognosis 192
— —, — of radiotherapy with and without Endoxan on survival 194
Extended field irradiation 177

Factor VIII activity after splenectomy 115, 116

Hashimoto goiters 45
Henle's method 56
Hepatic involvement in Hodgkin's disease 102 ff.
— — — —, aggregated type of — 102
— — — —, diffuse type of — 103, 104
— — — —, miliary type of — 102
Hepatic involvement in Hodgkin's disease, nodular type of — 102, 103
Hodgkin's disease 2, 51
— —, age and sex distribution 234
— —, bone marrow involvement and clinical stage in — 135
— —, — marrow involvement and histological type in — 135
— —, clinical and histological stage distribution 235
— —, — manifestation at the beginning 155
— —, — stage and bone marrow involvement in — 135
— —, — stage distribution 119
— —, — stage and histological type 237—238
— —, choice of treatment in — 184, 185
— —, continuous and discontinous affected groups of lymph nodes 156
— —, curabality of — 195 ff.
— —, disease-free survival rates 207 ff.—
— —, dose-time relationship for local cure 224
— —, duration of disease up to beginning of treatment according to stage, histological type 156
— —, effect of sex, age, systemic symptoms, mediastinal involvement and histological type of — on survival 192
— —, Epstein-Barr virus (EBV) in lymphoid cells from patients with — 59 ff.
— —, Evaluation of the extent of disease 152 ff.
— —, Extension after the first treatment in — 158 ff.
— —, frequency of mediastinal involvement 156
— —, histological classification of 182

Hodgkin's disease, histopathological type distribution 118, 119
— —, hiver, bone marrow parenchyma 2
— —, —, bone marrow parenchyma mesenchymal reactions and damage to 2
— —, hypothesis for the pathogenesis of 50, 51
— —, immunological phenomena in 48, 49
— —, indication for prophylactic irradiation depending on 177
— —, influence of histological type of — on survival 193
— —, — of radiotherapy with and without vinblastine in cases of — of the mixed cellularity type 193
— —, initial symptoms of — noted by patient 152
— —, location of primary involvement 154, 155
— —, post-mortem findings in — 160, 161
— —, presentation and progression of 152 ff.
— —, prognostic value of first remission in — 212 ff.
— —, — value of histological type in — 213
— —, — value of stage in — 213
— —, radiotherapy in — 177, 178
— —, results of laparotomy 157
— —, — of large field irradiation 229, 230
— —, — of local irradiation 229, 230
— —, — of radical radiotherapy of — Lund 1944 to 1956 and 1967—1971 223 ff.
— —, — of radiotherapy in relapses of — 216 ff.
— —, — of therapy concerning the Ann Arbor classification 208, 209
— —, — of therapy concerning the different forms of recurrences 214 ff.
— —, — of therapy concerning the different types of remission 212, 213
— —, — of therapy concerning the prognoses of the second remission 217, 218
— —, — of therapy concerning the survival and remission rates 209 ff.

Hodgkin's disease, results of therapy in — Freiburg i. Br. 1964—1971 206 ff.
— —, routes of spread in — 157
— —, site of relapse after mantle irradiation with and without vinblastine in stage I and II 192
— —, specific post-capillary venules of lymphoglandular tissue in 45
— —, survival for patients with Hodgkin's disease according to the number of intradiaphragmatic lymph node regions involved 91, 92
— —, — rates 207 ff., 235
— —, therapie results in stage I and II A, B after radiotherapy with and without vinblastine 190
— —, tumor dose 207, 238
— —, unspecific mesenchymal reaction in bone marrow 39 ff.
— —, — mesenchymal reaction of the liver 31
— —, — mesenchymal reaction of the liver, classification of the 31
— —, — mesenchymal reaction of the spleen 31

Immunity, cellular 48
—, humoral 48
Immunopathology of malignant lymphomas 48 ff., 61
Infectious mononucleosis 55
— — and Epstein-Barr virus (EBV) IgM antibodies 55

Laparoscopy 99 ff.
— different types of hepatic involvement 102 ff.
— in Hodgkin's disease 99 ff.
— indications for 105, 106
Laparotomy, exploratory 39
—, results of — in patients with Hodgkin's disease 157
Laparotomy secondary 121 ff.
— —, results of — depending on histology and time interval 127
— —, — of — depending on stage and time interval 127
— with splenectomy in patients previously treated for Hodgkin's disease 123 ff.
Liver scanning, results of — in malignant lymphoma 143
Lymphangio-adenogramm 64 ff.
Lymphangiography, alterations in pulmonary diffusion capacity 94 ff.

Lymphangiography, staging by 87 ff.
—, in clinical stage III Hodgkin's disease 89 ff.
Lymphangio- and adenography 64 ff.
Lymphatic system, afferent vessels 6
— —, — vessels, sinuses 6
— —, — vessels, sinuses intermediate 6
— —, — vessels, sinuses marginal 6
— —, anatomy of 5
— —, cross-connection between nodes 3
— —, descriptive anatomy 2
— —, efferent vessels, anastomoses of 3
— —, intraperitoneal organs 9
— —, — — function of viclial nodes 9
— —, lateral aortic nodes 9
— —, mesenteric nodes 9
— —, origin 3
— —, — chain formation 5
— —, — drainage area 5
— —, — primary (regional) nodes 5
— —, — secondary, tertiary nodes 5
— —, — tributary area 3
— —, — valveless capillary network 3
— —, — vein trunks 3
— — of pelvic organs 8, 9
— — — — anatomical and clinical investigations 8
— — — —, ascending lymphatics 9
— — — —, ascending lymphatics of testicle 9
— — — —, ascending lymphatics of utero-ovarian adnexa 9
— — — —, descending vessels 9
— — — —, efferent pathway 9
— — — —, function of inguinal nodes, common iliac nodes, external iliac nodes, internal iliac 7
— — — —, Hunter's gubernaculum 9
— — — —, ligamentum teves uteri 9
— — — —, lumbar nodes 9
— — — —, parauterine, parauageniak nodes 8
— — — —, viceral nodes 8
— —, röntgen anatomy of the — 64 ff
— —, segmental passing over 3

Lymphocytes 48, 51
—, 3H-cytidine-labeled — 51
—, thymus-derived (T) — bone-marrow-derived (B) — 48
lymphogranulomatosis (Syn-Hodgkin's disease) 1
—, chromosome abnormalities 2
—, Hodgkin cells 2
— malignancy, signs of 2
— new mistopathological classification 2
— Reed-Sternberg cells 2
Lymphographic differential diagnosis in malignant lymphomas 77 ff.
— — —, chronic lymphatic leukemia 83
— — —, diagnostic criteria of the lymph nodes in — 78, 79
— — —, diagnostic criteria of the lymph vessels in — 78
— — —, Fibrolipomatosis 83
— — —, Hodgkin's disease 83
— — —, Lymphadenitis 83
— — —, Lymphosarcomatosis 83
— — —, Sarcoidosis 83
— — —, Tuberculosis 83
— symptoms, Correlation of — with histological subgroups of Hodgkin's disease 85 ff.
lymphoma, anatomy of 5—17
—, classification of, immunological 27
—, — B-cell
—, — histocytic
—, — unclassifiable
—, histocytic medullary reticulosis 28
—, Hodgkin's disease 28
Lymphomas, Hodgkin 2, 3
—, Ann Arbor 3
—, etiology 2
—, Kye, New York 3
Lymphomas, malignant, age distribution 234
— —, B-Cells 22
— —, — —, Burkitt lymphoma 28
— —, — —, chronic lymphocytic leukemia 22, 25
— —, — —, follicular center cells 22, 23
— —, — —, follicular center cells, DNA Synthesis 23
— —, — —, follicular center cells, levels of transformation 25
— —, — —, follicular center cells, proliferation types 23
— —, — — immunoglobulin production 22
Lymphomas, malignant, techniques for identification 27
— —, chemotherapy 3, 182 ff.
— —, —, indications for 3
— —, classification of 20
— —, —, B-cell 20
— —, —, B-cell, location of 20
— —, — functional 18
— —, — functional immunology 18
— —, — immunological 27
— —, — T-cell 20, 27
— —, — T-cell, location of 20
— —, — U-cell 27
— —, Choice of treatment of 183 ff.
— —, chronic lymphocytic leukemia 27
— —, correlation between EBV infections and 55—58
— —, Curability of 182
— —, environmental and genetic factors of 51—52
— —, etiology 2
— — —, viral 2
— —, follicular-center-cell proliferation 18
— —, histiocytic lymphoma 18, 19, 26
— —, — B-cell proliferation 32
— —, — — follicular-center-cells 26
— —, — — macrophages 18
— —, — — reticulum-cell sarcoma 26
— —, histological classification of 182
— —, Hodgkin's disease 21
— —, — — detective T-cell surveillance system 21, 22
— —, — — development of 21
— —, — — hypersensitive responsiveness 21
— —, — — infections and infections mononucleosis 21
— —, — — influence of viral 55
— —, — — lymphocytic depletion 21
— —, — — morphology of 21
— —, — — Reed-Sternberg cells 21
— —, hypothesis of the development of 52, 53
— —, immune disorders 18
— —, — — alpha-chain disease 18, 26, 28
— —, — — immune deficiencies 18, 26, 28
Lymphomas, malignant, immunosuppression of patients for graft rejection 18, 26, 28
— —, — — Sjögren's syndrome 18, 26, 28
— —, immune pathology 1, 2
— —, immunoblastic Sarcoma 26
— —, — — alpha-chain-disease 26
— —, — — congenital immune defects 26
— —, — — reticulum-cell sarcoma 26
— —, — — Sjögren's syndrome 26
— —, immunology and immune reactions in 48
— —, immunpathology of 48—61
— —, investigative procedures in 62—152
— —, — — bone marrow biopsy 128, 131
— —, — — laparoscopy 99
— —, — — lymphangio-adenography 64, 77, 89
— —, — — Mediastinoscopy 62, 63
— —, — — Radioisotope investigations 139
— —, — — Splenectomy 107
— —, — — Staging laparotomy and splenectomy 118
— —, — — Thoraxscopy 63
— —, irradiation, total body 3
— —, leukemia 19, 21, 22, 27
— —, localization 1
— —, — and prognostic importance of post radiotherapy marginal recurrence of 240
— —, lymphogranulomatosis 12
— —, lymphomas of lymphocytes 18, 19
— —, lymphosarcoma 20
— —, methods of investigation 2
— —, — —, endoscopic and surgical measures with tissue biopsies 3
— —, — —, laparoscopy with hepatic and splenic biopsy 3
— —, — —, laparotomy with splenectomy 3
— —, — — mediastinoscopy 3
— —, — — open bone-marrow biopsy 3
— —, — — pharyngoscopy 3
— —, — — thorascopy 3
— —, morphology 1
— —, mycosis fungoides 27
— —, pathology of 18 ff., 47

Lymphomas pattern of organ involvement: per continuitatem (p. c.) and per disseminationem (p. d.) 169 ff.
— —, primary extend, later extension and stage as factors in therapy of 153 ff., 175
— —, radiotherapy 3, 176 ff.
— —, —, indications for 3
— —, — results 3
— —, —, reticulum-cell sarcoma 20
— —, —, reticulum-cell sarcoma 18, 19
— —, — reticulum-cell sarcoma, immunoblasts 18
— —, — Sézary's syndrome 27
— —, — spread 1
— — staging in — 167—175
— —, T-cells 21, 27
— —, — — acute lymphocytic leukemia 21
— —, — — Hodgkin's disease 21
— —, — — mycosis fungoides 21
— —, — — Sezary's syndrome 21
— —, — — Sternberg sarcoma 21
— —, — — techniques for identification 27
— —, terminology, problems of 20
— —, therapeutic results 195—239
— —, therapy 1
— —, treatment results 229, 233
— —, Waldenström's macroglobulinema 27
— modes of spread 3
— radiotherapeutic methods 3
— site of origin 3
— staging classifications 2, 3
Lympho- and reticulosarcomas prognostic influence of age in patients with 202
— —, results at 10, 15, 20 and 25 years for patients cured 5 years after treatment 202
Lymphoreticulosarcoma, Radiotherapy in 179—180
Lymphosarcoma 51
— age and sex distribution 234
— choice of treatment in — 185—189
—, clinical stage distribution 235
— disease free survival after curative irradiation 236
— histological classification of 182
Lymphosarcoma survival rates 235
Lymphoscintigraphy, ^{67}Ga accumulation and histological type Hodgkin's disease 145
—, results of bone scanning in malignant lymphoma 145
—, — of — compared with lymphography in malignant lymphoma 144
—, — of ^{67}Ga accumulation in malignant lymphoma 145
—, — of retroperitoneal in malignant lymphoma 144
Lymph nodes axillary 11—12
— —, bifurcation nodes cervical 11—13
— —, chains 3
— —, —, collector vessels 3
— —, —, embryonic development 3
— —, —, filter stations 3
— —, —, lymph vessels, afferent 3
— —, —, number of 3
— —, —, senile involution 3
— —, cross-connections between parallel chains 6
— —, — —, spread of metastases 6
— —, efferents, of hepatic nodes 9
— —, —, of the adrenal gland 8, 9
— —, —, of gastric nodes 9
— —, —, of the liver 9
— —, —, of lumbar, viceral nodes 9
— —, —, embryonic development 6
— —, gastric, hepatic, pancreato-lineal 9
— —, —, hepatic pancreato-lineal, initial position of 8, 9
— —, —, hepatic pancreato-lineal, results of organ relocation 8, 9
— —, Giant nodes 6
— —, head and neck 12, 13
— —, intercostal 10
— —, — pulmonary 11
— —, — parasternal 10
— —, — diaphragmatic 10
— —, lacunar 3
— —, — cervical 3
— —, — — involvement in diseases of the ovary, uterine tube, corpus uteri 4
— —, — common iliac 3
— —, — lumbar 3
— —, lumbar and visceral 9
— —, — —, thoracic duct 9—10
Lymph nodes axillary in the lymphardenogramm, acute or chronic inflammatory disease of the — 69
— — —, degenerative changes of the 67
— — —, initial stage of malignancy in the — 69—70
— — —, reactionary swelling of the 69
— — —, shape and size of the — 65
— — —, size and number of the — 65
— — —, volume of the — 65—66
— — of the mammary gland 11 ff.
— —, mediastinum 11, 12
— —, micro-nodes 6
— —, number and size 6
— —, primary 3
— —, regional, topography 6
— —, — chains 6
— —, — — intermediate 6
— —, — — lateral 6
— —, — — medial 6
— —, — iliac external, common 6
— —, — inguinal nodes 6
— —, — lumbar nodes 6
— —, — parietal node groups 6
— —, secondary 3
— —, senile involution 6
— —, — — effect on the medullary substance, the cortex 6
— —, — — formation on metastases 6
— —, tertiary 3
— —, topography of 3
— —, —, connection 3
— —, —, lymphography 3
— —, —, ways of drainage 3
— — of urogenital organs and adrenal gland 8
— —, vessels 6
— —, —, function of valves 6
— —, —, main outflow routes 6
— —, —, main outflow routes, bilateral connection between external, internal iliac nodes 7
— —, —, main outflow routes, crossing-over, right lumbar cord to left side 6
— —, —, main outflow routes, lateral chain 6
— —, —, main outflow routes, medial chain 6

Lymph nodes axillary main outflow routes, segmental passing over 6

Mediastinoscopy 62—63
MOPP-Chemotherapy 178
Morbus Hodgkin, disease free survival after curative irradiation 236
— —, — free survival after curative irradiation depending on clinical stage 236
— —, survival depending on clinical stage 236
— —, — rates 235

node groups, inguinal, iliac lumbar, topography and connections of cisterna chyli and thoracic duct 7
— —, common iliac 7
— —, deep inguinal 7
— —, external iliac (lacunar) 7
— —, internal iliac 7
— —, lumbar 7
— —, right and left lumbar lymph trunks 7
— —, superficial inguinal 7
Non-Hodgkin's lymphoma, bone marrow involvement and clinical stage in — 138
— — —, bone marrow involvement of nodular and diffuse type in — 138
— — —, bone marrow involvement and histological type in — 138
— — —, Frequence of bone marrow involvement in — 138
— — —, Frequency of bone marrow involvement detected by biopsy and by aspiration in — 138
— — —, staging laparotomy 3

Patterson dose-time curve for orthovoltage radiation 224
— — — curve for supervoltage radiation 224
Patterns of involvement in Hodgkin's disease 118—122
Platelets count after splenectomy 113—115
Post-capillary high endothelium 45
— — — endothelium in chronic lymphatic leukemia 46
— — — endothelium in Hodgkin's disease 46
— — — endothelium in Lymphosarcoma 46
— — — endothelium in reticulum cell 46
Post-capillary high endothelium sarcoma 46

Radioisotope Investigations in malignant lymphoma 141 ff.
— —, — lymphoma, methods 141
— —, — lymhoma, results 142
Radiotherapy in Lymphosarcoma and reticulum cell sarcoma 185 ff.
— of malignant lymphoma 176 ff.
—, results and dose-time relationship — in reticulum cell sarcoma 221—224
Recurrence of malignant lymphoma, criticism 203 ff.
Recurrences, the different kinds of — in Hodgkin's disease 214
—, the prognostic value of — in Hodgkin's disease 214—217
Remission, the different kind of —, complete, partial, without 213
—, the prognostic value 212, 213
Reticulosarcoma and Lymphosarcoma, 5-years survival 165
— —, pattern of relapse and spread 163—166
— —, possible benefit of prophylactic irradiation 165
— —, radiation dose (in rad) and time relation for local cure 164
— —, Rye classification 163—165
Reticulum cell sarcoma, age distribution 223, 230
— — —, age and sex distribution 234
— — —, choice of treatment in 185 ff.
— — —, clinical stage distribution 235
— — — disease free survival after curative irradiation 236
— — —, dose-time relationship for local cure 223, 224
— — — histological classification 183
— — —, prognosis depending on age 202
— — —, prognosis depending on anamnesis time 230
— — —, prognostic value of involvement of Waldeyer's ring 221
Reticulum cell sarcoma, radiotherapeutic doses for treatment 221
— — —, radiotherapy — 221 ff.
— — —, site of primary manifestation in patients with 222
— — —, survival rates 235
— — —, survival rates in — depending on therapy 231
— — — "Therapyfactor" 231
Röntgenanatomy of the lymphatic system 64 ff.

Scott dose-time curve for orthovoltage radiation 224
Skin cancer, dose-time relationship for local cure (Strandquist) 224
Spleen scanning, results of — in malignant lymphoma 143
Splenectomy, changes in blood coagulation after — 113—117
— in Hodgkin's disease 107 ff.
— — —, diagnostic value — 110, 111
— — —, intra- and postoperative complications 109, 110
— — — technique — 108, 109
Staging in Hodgkin's disease classification according to Jelliffe 156
— — — Rye classification 168
— laparotomy 118
— —, association of liver and bone marrow involvement with spleen and para-aortic nodes involvement after — 122
— —, — of subdiaphragmatic involvement at — with preoperative patterns 121
— —, histopathology and frequency of para-aortic and splenic involvement after — 119
— —, influence of — on final stage 120
— —, Stage distribution — 119
— — in the non-Hodgkin Lymphoma 128—132
— — in the non Hodgkin Lymphoma histopathological findings and influence on treatment planning after — 129
— — in the non Hodgkin Lymphoma influence of extensive biopsy sampling 128—132
— — and splenectomy 107, 118
— by lymphography 87, 88

Staging in malignant lymphoma Ann Arbor classification 171
— — —, classification according to Musshoff et al. 170
— — —, Hodgkin's disease and non-Hodgkin lymphomas 167 ff.
— — —, Paris classification 168
— — —, Rye classification 168
— — —, clinical 173
— — —, pathological 172, 173
— — —, pathological staging symbols 172
Strandquist dose-time curve 224

Therapeutic results in malignant lymphoma 195 ff.
Therapie of malignant lymphoma 176 ff.
— — —, chemotherapy 182 ff.
— — —, radiotherapy 176 ff.
Thoracoscopy 63
Total body irradiation 179
— nodal irradiation 177
Transformation of cells 55
Tumor myelopathy- and histological subgroups 41
— — — — and clinical classification 41
— — — — immunology
— — — — and lupus erythematosus 42
— — — — and malignant lymphomas 42
— — with vascular obliteration and mesenchymal sclerosis 43
Tumor myelopathy with vascular obliteration and mesenchymal sclerosis, anemia 43
— — with vascular obliteration and mesenchymal sclerosis, granulocytopenia 43
— — with vascular obliteration and mesenchymal sclerosis, thrombocytopenia 43

Uterine cervix cancer, prognostic influence of age in patients with — 203
— — —, results at 10, 15, 20 and 25 years for patients cured years after treatment 203

32 NELSON, R. S: Endoscopy in Gastric Cancer. Cloth DM 53,00; US $ 21.70

33 Experimental and Clinical Effects of L-Asparaginase. Edited by E. GRUNDMANN and H. F. OETTGEN (Symposium). Cloth DM 64,00; US $ 26.20

34 Chemistry and Biological Actions of 4-Nitroquinoline 1-Oxide. Edited by H. ENDO, T. ONO, and T. SUGIMURA. Cloth DM 36,—; US $ 14.70

35 PENN, I.: Malignant Tumors in Organ Transplant Recipients. Cloth DM 26,50; US $ 10.90

36 Current Concepts in the Management of Lymphoma and Leukemia. Edited by J. E. ULTMANN, M. L. GRIEM, W. H. KIRSTEN, and R. W. WISSLER (Symposium). Cloth DM 48,—; US $ 19.60

37 CHIAPPA, S., R. MUSUMECI, and C. USLENGHI: Endolymphatic Radiotherapy in Malignant Lymphomas. With contributions by G. BONADONNA, B. DAMASCELLI, G. FAVA, F. PIZZETTI, U. VERONESI. Cloth DM 48,—; US $ 19.60

38 KOLLER, P. C.: The Role of Chromosomes in Cancer Biology. Cloth DM 48,—; US $ 19.60

39 Current Problems in the Epidemiology of Cancer and Lymphomas. Edited by E. GRUNDMANN and H. TULINIUS (Symposium). Cloth DM 58,—; US $ 23.70

40 LANGLEY, F. A., A. C. CROMPTON: Epithelial Abnormalities of the Cervix Uteri. Cloth DM 58,—; US $ 23.70

41 Tumours in a Tropical Country. A Survey of Uganda (1964—1968). Edited by A. C. TEMPLETON. Cloth DM 72,—; US $ 29.40

42 Breast Cancer: A Challenging Problem. Edited by M. L. GRIEM, E. V. JENSEN, J. E. ULTMANN, and R. W. WISSLER (Symposium). Cloth DM 48,—; US $ 19.60

43 Nomenclature, Methodology and Results of Clinical Trials in Acute Leukemias. Edited by G. MATHÉ, P. POUILLART, and L. SCHWARZENBERG (Symposium). Cloth DM 58,—; US $ 23.70

44 Special Topics in Carcinogenesis. Edited by E. GRUNDMANN (Symposium). Cloth DM 58,—; US $ 23.70

45 KOLDOVSKÝ, P.: Carcinoembryonic Antigens. Cloth DM 38,—; US $ 15.50

46 Diagnosis and Therapy of Malignant Lymphoma. Edited by K. MUSSHOFF (Symposium). Cloth DM 62,—; US $ 25.30

Special Supplement: Biology of Amphibian Tumors. Edited by M. MIZELL. Cloth DM 96,00; US $ 39.20

In Production

47 Investigation and Stimulation of Immunity in Cancer Patients. Edited by G. MATHÉ and R. WEINER (Symposium)

48 Platinum Compounds in Cancer Chemotherapy. Edited by T. A. CONNORS and J. J. ROBERTS (Symposium)

49 Complications of Cancer Chemotherapy. Edited by G. MATHÉ and R. K. OLDHAM (Symposium)

Prices are Subject to change without notice

MIX
Papier aus verantwortungsvollen Quellen
Paper from responsible sources
FSC® C105338

If you have any concerns about our products,
you can contact us on
ProductSafety@springernature.com

In case Publisher is established outside the EU,
the EU authorized representative is:
Springer Nature Customer Service Center GmbH
Europaplatz 3, 69115 Heidelberg, Germany

Printed by Libri Plureos GmbH
in Hamburg, Germany